D1011502

×3.00

Stains on edges 2/02

DATE DUE   1/02

Checked - OR ILL 8-11-03			
GAYLORD			PRINTED IN U.S.A.

THE INVISIBLE PLAGUE

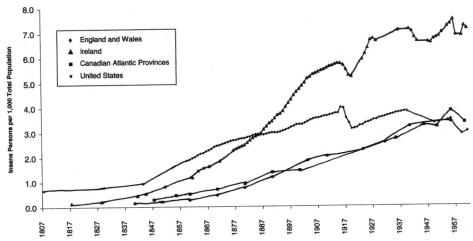

Insane Persons per 1,000 Population in England and Wales, Ireland, Canada (Atlantic Provinces), and the United States, 1807–1961.

THE INVISIBLE PLAGUE

The Rise of Mental Illness
from 1750 to the Present

E. Fuller Torrey, M.D.

Judy Miller

Rutgers University Press

New Brunswick, New Jersey, and London

Library of Congress Cataloging-in-Publication Data

Torrey, E. Fuller (Edwin Fuller), 1937–
    The invisible plague : the rise of mental illness from 1750 to the present / E. Fuller Torrey, Judy Miller.
        p. cm.
    Includes bibliographical references and index.
    ISBN 0-8135-3003-2 (alk. paper)
        1. Psychiatric epidemiology.   2. Mental illness—History—18th century.   3. Mental illness—History—19th century.   4. Mental illness—History—20th century.   I. Miller, Judy, 1949–   II. Title.

RC455.2.E64 T67   2002
616.89'009—dc21

                                                                                        2001019840

British Cataloging-in-Publication information is available from the British Library.

The poems "The First Day's Night had come," "I felt a funeral in my brain," "I felt a cleaving in my mind" by Emily Dickinson are reprinted with permission of the publishers and the Trustees of Amherst College from *The Poems of Emily Dickinson*, Ralph W. Franklin, ed., Cambridge, Mass.: The Belknap Press of Harvard University Press. Copyright©1998 by the President and Fellows of Harvard College. Copyright©1951, 1955, 1979 by the President and Fellows of Harvard College.

Manufactured in the United States of America
Design by John Romer

For Chris, Martha, Lucas, and Olivia,
who will carve a future out of our past.

For Ron, Jonathan, Carl, Lizzy, and Jenny,
with thanks for their love and support.

CONTENTS

PREFACE *ix*

ACKNOWLEDGMENTS *xiii*

1. Introduction: Why Is the Epidemic Important? *1*

2. The Birth of Bedlam: Insanity Prior to 1700 *6*

3. The "English Malady" Appears: England, 1700–1800 *23*

4. "The Clap of Tortured Hands": England, 1800–1850 *43*

5. "A Mania for Madness": England, 1850–1890 *73*

6. "A Great and Progressive Evil": England, 1890–1990 *103*

7. The Road to Grangegorman: Ireland, 1700–1990 *124*

8. "A Constantly Increasing Multitude":
   Atlantic Canada, 1700–1990 *161*

9. "The Disease Whose Frequency Has
   Become Alarming": The United States, 1700–1840 *193*

10. An Apostle for Asylums: The United States,
    1840–1860 *215*

11. "A Very Startling Increase": The United States,
    1860–1890 *244*

12. "The Apocalyptic Beast": The United States,
    1890–1990 *276*

13. Why Is the Epidemic Forgotten?
   The Politicalization of Insanity   300

14. Possible Causes of Epidemic Insanity   314

APPENDIX A: What Is Insanity?   335

APPENDIX B: The Baseline Rate of Insanity   339

APPENDIX C: Tables of Insanity Rates   345

NOTES   351

SELECTED REFERENCES   391

INDEX   397

PREFACE

Insanity, in one disguise or another, has always been with us, an occasional unbidden guest in life's masquerade. In recent centuries, however, it has appeared in previously unseen masks and in much greater numbers. For many of those afflicted, insanity not only ruins festivities, it destroys life itself.

Delusions, hallucinations, mania, and other symptoms of insanity can be caused by a variety of medical conditions, ranging from brain tumors and brain infections to toxic and metabolic disorders. Throughout history, these medical conditions, by themselves, have produced only relatively few cases of insanity. These are discussed in detail in appendix B, and their number is referred to as the "baseline rate of insanity." Throughout history this rate of insanity was approximately one case per 1,000 adult population, or 0.5 cases per 1,000 total population, since insanity occurs only rarely in children.

Clinically, the increasing number of new cases of insanity have looked like the old cases, with two exceptions. First, the new cases began more often in younger adults; and second, those who were affected often did not recover as quickly. Increasing numbers, in fact, have not been recovering at all.

Initially, the increase in new cases of insanity caused little notice. A few observers in the seventeenth century expressed concern, but the prevalence of insanity remained low compared with what was to come. By the eighteenth century, the stream of insanity had begun to gather force, and cases appeared with increasing frequency. Members of the public now noticed and asked why. Physicians expressed concern. Was the increase being caused by excess alcohol consumption? Moral degeneration? Consanguineous marriages? The stresses of industrialization or urban living? Nobody could say for certain.

By the nineteenth century, it was no longer possible to ignore the increasing number of the insane, and it became a major topic of discussion for medical professionals, the public, and writers. The prevalence of insanity, which historically had been considerably less than 1 case per 1,000 total population, passed 2 cases per 1,000, then 3 cases per 1,000 in the 1800s. Yet, it still continued to increase, and during the twentieth century the rate passed 5 cases per 1,000, then climbed even higher. What had once been a small stream of insanity had become a mighty river. And for many of those afflicted it was the River Styx.

Proving that such an epidemic has taken place, and is apparently continuing to take place, is a daunting task. We cannot exhume insane persons from past centuries to ascertain whether or not they meet the present diagnostic criteria for insanity, now officially called schizophrenia or manic-depressive illness. Nor can we transport ourselves back in time to carry out prevalence surveys using techniques comparable to those used today.

We must instead rely on the historical record and on epidemiological associations. Bradford Hill, a leading American epidemiologist, said that such associations should be evaluated on their strength, temporal relationships, consistency, and specificity.[1] We have mined the historical records for all available indicators of insanity's prevalence and have supplemented these records with commentaries from contemporary publications and writers. No single piece of evidence has proven that insanity has been increasing. Instead, it is the cumulative record that must be assessed and then compared to the existing—and almost universally shared—belief that there has been no real increase in insanity in hundreds of years, if ever.

To assess the prevalence of insanity over time, we have chosen for detailed analysis England (often including Wales), Ireland, the Atlantic provinces of Canada, and the United States, emphasizing especially Massachusetts, Connecticut, New York, Pennsylvania, South Carolina, and California. Our choices were determined by the availability of research material in the English language. There also appear to be good records in Scotland, in the Canadian province of Ontario, and in several U.S. midwestern states. Among non-English-speaking countries, France and Germany have excellent archives, and apparently also Russia and Scandinavia. In each case, the records appear to tell the same story we are telling here.

To simplify the analysis of data, we have standardized all rates to prevalence per 1,000 total population and first admissions per 10,000 total population. We recognize that such standardizations are imperfect, since the age distributions of populations vary. Thus, for a disease like insanity, which occurs primarily in adults, if the rates are age corrected, a rate of 5 per 1,000 total population in Ireland, where a large percentage of the population is under age eighteen, is actually higher than a rate of 5 per 1,000 total population in England, where a smaller percentage of the population is under age eighteen.

To simplify comparisons, we have translated money to 1997 British pounds and 1997 American dollars. We have also used "insanity" as a generic term for what we now call schizophrenia and manic-depressive illness. The term was widely used until the early years of the twentieth century and seems satisfactory in the context of this book, especially in view of the fact that we are increasingly uncertain whether our current divisions of insanity represent separate diseases or merely different manifestations of a single disease. Similarly, we have used the term "idiot" to refer to mentally retarded individuals, as it was used in centuries past.

It has now been almost thirty years since one of us—E. Fuller Torrey—submitted a paper for publication suggesting that epidemic insanity was a recent phenomenon. Entitled "Is Schizophrenia of Recent Origin?" the paper was summarily rejected as fanciful by all journals to which it was submitted, and it was never published. One anonymous reviewer even commented, "I cannot grant a thing to this paper." This book is in part a very belated and detailed response to those critics, in the hope that they are still alive to read it.

In the final analysis, the reader must assess the evidence and decide whether or not an epidemic of insanity is truly taking place. The evidence is admittedly, and of necessity, circumstantial. However, as Henry David Thoreau once noted, "Some circumstantial evidence is very strong, as when you find a trout in the milk."[2]

ACKNOWLEDGMENTS

Our analysis of historical material has been possible only because of the kind assistance of many people. Foremost among those to whom we are indebted are Herb, Kirk, and Andrew MacDonald, Faith Dickerson, Christine Miller, Hugh Freeman, Robert Yolken, Mischa Myslobodsky, and especially Barbara Torrey, who all helped with research and/or reading portions of the manuscript. We are also grateful to Ken Niles and the staff of the History of Medicine Division at the National Library of Medicine and to Paul Baker and Tony Mullan at the Library of Congress, who provided essential help.

For England, we were assisted by Catherine Bergin, Debbie Bloxam, and Roy Porter at the Wellcome Institute for the History of Medicine; Michelle Webb at the British Library; Naomi Blake and Martin Guha at the Kings College School of Medicine Library; Marie Ford at the St. Helens and Knowsley Health Center; John Bartlett at the Department of Health; Sarah Millard at the Bank of England; Peter Cox with the John Clare Society; Peter Jones with the Department of Psychiatry, Cambridge University; Rajendra Persaud with the Institute of Psychiatry; and A. G. Gordon.

For Ireland, we received help from Donall O Luanaigh and the staff of the National Library of Ireland; Bill Fowler with the Department of Health and Children; and Tony O'Brien with the Department of Health and Social Services in Northern Ireland.

For Canada, the following individuals were helpful: Charlotte

Stewart and Marilyn Bell in the Public Archives and Records Office, Prince Edward Island; Jeanne MacDonald at Statistics Canada; and Brien St. Jacques with the Canadian Embassy Library in Washington, D.C.

For the U.S. data, we are indebted to Jackie Richardson and Scott Nelson, who made available the library at St. Elizabeths Hospital; the staff of the library at American University; Joy Gilchrist Stalnaker at Weston State Hospital; Steve Green at the Northeast Archives of Folklore and History; and Charles Pridgeon at Marietta College.

Khoi Nguyen and Shen Zhong saved our computerized files from cyberspace death on numerous occasions.

Helen Hsu welcomed the manuscript into her home at Rutgers University Press, while Suzanne Kellam and Alice Calaprice made sure that it was properly fed and editorially clothed.

A special thanks goes to Gerald Grob for his generosity and time. Finally, we wish to acknowledge the intellectual contribution and friendship of the late Edward Hare; may the book serve partially to perpetuate his memory and his important contributions to psychiatric history.

THE INVISIBLE PLAGUE

Here, where men's eyes were empty and as bright
As the blank windows set in glaring brick,
When the wind strengthens from the sea—and night
Drops like a fog and makes the breath come thick.

By the deserted paths, the vacant halls,
One may see figures, twisted shades and lean,
Like the mad shapes that crawl an Indian screen,
Or paunchy smears you find on prison walls.

Turn the knob gently! There's the Thumbless Man;
Still weaving glass and silk into a dream,
Although the wall shows through him—and the Khan
Journeys Cathay beside a paper stream.

A Rabbit Woman chitters by the door—
—Chilly the grave-smell comes from the turned sod—
Come—lift the curtain—and be cold before
The silence of the eight men who were God!
             Stephen Vincent Benét,
             "Ghosts of a Lunatic Asylum," 1918

CHAPTER 1

Introduction

Why Is the Epidemic Important?

Such a disease, which disorders the senses, perverts the reason, and breaks up the passions in wild confusion;—which assails man in his essential nature,—brings down so much misery on the head of its victims, and is productive of so much social evil—deserves investigation on its own merits, by statistical as well as other methods.

—WILLIAM FARR, "Report upon the
Mortality of Lunatics," 1841

A Plague is a formidable Enemy, and is arm'd with Terrors, that every Man is not sufficiently fortified to resist, or prepar'd to stand the Shock against.

—DANIEL DEFOE, *A Journal of the Plague Year,* 1722

Some epidemics are obvious. In September 1918, 12,000 Americans died. The following month, 195,000 died. Four months later, the death toll had reached 675,000. Coffins were no longer available, so steam shovels dug mass graves. People hid in their homes, terrified, reluctant to go out even for food. It struck so rapidly and killed so appallingly: "One moment a person was fine, the next incapacitated, delirious, dying. Wrenching coughs produced pints of greenish sputum. Blood gushed from the nose. Body temperature soared to 104 or 105 degrees. Oxygen-starved skin turned blue, purple, or deep mahogany brown. Massive pneumonia set in. In the end, patients literally drowned in their bloody, fluid-filled lungs. It was a savage, swift, terrifying death."[1] By the time it had run its course, the influenza pandemic had infected one-fifth of the world's population and killed 25 million people, mostly young adults in the prime of their lives.

Some epidemics are less obvious, especially in their early stages. In 1981 a medical journal reported four cases of pneumonia in young men caused by *pneumocystis carinii*, rarely known to cause such pneumonia. Simultaneously, cases were also being reported of a rare skin cancer, Kaposi's sarcoma, in young men. Homosexuality or intravenous drug use appeared to be common denominators among most of the early cases. Slowly, the picture of underlying immune system deficiency came into focus, and the disease was christened "acquired immunodeficiency syndrome" (AIDS). Retroviruses were indicted, then convicted, and led to a newly discovered human immunodeficiency virus (HIV). The linking of the virus to the epidemic was complicated because there was a latent period of several years between the initial infection and the symptoms of AIDS.

It took a few years to fully comprehend the AIDS epidemic. Today, almost one million people are infected with HIV in the United States, and at least 32 million are infected worldwide, mostly young adults in the prime of their lives, almost all of whom will die. AIDS, the wasting disease, kills slowly by recurrent infections. Worldwide there are approximately 16,000 new cases each day.[2]

Some epidemics are not obvious at all. Imagine, for example, an epidemic that begins not over a few weeks or a few years but over a few decades. Imagine an epidemic that does not cause cupfuls of sputum, skin cancers, or a 60-pound weight loss but rather affects the brain, causing people to have strange beliefs, extreme mood swings, and illogical thinking, to hear voices that others cannot hear, and to exhibit bizarre behavior in response to their strange beliefs and illogical thinking. Imagine an epidemic that does not quickly kill a large percentage of those affected, but instead slowly kills 15 percent by suicide. Imagine an epidemic that is so insidious and ingratiating that, two centuries after it has begun, it is barely noticed, so blended into the fabric of people's lives that a few otherwise intelligent people even deny that the disease exists. Imagine an epidemic that affects over 4 million Americans, most of them in the prime of their lives, and will continue to affect more than one in every one hundred people born, but that is not recognized as a major public health problem and is largely ignored by officials overseeing the nation's health.

This is the epidemic of insanity.

Insanity is an invisible plague. There are no body counts with which one can compare the present with the past. In most countries, there are remarkably few statistics that can be used to assess insanity's prevalence over time. Professional textbooks assume that insanity has always been present in approximately the same numbers as now. The textbooks seem unaware of the milieu of the mid–nineteenth century, when, according to one writer, "the terror of madness and of the sinister alienist with his lunacy certificates haunted the age much like the terror of AIDS and other 'plagues' haunt the late twentieth century."[3]

A major impediment to understanding the epidemic of insanity is the fact that its onset occurred over so many years. Few people lived long enough to fully appreciate what was happening. Those who did raise an alarm were largely ignored since the specter of increasing insanity clashed with both professional self-esteem and national pride. Some observers said that insanity *could* not be increasing because it *should* not be increasing. Even today, the suggestion that we are living in the midst of an epidemic of insanity, a plague of brain dysfunction that hides behind labels such as schizophrenia and manic-depressive illness, strikes most people as unbelievable.

But there are consequences of our failure to appreciate epidemic insanity. From a purely historical viewpoint, we fail to understand what has been taking place. What role, for example, did the earliest increase in insanity in Massachusetts play in precipitating the Salem witchcraft trials when Cotton Mather and other authorities became concerned about the apparent increase in insanity? To what degree were the late-nineteenth-century eugenics movement and ethnic discrimination against Irish and Eastern European immigrants in the United States fueled by rapidly rising insanity? Would the mental hygiene movement have taken root in the early twentieth century if insanity had not been increasing exponentially?

Much more important, however, is the fact that by misunderstanding the past, we also misunderstand the present. Authorities in

England, Ireland, Canada, the United States, and many other countries seem genuinely puzzled by the legions of insane persons who now roam the streets, sleeping in parks and crowding public shelters, threatening passersby, and occasionally committing mayhem. Authorities seem equally perplexed by the continuing increase of insane individuals in jails and prisons, and by the increasing acts of public violence perpetrated by insane persons who are not being treated. There is no understanding of the fact that these developments are inevitable complications of epidemic insanity, that earlier versions of these problems were observed 150 years ago, and that their occurrence at that time led to decisions to put most insane persons into asylums.

If we had understood that insanity was an increasing epidemic of brain dysfunction, we would have made different decisions following World War II. We would not have been seduced by the writings of Michel Foucault, Thomas Szasz, Ronald Laing, and their brethren. We would not have emptied the insane asylums, the mainstay for containing the epidemic for a century and a half, without first ensuring that the individuals were going to receive the treatment needed to control the symptoms of their illness. We would not have confused civil liberty with the right to remain insane. And we certainly would have demanded much more research to determine the causes of epidemic insanity and to develop better treatments for it.

Our failure to understand the epidemic of insanity becomes even more incomprehensible when its costs are considered. In England in 1992, schizophrenia alone was estimated to amount to £652 million per year just for hospitalization, 5.4 percent of all National Health Service (NHS) hospital costs. The NHS direct costs for schizophrenia and manic-depressive illness together that year were more than twice that for Alzheimer's disease and other dementias. When indirect factors such as lost wages, social services, courts, and family costs were added in, the total annual cost of insanity in England was at least £3 billion.[4] In Canada, a recent estimate for the costs of schizophrenia alone was $2.3 billion (Canadian dollars), including $1.1 billion in direct and $1.2 billion in indirect costs.[5]

In the United States in 1991, it was estimated that schizophrenia alone cost $65 billion ($19 billion in direct and $46 billion in indirect costs). Similarly, in 1991 it was estimated that manic-depressive illness alone cost over $45 billion ($7.6 billion in direct and $37.6 billion in indirect costs). Thus, together in 1991, insanity cost the United States $110 billion, and this included the single largest disease category for federal payments under the Supplemental Security Income (SSI) and Social Security Disability Insurance (SSDI) programs.[6] It seems extraordinary that an epidemic that costs so much has been so ignored by so many.

What of the future? If insanity is still increasing in Europe and North America, how long is this likely to continue? Should we resurrect the eschatological predictions of the last century to estimate in which year half the total population will be insane? And what of India, China, and the other developing nations of the world? If the pattern of the epidemic continues, insanity should increase dramatically in these countries as urbanization takes place. The number of people who live in cities is currently increasing at a rate of 68 million each year, mostly in developing nations. If the epidemic of insanity in developing nations follows the pattern set in developed nations, insanity will become an even more formidable disease burden worldwide.

At the end of the seventeenth century, insanity was of little significance and was little discussed. At the end of the eighteenth century, it was perceived as probably increasing and was of some concern. At the end of the nineteenth century, it was perceived as an epidemic and was a major concern. And at the end of the twentieth century, insanity was simply accepted as part of the fabric of life. It is a remarkable history.

We believe, therefore, that insanity has been an important but neglected actor on the stage of recent history in the Western world. As historian Mary Ann Jimenez said in her book *Changing Faces of Madness*, we are writing with "the assumption that madness has a force, an impact of its own."[7]

CHAPTER 2

The Birth of Bedlam

Insanity Prior to 1700

Till now, madness has been thought a small island in an ocean of sanity. I am beginning to suspect that it is not an island at all but a continent.

—J. M. MACHADO, *The Psychiatrist,* 1881

The first Person that died of the Plague was in *December* 20th, or thereabouts 1664, . . . But after this we heard no more of any Person dying of the Plague . . . till the 9th of *February;* . . . Then it was hush'd, and we were perfectly easy as to the publick, . . . till the 22d of *April,* when there was 2 more buried not out of the same House, but out of the same Street; . . . and after this we had No more till a Fortnight, and then it broke out in several Streets and spread every way.

—DANIEL DEFOE, *A Journal of the Plague Year,* 1722

Occasional insanity as it existed for thousands of years had certain characteristics consistent with its medical and neurological origins. It might affect adults of any age, it was usually of brief duration, and the affected person was expected to either recover or die. The symptoms of insanity were often described in conjunction with other symptoms of the person's illness. Finally, visual hallucinations were more frequently reported than were auditory hallucinations. Such characteristics allow us to separate many cases of insanity in the past from the more common contemporary forms of insanity that we call schizophrenia and manic-depressive illness.

Mesopotamian tablets, dating to the second millennium B.C.E., provide the earliest known descriptions of human diseases and include symptoms of mania, depression, and paranoid delusions. There are also occasional references to insanity in the Hebrew Bible. For example, Deuteronomy 28 warns, "The Lord will smite you with madness and blindness and confusion of mind [for breaking his commandments]." Daniel 4 describes King Nebuchadnezzar's seven-year exile by God, during which the king "did eat grass as oxen." Some observers have contended that King Saul's affliction described in I Samuel 16 was a case of manic-depressive illness. Others have cited Ezekiel, who experienced auditory and visual hallucinations, as "the finest example of a case of schizophrenia in biblical times."[1] The New Testament includes multiple references to hearing voices or seeing visions, although these are presented in a context as having come from God.

Occasional references to insanity are also found in early Indian texts on Ayurvedic medicine. The most complete such description, according to C. V. Haldipur, is in the *Charaka Samhita* from the first century C.E. The chapter on insanity describes mania ("confusion of intellect, extreme fickleness of mind . . . [and] incoherence of speech") but not hallucinations. Such insanity is said to occur in people who are "wasted in body" and who also have physical symptoms such as fever, jaundice, "agitation of the eyes," and "unsteadiness," thus suggesting that the symptoms of insanity were being caused by medical illnesses.[2]

Insanity can also be found in the literature of the ancient Greeks and Romans. Hippocrates, the most astute physician of his day, described insanity following childbirth (postpartum psychosis) and insanity accompanying epilepsy. He also described delirium that was secondary to high fevers ("phrenitis"). The Greeks regarded insanity "as a form of punishment by the gods," and many characters in Greek mythology were visited by madness. However, as Bennett Simon observed, "The Greek stereotypes of madness emphasize visual distortions. . . . There is greater emphasis on visual disturbances than on auditory ones."[3]

With the collapse of the Roman Empire in the fifth century C.E., the study of medicine went into decline. It was revived in the seventh and eighth centuries by the rise of Islamic culture, whose most famous physicians, Al-Razi (Rhazes) and Ibn Sina (Avicenna), described insanity in their writings. Al-Razi provided an extensive discussion of nine subtypes of melancholia. He also differentiated smallpox from measles and documented the association of delirium with fevers and infectious diseases. Ibn Sina discussed mania and believed that rabies was a type of mania. He also described a patient having delusions of being a cow, who recovered completely when he received proper nutrition. During the height of Islamic medicine, wards for the treatment of insane patients were operational in hospitals in Cairo, Alexandria, Damascus, Aleppo, Baghdad, and Fez.[4]

"God's Minstrels"

During the Middle Ages in Christian Europe, there was virtually no systematic study of medicine. It has been widely assumed that those cases of insanity that did exist were attributed to God's punishment for sins, but Jerome Kroll and Bernard Bachrach have disputed this. After extensively examining medieval documents, they concluded that physicians at that time were "well aware of the proximate causes of mental illness, such as humoral imbalance, intemperate diet and alcohol intake, overwork, and grief."[5]

Kroll and Bachrach also analyzed 134 instances of visual hallucinations reported in medieval documents. In sixty-one cases, the hallucinations occurred during sleep or as the person was awakening (hypnagogic hallucinations). In thirty-seven cases, the hallucinations were associated with physical illnesses, fasting, or starvation, including one case of alcoholic hallucinosis. In fifteen cases, the hallucinations occurred during stressful circumstances, such as the "mass psychic phenomena" during the Crusaders' siege of Jerusalem. In eighteen cases, the visual hallucinations occurred with "no special or unusual mental state or circumstances." In only three out of the 134 cases were the visual hallucinations associated with mental illness. One occurred during a brief depression from which the person completely recovered. A second case occurred in a young man who "loses his wits" but was also eventually cured. The final case was "an unrepentant penitent who cuts off his penis and slashes his throat in response to the command of the devil," an example of severe insanity.[6]

Jeste and colleagues also analyzed twenty-two cases of illness from twelfth-century records "that could be considered neurological or psychiatric in nature." They reported that in four of the cases, symptoms of insanity were present and therefore "a diagnosis of schizophrenia may be considered." However, in one of their cases, the person was "foaming at the mouth" and had "unrestrained gesture of her limbs," and in another the person's "eyes were sometimes rolled upward" and she became paralyzed, thus suggesting epilepsy or other medical causes of the insanity. In addition, all four cases were also said to be "cured within a short period of time," making a diagnosis of schizophrenia very unlikely.[7]

As the Middle Ages in Europe gave way to the Renaissance, insanity became more visible. A major reason for this was the illness of King Charles VI in France and the subsequent insanity of his grandson, King Henry VI, in England. Charles VI had a sudden onset of insanity in 1392, when he was twenty-four, then proceeded to have a series of remissions and relapses for the next thirty years. Henry VI had the onset of his insanity in 1453 at the age of thirty-one, with "no known prodromal signs."[8] He had a prolonged course of relapses and remissions with delusions, auditory and visual hallucinations, and catatonic behavior. In 1461 he was deposed and imprisoned, and ten years later he was executed during the political struggles of the War of the Roses.

The first English-language autobiographical account of insanity was dictated by Margery Kempe in 1438. She had originally become ill in 1394 following the birth of a child and eight weeks of severe pain that "afflicted various portions of her anatomy including her head." There followed a period of ten years, during which Kempe had episodes of rolling on the floor with "great fits of weeping and shrieking, especially during mass."[9] In her autobiographical account, Kempe described both auditory and visual hallucinations, which she believed came from God.

Religious interpretations of insanity's symptoms continued to be common in the fifteenth century, and prayer was the accepted form of treatment. As early as the thirteenth century, two windows in Canterbury Cathedral depicted an insane man in a before-and-after sequence: "Mad he comes" and "He prays. Sane he goes away." The popular epic poem *Piers Plowman,* written in 1377, refers to insane persons as "God's minstrels." Prayer was a relatively benign treatment compared with the alternative bloodlettings and purgatives used at that time. Among the more unusual treatments promoted for curing insanity were toasted silk and "a roasted mouse eaten."[10]

It was also during the fifteenth century that Bethlem Hospital emerged as an institution exclusively devoted to treating the insane. Monasteries had accepted occasional insane persons for board and care throughout the Middle Ages, and early hospitals in Spain, Italy, and the Islamic world had admitted insane persons along with individuals with other medical problems. It was therefore not unusual in the late fourteenth century for St. Mary's priory in London to admit both persons with medical problems and those with insanity. In 1403 the priory housed six men who had "fallen owte of hyr wytte,"[11] and it subsequently evolved into Bethlem. In 1547, as part of King Henry VIII's policy of dissolving the monasteries, he assigned Bethlem Hospital to the city of London for use by insane poor persons. By that time, Bethlem Hospital was also being widely referred to simply as Bedlam.

"There the Men Are as Mad as He"

The earliest suggestion of an increasing public interest in insanity seems to have occurred in late-sixteenth-century England. As summarized by Michael MacDonald in his book *Mystical Bedlam:* "During the late sixteenth and early seventeenth centuries, the English people became more concerned about the prevalence of madness, gloom, and self-murder than they had ever been before, and the reading public developed a strong fascination with classical medical psychology. . . . Interest in insanity quickened about 1580, and madmen, melancholics, and suicides became familiar literary types. Scientific writers popularized medical lore about melancholy, and clergymen wrote treatises about consoling the troubled in mind."[12]

At this time, there also appeared to be an increasing visibility of violent acts committed by insane persons. In 1565, for example, a Sussex man killed his wife with an axe and was judged at his trial to be insane. Highly publicized was the 1573 case of Peter Berchet, who stabbed Sir John Hawkins, a member of the House of Commons and a favorite of Queen Elizabeth I. Berchet, overtly insane, was imprisoned in the Tower of London, where he promptly killed a guard. He was then publicly executed near the spot where he had attacked Hawkins, and "his right hand [was] cut off and nailed to the gibbet."[13]

One measure of the increasing popular interest in insanity was the number of ballads written about it. According to a historian of English popular culture: "Amongst many individual songs and verses, two principal song-families stand out: 'Bedlamite' verses and 'mad songs.' The former, dating from the sixteenth century and much in vogue in the later seventeenth, use the theme of the beggar released from Bethlem." These ballads were printed on single sheets, or "broadsides," and sold for a penny apiece. They could be read (approximately half of London's males were literate at that time), or they could be sung in the streets or at fairs and were "the cheapest and probably the most widely distributed form of popular literature of the time."[14]

Many of those ballads described Bethlem Hospital and the reasons why people became insane. Unrequited love was a popular theme:

> As I was a-walking one morning in Spring,
> I heard a maid in Bedlam so sweet-i-ly she sing,
> Her chains she rattled with her hands and this she sigh and sing,
> "I love my love because I know he first love me."

Another ballad, dating to at least 1637, was titled "Love's Lunacie":

> This Bethlem is a place of torment;
> Heere's fearfull notes still sounding;
> Heere minds are fil'd with discontent,
> And terrors still abounding.
> Some shake their chaines in wofull wise,
> Some sweare, some curse, some roaring,
> Some shrieking out with fearfull cries,
> And some their cloaths are tearing.[15]

The largest number of Bedlamite ballads, however, described patients who had been released from Bethlem and were licensed to beg. Since antivagrancy laws prohibited all other forms of begging, it became common for sane beggars to feign insanity in order to ply their trade. The released patients were widely known as Toms o' Bedlam and became ubiquitous in the ballads of the seventeenth century:

> *From forth my sad and darksome cell,*
> *And from the deep abyss of hell*
> *Poor Tom is come to view the world again,*
> *To see if he can ease distempered brain.*
> *Fear and despair possess his soul,*
> *Hark how the angry furies howl!*

Other songs dating to this period include "The Bedlamite," "Bess of Bedlam," "The Maniac," "The Lunatic Love," and "The Mad-man's Song."[16]

In her history of English psychiatry, Kathleen Jones says that "up to the middle of the seventeenth century, 'Toms o' Bedlam'—discharged patients with a recognizable badge which gave them license to beg in order to pay their arrears—were a familiar sight in towns and villages throughout England." Bishop Thomas Percy claimed in 1763 that "the English had more songs and ballads on the subject of insanity than any of their neighbors. . . . We certainly do not find the same in the printed collections of French and Italian songs." And according to David Mellett: "It would be a logical assumption to consider them [Bedlamite songs] as evidence of contemporary popular imagery, and an imagery which they reinforced as well as reflected."[17]

A second measure of the increasing popular interest in insanity was the use of insanity in plays of that period. William Shakespeare, of course, is the best-known playwright, and, according to Thomas Dalby, "in at least 20 of his 38 plays (and many of his sonnets) he comments on the nature of madness and its causes."[18]

The title character of *Hamlet*, written in 1601, has received extensive psychiatric analysis; Joseph Collins suggests that "the mentality of the latter [Hamlet] has probably occupied more printed space than that of any other person, real or imaginary." Opinions regarding whether Hamlet was feigning insanity or was truly insane have been approximately evenly divided, with many prominent psychiatric professionals having written on the subject, including John Conolly, John

Bucknill, Henry Maudsley, Forbes Winslow, Isaac Ray, Amariah Brigham, Sigmund Freud, Otto Rank, Ernest Jones, and Eliot Slater.[19]

King Lear, written in 1606, illustrates a type of senile dementia in the eighty-year-old king but also provides a clear demonstration of feigned insanity when Edgar disguises himself as a mad Tom o' Bedlam. Nigel Bark has cited this as evidence that Shakespeare was familiar with the syndrome of schizophrenia.[20] Whether or not schizophrenia even existed in 1600 is unclear; what is clear is that Shakespeare, like most educated men of his generation, was knowledgeable about and intrigued by insanity, as represented by the patients discharged from Bethlem Hospital.

There is also a suggestion in Act V of *Hamlet* that Shakespeare may have believed that insanity was increasing in England, although, as in much of Shakespeare, it is difficult to differentiate serious thought from jest:

> HAMLET: . . . How long hast thou been a grave-maker?
> FIRST CLOWN: Of all the days i' the year, I came to't that
>   day that our last king Hamlet overcame Fortinbras.
> HAMLET: How long is that since?
> FIRST CLOWN: . . . it was the very day that young Hamlet
>   was born; he that is mad, and sent into England.
> HAMLET: Ay, marry, why was he sent into England?
> FIRST CLOWN: Why, because he was mad; he shall recover
>   his wits there; or, if he do not, 'tis no great matter there.
> HAMLET: Why?
> FIRST CLOWN: 'Twill not be seen in him there; there the
>   men are as mad as he.

Shakespeare was one of many playwrights writing for the Elizabethan and Jacobean stage. Karin Coddon noted that "Jacobean drama is noteworthy for its ubiquitous lunatics," and Thomas Dalby similarly said, "The depiction of madness was ubiquitous during plays of this [Elizabethan] time." Michael MacDonald added: "The Jacobean stage teemed with idiots and lunatics. . . . The fascination with madness was so strong that it minted new words and . . . at least twenty-seven proverbs." Robert Reed wrote an entire book about Bedlam on the Jacobean stage, in which he said: "The Jacobean stage was, and remains, distinguished by unusual abnormality, extravagancy, and bombastic utterance; its average temperature, figuratively speaking, was not a great deal short of madness."[21]

The examples of insanity in Elizabethan and Jacobean drama are many. In Christopher Marlowe's *Tamburlaine,* Zabrina becomes insane after discovering her husband's suicide. In Ben Jonson's *Bartholomew Fair,* Dame Purecraft is told that she must marry a mad-man and visits Bethlem to select one. In John Webster's *The Duchess of Malfi,* Ferdinand brings patients from Bethlem to dance and sing before his sister to try to drive her insane, while in Philip Massinger's *A New Way to Pay Old Debts,* Sir Giles Overreach becomes insane and is treated by physicians from Bethlem. The character Memnon in John Fletcher's *The Mad Lover* becomes insane when he is rejected by Calis but then recovers his sanity when she accepts him. Thomas Dekker's *The Honest Whore* includes a visit to Bethlem and a description of various patients therein. And Thomas Middleton's *The Changeling* takes place in a madhouse run by a doctor who is himself insane. All of these perhaps coalesce in Hieronimo's remark in Thomas Kyd's *Spanish Tragedy;* when his son is killed, Hieronimo becomes insane and says: "O no, there is no end: the end is death and madness!"[22]

"A Rare Diversion"

The increasing public interest in insanity, first noted in the late six-teenth century, became more intense in the seventeenth century. The most direct measure of this change was the number of public visitors to Bethlem Hospital. As early as 1610, Lord Percy had recommended "the shew of Bethlem" as a London attraction, along with "the fireworks at the Artillery Garden." Beginning in the middle of the seventeenth cen-tury, visits to Bethlem Hospital increased markedly. In the 1650s, there were complaints that visitors were harassing the patients by "jest" or "knavery," and Sunday visitations were banned. In 1619 Samuel Pepys told his cousin's children "to see Bedlam" during their visit to London, and nine years later, James Yonge, visiting from Plymouth, included a visit to Bethlem "with all that was curious in London."[23]

By the closing years of the seventeenth century, Bethlem Hospi-tal had become "a rare Diversion" visited by "Swarms of People," espe-cially on holidays. In 1681 the hospital's board of governors expressed concern about "the greate quantity of persons that come daily to see the said Lunatickes." In 1676, Bethlem Hospital had been moved to a new, larger, and architecturally splendid building, which further increased its appeal. The hospital had become a "zoo and freakshow . . . in which the inmate was regarded as a beast or monster." The "visitors themselves exploited the patients by getting them drunk, while hucksters hawked 'Nutt Cake [and] . . . fruite' to the patients and visitors, contributing to the fairground atmosphere." "Drunken" visitors were recorded as regularly harassing the patients and then "Laughing and Hooting" at the "Raving . . . Cursing and Swearing" that they provoked. In 1690 precautions were even instituted "to prevent sexual contact between visitors and women patients." Edward O'Donoghue, who wrote a history of Bethlem Hospital, summarized this period as follows: "Everybody who lived in London or ever came to London visited Bethlem as a matter of course."[24]

The reason for the increasing public interest in insanity, beginning in the late sixteenth century and intensifying in the second half of the seventeenth century, is not immediately apparent. Historians of psychiatry have almost universally assumed that no major change in the prevalence of insanity occurred during this time, and they claim that most insane persons were kept at home or wandered the streets of towns and cities. If that were true, most people would have been exposed to insane persons on a regular basis, as people in Europe and North America today are exposed to the homeless mentally ill in the postdeinstitutionalization age. And if that were the case, why would London's residents and its visitors have found a visit to Bethlem so appealing? Clergymen promoted a visit to Bethlem as a moral lesson to those who might be tempted by sin, but the accounts of the visitations make clear that most people came for pure entertainment.

The interest in insanity in general, and Bethlem Hospital in particular, becomes even more extraordinary when it is realized that Bethlem contained relatively few patients. In the early 1600s, when Elizabethan and Jacobean playwrights were focusing their attention on it, Bethlem Hospital had only twenty to thirty patients at any one time. By midcentury, their number was still less than fifty, and by the end of the seventeenth century, after the opening of the new building in 1676, there were approximately one hundred and thirty patients. On many holidays, there must have been more visitors than there were patients.

Some historians have suggested that the seventeenth-century public fascination with madness had social origins and was "an aspect of the contemporary perception that the world itself had gone mad."[25] It was a socially and politically unstable century in England, with a civil war, an unstable monarchy, and periodic visitations of the plague, which in 1665 killed one-quarter of London's population. It is, of course, possible that there is a relationship between this instability and an increasing interest in insanity, but such a relationship has not been observed during other periods of instability in England or in other nations.

Another possible reason for the increasing public interest in insanity at this time was the dissolution of English monasteries by Henry VIII in the mid–sixteenth century. The monasteries had been the main locus of support for the poor and insane, and suddenly they were closed. According to one observer, as a consequence of this, "the idle and dissolute were suffered to wander about the country, assuming such characters as they imagined were most likely to insure success to their frauds. . . . Among other disguises, many affected madness, and were distinguished by the name of Bedlam Beggars."[26]

An additional explanation we must consider for the increasing interest in insanity in seventeenth-century England is that insanity was beginning to change in its course, severity, and prevalence. If, for example, most cases of insanity had always been relatively brief and time limited and suddenly more chronic cases began to appear, it would have been noteworthy. Or, if most cases of insanity had been relatively mild and then more severely insane persons had begun to appear, this change would also have been noteworthy. And finally, if insanity was becoming more common, that certainly would have been noteworthy as well.

The population of London was increasing rapidly during the seventeenth century, tripling between 1600 and 1700 to a total of approximately 600,000 inhabitants. It was, in fact, the fastest-growing city in Europe.[27] Recent studies have reported that being born or raised in an urban area increases one's risk for developing schizophrenia (see chapter 14), so London's seventeenth-century population explosion in some way may have been causally related to an increasing prevalence of insanity.

Richard Napier of Buckinghamshire

Data that can be used to estimate the prevalence of insanity in seventeenth-century England are valuable resources. One such treasure trove is the remarkably detailed casebooks of Richard Napier, who practiced medicine in Buckinghamshire from 1597 to 1634. Napier's patients came from Bedfordshire and Northamptonshire as well as Buckinghamshire, rural counties north of urban London and slightly east of Stratford-upon-Avon, the birthplace of Napier's contemporary, William Shakespeare.

Napier was a clergyman by training, educated at Oxford and rector of the parish at Great Linford. Like many clergymen of his era, he practiced general medicine, utilizing an assortment of treatments derived from alchemy and astrology. During his thirty-seven-year practice, he saw approximately 60,000 patients, mostly drawn from the rural villages of the surrounding counties. According to Michael MacDonald's extensive analysis of Napier's case notes, published as *Mystical Bedlam*, Napier treated patients from all socioeconomic levels of the population, although disproportionately fewer came from the lowest quarter. According to MacDonald, "his fees were rather small, and he forgave them for the poor."[28]

In the early seventeenth century, Napier's reputation grew and, according to MacDonald, he "became a famous healer." "By the last decade of his life he counted earls among his clients and knights and baronets among his friends." He was known as someone who had special expertise in treating mental disorders and was asked by the Duke of Buckingham to treat the duke's insane brother. Nearly 80 percent of the mentally disturbed patients seen by Napier came from the three surrounding counties, which had a total population of approximately 200,000. A few patients came from London and from as far away as Yorkshire and Dorset, drawn by Napier's reputation.

In his assessment of Napier's detailed case notes, MacDonald categorized 2,039 patients as having "evidence of mental or emotional disturbance." Within this group, Napier himself diagnosed only 139 of them as being "mad" or "lunatic," terms he used interchangeably. As MacDonald noted, "It is plain that extravagant mental disorders were comparatively rare."[29]

The case notes of the 2,039 patients with "mental or emotional disturbance" were given by MacDonald to Michael Shepherd, a senior English psychiatrist, for analysis by twentieth-century diagnostic standards. Shepherd identified "at least 20" cases as meeting criteria for schizophrenia and an additional, unspecified number that could be diagnosed as manic-depressive illness. As an example of schizophrenia, Shepherd cited the case of a nineteen-year-old woman with the sudden onset of delusions, bizarre behavior, and inappropriate affect ("will smile at everything"), who continued to be insane two years later. Napier characterized such patients as "like a Bedlam" or "stark Bedlam mad."

In addition to the cases of schizophrenia and manic-depressive illness diagnosed by Shepherd among Napier's "mad" and "lunatic" patients, many others apparently suffered from medical causes of insanity. One, for example, was "a strong maddish fellow" who "was frightened with [by] two fellow that fell upon him and wounded him in the head." Another was suffering from "smallpox and frenzy, frantic and unruly [for] about three weeks." According to MacDonald, Napier, unlike most of his colleagues at that time, did not differentiate "frenzy" (insanity with a fever) from insanity without a fever, which would have led him to categorize many cases of infectious disease with delirium as insanity.[30]

In summarizing the psychiatric findings from Napier's practice, Michael MacDonald noted that "the most flamboyant and recognizable kinds of insanity . . . are comparatively scarce. . . . The distinctive features of the contemporary concept of utter insanity, madness, or lunacy will thus be found in only a tiny proportion of the total number of psychiatric consultations." MacDonald also searched for cases of insanity not treated by Napier and identified twenty-eight others in court records of the three counties during the years Napier was practicing. Even with these additions, MacDonald concludes that "it is plain that extravagant mental disorders were comparatively rare. . . . One would have to conclude that madness was not a common phenomenon."[31]

Since it is not known how many additional insane individuals among the population of 200,000 were being treated by other medical practitioners, it is not possible to estimate the prevalence of insanity with any degree of precision. Napier treated 139 cases of insanity, and

MacDonald identified 28 additional cases, thus totaling 157 cases. Since most of these people were insane for a limited period of time—and in cases of frenzy, for only days or weeks—only a small proportion of the total cases would have been insane at any given time during the thirty-seven-year period. In order to achieve the baseline insanity rate of 0.5 per 1,000 total population discussed in appendix B, there must have been at least one hundred persons insane at any given time among this population of 200,000. Napier's case notes suggest that the prevalence of insanity was almost certainly lower than that.

Except for Napier's case notes, no other seventeenth-century data are sufficiently detailed to give a reasonable estimate of the prevalence of insanity. The records that do exist are mostly those of local justices of the peace and the Court of Wards and Liveries. These officials "were responsible for all important judicial, financial, and administrative matters pertaining to idiots and lunatics." In recent years, scholars such as A. Fessler, Richard Neugebauer, Peter Rushton, and Akihito Suzuki have analyzed these seventeenth-century records.[32]

What the records show is that the local courts were usually humane and tried to avoid the confinement of insane persons except when necessary because of violent behavior. As Neugebauer noted: "Government involvement with Court of Wards cases was designed to protect the disturbed person and his property." In contrast to the picture Michel Foucault painted in *Madness and Civilization*—of mass deportations of insane persons on ships of fools, and of a governmental conspiracy to lock up all deviant individuals—the actual records depict a different and much more humane reality. Andrew Scull has called the ships of fools "simply a figment of [Foucault's] overactive imagination," and Eric Midelfort has added: "Nowhere can one find reference to real boats or ships loaded with mad pilgrims in search of their reason." Suzuki similarly noted that the impetus to confine violent insane persons came from the "family, relatives and neighbors of the dangerous lunatic," not from the government. "If there was any conspiracy concerning the confinement of dangerous lunatics in pre-asylum England, it was not of the ruling class against the plebs, but of the sane against the insane."[33]

Insane persons in the seventeenth century, then, were kept at home whenever possible. The court records "suggest that it was considered normal for a lunatic to be kept, maintained and governed by the able head of the household." When this was not possible, the insane person was often boarded with another family, or someone was employed to care for the person in his or her own home. For example, when the Reverend George Trosse became insane in 1656, he was boarded with a physician until he recovered. Trosse's illness, the details of which he published in autobiographical form in 1690, has been cited as an early example of schizophrenia by some writers, but Edward Hare cast doubt on this speculation, noting the large role of Trosse's alcoholism in causing his psychiatric symptoms.[34]

Confinement of insane persons in the seventeenth century was thus reserved for those who were violent or otherwise dangerous. Such cases were relatively uncommon; for example, in Rushton's examination of court records in northern England, violence was "mentioned in less than a tenth of the total" cases. Violent behavior associated with insanity in the seventeenth-century cases ranged from breaking glass windows (which were very expensive at that time) and setting fires (e.g., an insane woman in Somerset was feared by her neighbors because "she should set on fire where she dwelleth") to being dangerous to self or others (e.g., an insane woman in Lancashire "hath lately pulled out one of her eyes and is wandering about and offers violence to her own children").[35]

In such cases of dangerousness, the insane individual was usually remanded by the courts to Bethlem Hospital, the local jail, or, if the person's family was wealthy, to one of the few but growing number of private psychiatric hospitals. As Suzuki noted, "Those lunatics who were sent to Houses of Correction were perceived as dangerous, and JPs [justices of the peace] did not put lunatics indiscriminately into the institution."[36] Then, as now, authorities sought the least expensive solution to the problem of insanity, and that solution was usually to leave the persons at home or board them with another family.

Thus, an examination of the records of insane persons in seventeenth-century England shows an increasing public interest in insanity but does not reveal an unusually high prevalence of it. It certainly existed and was handled as expeditiously and inexpensively as possible, but it does not appear to have been a problem of anywhere near the magnitude that it was to become two centuries later.

Three other impressions emerge from seventeenth-century English records and writings on insanity. First, many of the cases appear to have been caused by medical conditions and were indeed assumed to be diseases by the populace. Neugebauer, for example, noted that the seventeenth-century court petitioners on insanity cases "most commonly . . . ascribed the mental disturbance to some prior physical illness." Second, most of the court decisions on insanity cases were "intended to be temporary settlement and once individuals were, in the eyes of the court, 'sane mentis,' they could regain custody of their possessions." The expectation, therefore, was that most insane persons would recover in a relatively short time, and apparently a large percentage of them actually did so. Boarding insane individuals with families or sending them to jail was usually viewed as a temporary solution that could be reversed as soon as the person got well. Even the severest cases, which were sent to Bethlem Hospital, were considered curable; a study of all such admissions between 1694 and 1718 found that 60 percent of them were discharged in less than a year. Insanity was thus usually a temporary state, which is consistent with most cases that are caused by medical conditions.[37]

Finally, it is also noteworthy that prominent English physicians who wrote about mental illness and brain dysfunction in the seventeenth century paid remarkably little attention to insanity, suggesting that it was not a major problem at that time. For example, Robert Burton, who published his epic *Anatomy of Melancholy* in 1621, defined insanity as a "raving without a fever, far more violent than melancholy," but then dismissed it from further discussion. Thomas Sydenham similarly differentiated madness from phrenitis by the absence of a fever but concentrated his professional efforts on the first complete description of hysteria and on the childhood chorea that now bears his name.[38] In the closing years of the seventeenth century, Thomas Willis published his seminal work on brain anatomy and the first description of general paresis, the neurological and psychiatric syndrome caused by syphilis. Willis subscribed to the general belief that insanity could be differentiated from phrenitis by the absence of fever, and in 1683 he described a form of illogical thinking that occurs in some cases of insanity, but insanity does not appear to have been a major concern in his work.

Probably the most useful seventeenth-century English contribution to understanding insanity, however, came from a philosopher not a physician. In his 1690 "Essay Concerning Human Understanding,"

John Locke differentiated idiots ("natural fools") from insane persons. The latter, he said, "do not appear to me to have lost the faculty of reasoning, but having joined together some ideas very wrongly, they mistake them for truths; and they err as men do that argue right from wrong principles."[39] Locke thus defined delusions as the hallmark of insanity, setting the standard for thinking about insanity for the next century.

CHAPTER 3

The "English Malady" Appears
England, 1700–1800

There is no disease more to be dreaded than madness. For
what greater unhappiness can befall a man than to be deprived
of his reason and understanding.

—RICHARD MEAD, *Medical Precepts and Cautions,* 1751

And here I must observe also, that the Plague, as I suppose all
Distempers do, operated in a different Manner, on differing
Constitutions; some were immediately overwhelm'd with it,
. . . while others, as I have observ'd, were silently infected.

—DANIEL DEFOE, *A Journal of the Plague Year,* 1722

The eighteenth century in England opened with Queen Anne's
ascension to the throne. Tragically, she had lost all fifteen of her
children—ten by miscarriage or stillbirth, four in infancy, and
one at age eleven. The century closed with King George III on the
throne. In 1783 he had lost all thirteen American colonies, and five
years later he lost his mind as well. By this time, insanity had become
more prominent in England, the King's madness being a coincidental,
if ironic, sovereign sanction of the emerging "English malady."

An official suggestion that insanity was a developing problem in
the early eighteenth century was the Vagrancy Act of 1714, passed by
Parliament shortly before Queen Anne's death. Although legislation

had previously been enacted regarding paupers, this was the first law that differentiated "pauper lunatics" from "rogues, vagabonds, sturdy beggars and vagrants." The law empowered justices of the peace to apprehend individuals "who, by lunacy, or otherwise, are furiously Mad, and dangerous to be permitted to go Abroad" and to see that such individuals were "kept safely Locked up in such secure place within the County where such Parish or Town shall lie . . . and (if such Justices find it necessary) to be there Chained." An example of such a case was James Hey of Lancashire, who was confined in 1720 upon a complaint of his wife, who said that "he is not only lunatick but very often distracted and outrageous and so furiously mad and distracted at this time that she is constrained to get three or four men at the present time to attend him, therefore to prevent mischiefe to herselfe and children and to others also." The cost of the confinement was to be paid by the parish or town from which the person came, and confinement could be continued as long as "such Lunacy or Madness shall continue."[1]

Since there were virtually no hospital beds for the insane in the early eighteenth century, confinement under the Vagrancy Act usually took place in local jails. Bethlem Hospital, which had been the sole psychiatric hospital in England for more than three hundred years, had provision for only 150 beds. When the new hospital building had opened in 1676, these had been thought sufficient to meet England's needs for many years to come. Yet by 1720, Bethlem's wards could no longer accommodate all admissions, and the hospital had to be further enlarged. Increasing hospitalization of England's insane was under way, a process that would not stop for 250 years.

Some historians have claimed that the increasing confinement of the insane in the eighteenth century was due primarily to broadening diagnostic boundaries for those who could legitimately be confined. An analysis of admissions to Bethlem in the eighteenth century does not support this thesis. In *A Survey of the Cities of London and Westminster,* published in 1720, John Strype noted that "those are judged the fittest Objects for this Hospital [Bethlem] that are raving and furious and . . . likely to do mischief to themselves or others." Specifically excluded from admission were "those that are only Melancholik . . . or Ideots . . . these the Governors think the House [Bethlem] ought not be bothered with." Similarly, in *A History of Bethlem,*

Jonathan Andrews said that "Bethlem was primarily a place for keeping lunatics who were a menace to themselves or others. . . . The strict admissions criteria seem to have been effective in keeping numbers low."[2]

A study of patients admitted to Bethlem Hospital between 1772 and 1787 also reported that "above one half of the patients . . . have attempted some mischief against themselves or others. . . . There are above a score of atrocious murderers: there are parricides, and butchers of their own offspring." Bethlem's beds were continuously full, and "by the 1780s there were 200 patients every year on the waiting-list." For readmissions, "Nearly two-thirds were forced to wait between five and nine years from the time their petitions were read before they were readmitted."[3]

During the early eighteenth century, as Bethlem Hospital was expanding and experiencing increased crowding, the hospital became an even greater tourist attraction than it had been in the seventeenth century. English essayist Richard Steele took his three younger brothers "to show 'em . . . Bedlam" and later sarcastically wrote that he had consulted "the Collegiates of Moorfield," the part of London where Bethlem Hospital was located. Nicholas Blundell, visiting from Lancashire in 1703, "walked to Bedlom [*sic*]" and on two subsequent visits to London returned to the hospital to show his wife and daughters. Literature of this period also mentioned visits to Bethlem, including Ned Ward's *The London Spy* (1699) and George Farquhar's *Love and a Bottle* (1697), in which a London visitor wishes to see "the Rarities of the Town," including Westminster Abbey and Bethlem Hospital.[4]

Bethlem was a major attraction for foreign visitors as well. Travel guides such as *Les Délices d'Angleterre* (1707) and *Travels in London* (1710) listed Bethlem as a major attraction. A German traveler at this time was intrigued by a patient "who is said to have crowed all day long like a cock."[5]

By the 1730s, the crowds at Bethlem included England's foremost aristocrats. The Prince of Wales visited in 1735, the same year in which William Hogarth painted the eighth and final scene of *The Rake's Progress* on a Bethlem ward, showing an insane Thomas Rakewell being looked down upon by two noble ladies. In 1741 Samuel Richardson published *Familiar Letters on Important Occasions,* intended to provide "the requisite style and forms" for "letters written to and for particular friends on the most important occasions." One of the model letters was "from a young Lady in Town to her Aunt in the Country Describing Bethlem Hospital": "I have this afternoon been with my cousins to gratify the odd curiosity most people have to see Bethleham [*sic*] or Bedlam Hospital. A more affecting scene my eyes never beheld. . . . For there we see man destitute of every mark of reason and wisdom, and levell'd to the brute creation, if not beneath it."[6]

By 1742 the flow of visitors to Bethlem had become a constant stream. The hospital governing board estimated "about nineteen thousand visitors" each year to observe the approximately two hundred patients. That same year, the hospital governing board decided to appoint the hospital porter as a constable "to prevent disturbances . . . at Holiday times." The crowds continued to increase and included such individuals as the young lady who in 1752 came "down from the country" to "see the Tower, the [Westminster] abbey, and Bedlam, and two or three plays." By 1764 it became necessary to assign "four constables and also four Stout Fellows as Assistants in each Gallery" because "great Riots and Disorders have been Committed in this Hospital during the Holidays." Because of the continuing disorder, two years later Bethlem Hospital was closed to all visitors on major holidays, and in 1770 it was closed to all visitors except those who had a ticket signed by the hospital's governor.[7]

The interest in viewing the insane in eighteenth-century England was quite extraordinary. A few visitors came out of "a moral duty, painful and distressing, yet pointing useful lessons. . . . A sight of Bethlem might be recommended as a peculiarly effective deterrent to the wayward inclinations of children." Most visitors, however, came to see the patients as "curiosities," "remarkable characters," and "very amusing objects." It was the titillation of a freak show, of viewing exotic human specimens not previously seen. Bethlem Hospital was thus regarded as a kind of human zoo, reminiscent of public exhibitions of lions, elephants, and other exotic creatures put on display by English explorers as they returned from Africa and Asia. In Henry Mackenzie's 1771 novel *The Man of Feeling*, Harley, the protagonist, described a visit to Bethlem Hospital, made because it was one of "those things called Sights in London, which every stranger is supposed desirous to see." During the visit the guide told Harley, "in the phrase of those that keep wild beasts for show," that patients in one ward "were much better worth seeing than any they had passed, being ten times more fierce and unmanageable."[8]

"No Cure—No Money"

As pressure for admission to Bethlem's limited number of beds increased, other psychiatric beds, both public and private, were being made available. In Norwich, one of the largest cities outside of London, Mary Chapman left funds upon her death in 1724 to endow a public hospital for "distrest lunaticks." Chapman, the daughter of one of the city's wealthiest men, had had "lunacy . . . afflict some of my nearest relacons and kindred" and founded the hospital "as a monument of my thankfulness to God" for having "blessed me with the free use of my reason and understanding." In 1725 London bookseller and member of Parliament Thomas Guy left funds in his will to create a "lunatic house" in what would be called Guy's Hospital. In 1751 London's St. Luke's Hospital was opened by public subscription; a pamphlet entitled "Reasons for Establishing St. Luke's" noted Bethlem Hospital's overcrowding and long waiting list. In its first ten years, St. Luke's admitted 749 patients, and by 1800 it had three hundred beds, surpassing Bethlem in size. Additional psychiatric hospitals using public subscriptions were opened in 1764 in Newcastle, in 1766 in Manchester, in 1777 in York, in 1795 in Liverpool, and in 1801 in Oxford. Most of these facilities were small, with accommodations for thirty or fewer patients, but they represented a beginning for the increasing number of mentally ill individuals who were considered in need of hospitalization.[9]

It is noteworthy that subscribers who contributed funds for these hospitals did so specifically in response to perceived needs: for example, the founders of the Manchester Lunatic Hospital voted to raise the necessary funds for the hospital in order to provide care for "the Number of distressed Objects of this kind, with which this Kingdom unhappily abounds . . . no Cases could be more truly deplorable than those of Poor Lunaticks, who had in common no Prospect of a Cure and who . . . continued public Spectacles of the deepest Misery, if not Terror, to the Neighbors." Similarly, the Yorkshire Asylum was opened because of a belief that "something should be done for the relief of those unhappy sufferers who are the objects of terror and compassion to all around them and whose cases lay a just claim to the benevolence of their fellow creatures." According to Nigel Walker and Sarah McCabe, "an unmistakable phenomenon of this period was a growing public awareness of the special nature of the social problem posed by the mentally disordered," which showed itself "in the foundation by voluntary subscription of hospitals for the insane." Also representative of this growing public awareness was a sermon preached at St. Bridget's Church in London during Easter Week of 1759: "The Case of Incurable Lunaticks, and the Charity Due to Them, Particularly Recommended."[10]

Since public psychiatric hospitals admitted primarily, or exclusively, paupers in the eighteenth century, private hospitals opened to provide care for patients who could pay. A few such facilities had come into existence in the late seventeenth century, and their number grew in parallel with the foundation of public hospitals. By 1807 these private hospitals numbered forty-five, although most were very small, and they were variously referred to as private madhouses, private asylums, or, at the end of the eighteenth century, private licensed houses. Their claims were often immodest, as illustrated by an advertisement in 1700 in which a private madhouse claimed to be able to cure "all lunatick, distracted or mad people" in three months or less. "Several," it continued, "have been cur'd in a fortnight, and some in less time." The advertisement finished with an appealing guarantee: "No cure— no money."[11] The best known of the eighteenth-century private madhouses was the York Retreat, founded in 1792 by William Tuke, a Quaker tea and coffee merchant, in response to the death, presumably due to neglect, of a Quaker woman in the public Yorkshire Asylum. Another possible reason for Quaker interest in the treatment of insanity was cited by an American who traveled in England in 1810, who was told "by a well-informed person, born a Quaker, that there are more instances of insanity among that persuasion than among other people." When Tuke proposed the idea of a private asylum to his wife, she is said to have replied: "Thee has had many wonderful children of thy brain, dear William, but this one is surely like to be an idiot." In fact, the York Retreat became a widely emulated model for other psychiatric hospitals both in England and abroad, including the Quaker-founded Pennsylvania Hospital in Philadelphia.[12]

Until passage in 1774 of the Act for Regulating Madhouses, the main problem with private madhouses was the absence of licensing or inspection. Before that time, anyone could open a madhouse and advertise for patients, leading to inevitable abuses. As early as 1706 Daniel Defoe, journalist and novelist, publicized the case of a young woman who had been wrongfully confined in a private madhouse and urged that they be publicly regulated. After publishing his books *Robinson Crusoe, Moll Flanders,* and *A Journal of the Plague Year,* Defoe returned to the subject of madhouse abuse in his 1728 treatise *Augusta Triumphans.* "Of all Persons who are Objects of our Charity," said Defoe, "none move my Compassion like those . . . deprived of Reason to act for themselves." He went on eloquently to condemn "the Vile practice now so much in vogue among the better Sort" of husbands sending their wives to madhouses so that the men would be free to live with their mistresses. "How many," asked Defoe, "grow weary of the pure Streams of chaste Love, and thirsting after the Puddles of lawless Lust, buries his vertuous Wife alive, that he may have the greater Freedom with his Mistresses?"[13]

How often such private madhouse abuses actually happened in the eighteenth century is less clear. Patricia Allderidge suggests that "such cases were not frequent but were well publicized." William Parry-Jones, author of the definitive *The Trade in Lunacy,* also concludes that "despite the view that such abuses were widespread, surviving evidence for this is limited and often is based upon sensational accounts by persons of doubtful reliability."[14]

Wrongful confinement of sane persons in private madhouses was thematically used in several novels of the period, including Samuel Richardson's *Pamela; or, Virtue Rewarded* (1740) and *Clarissa Harlowe* (1748), Tobias Smollett's *The Adventures of Sir Launcelot Greaves* (1760), and Mary Wollstonecraft's *Maria* (1798). Several individuals who believed they had been wrongfully confined also published personal accounts, including Alexander Cruden (*The Adventures of Alexander the Corrector,* 1754) and Samuel Bruckshaw (*The Case, Petition and Address of Samuel Bruckshaw,* 1774). Both of these personal accounts include suggestions that the writers were indeed legitimately insane at the time of their involuntary confinement, despite their protestations to the contrary.

Stimulated by such public accounts, Parliament in 1763 appointed a Select Committee to examine possible abuses in private

London madhouses, and the committee recommended that the mad-houses be brought under official regulation. It took until 1774 for such legislation to be enacted. The law provided for the licensing and inspection of private madhouses and restricted involuntary admissions to cases approved by both a justice of the peace and a physician to confirm that the person was truly insane and not merely being confined for nefarious reasons. However, it would be many years before these regulations would be enforced, and examples of private madhouse abuses continued to surface periodically.

"Moody Madness Laughing Wild"

The second half of the eighteenth century in England gave birth to both industrialism and a middle class. Advances in the smelting of iron, the invention of the steam engine, power loom, and spinning jenny, the introduction of agricultural techniques such as crop rotation, and increasing trade with England's colonies combined to bring prosperity to an increasingly broad group of people. According to Roy Porter, "England came to boast a broad and ever-expanding middling class of merchants, tradesmen, shopkeepers, clerks, farmers, skilled craftsmen and the like, with money to spare after the necessities of life had been supplied."[15] Books were one of the luxuries increasingly purchased by this expanding middle class, and England's literary establishment grew proportionately.

Insanity was a frequent subject in these books. In Henry Fielding's *The Intriguing Chambermaid* (1733), Mr. Goodall is told that he is "a poor distracted wretch, and ought to have an apartment in a dark room, and clean straw." In Tobias Smollett's *Count Fathom* (1753), Elenor becomes insane and is sent to Bethlem Hospital to recover. In Laurence Sterne's *Tristram Shandy* (1760), Maria is also insane, and the book was so popular that "Maria had inspired more than thirty paintings by the start of Victoria's reign." In Frances Sheridan's *Memoirs of Miss Sydney Biddulph* (1767), the protagonist is driven insane by guilt and confined to an asylum for the remainder of his life. And in Henry Mackenzie's *The Man of Feeling* (1771), the hero encounters an insane woman in Bethlem, "the most pathetic and attractive inmate of the asylum," and weeps for her. Insanity appeared increasingly as a topic in eighteenth-century poetry as well, as in Thomas Gray's "Ode on a Distant Prospect of Eton College" (1742), his first published poem: "And moody Madness laughing wild/Amid severest woe."[16]

Perhaps the most striking aspect of literary England in the second half of the eighteenth century, however, is how many of its best writers themselves became insane. The list includes William Collins, Christopher Smart, William Cowper, Charles Lamb, and probably Thomas Chatterton. As George S. Rousseau noted in 1969, "It is an ironic contrast that the supposed 'Age of Reason' should have produced so many cases of insanity among its writers."[17]

William Collins, born in 1721, was a poet of nature and a friend of Samuel Johnson's. In his *Lives of the English Poets* (1779–1781), Johnson describes Collins's work as follows: "He loved fairies, genii, giants, and monsters; he delighted to rove through the meanders of inchantment, to gaze on the magnificence of golden palaces, to repose by the water-falls of Elysian gardens." At age thirty-two, Collins was "confined in a house of lunaticks" because of "that depression of mind which enchains the faculties without destroying them, and leaves reason the knowledge of right without the power of pursuing it." Johnson also noted that Collins "puts his words out of the common order, seeming to think, with some later candidates for fame, that not to write prose is certainly to write poetry." Following discharge from the madhouse, Collins lived with his sister and died at age thirty-eight.[18]

Christopher Smart, born in 1722, was a poet who, according to Russell Brain, was "unique in that his poetry was improved by his madness." Smart himself acknowledged, "I have a greater compass both of mirth and melancholy than another,"[19] and at age thirty-four he began an almost continuous seven-year hospitalization for what appears to have been manic-depressive illness. One of his poems, "Jubilate Agno," was written while he was hospitalized and demonstrates some classic features of psychotic thinking:

> *For the cymbal rhimes are bell well toll soul & the like.*
>
> *For the flute rhimes are tooth youth suit mute & the like.*
>
> *For the dulcimer rhimes are grace place beat heat & the like.*
>
> *For the Clarinet rhimes are clean seen and the like.*
>
> *For the Bassoon rhimes are pass, class and the like.*
>
> *God be gracious to the Baumgarden.*

His best-known poem, "A Song to David," was written while he was still in the private asylum but was recovering from his illness.

William Cowper, born in 1731, developed a "morbid religious mania" at age twenty-four. He told a friend that he was "hunted by spiritual hounds in the night-season" and wrote: "Satan plied me closely with horrible visions, and more horrible voices. My ears rang with the sound of torments, that seemed to await me."[20] After failing in several attempts to kill himself by poison, drowning, and hanging, Cowper was sent by his brother to Nathaniel Cotton's private mad-house at St. Albans, where he remained for eighteen months. Dr. Cotton's establishment was one of the most exclusive private asylums of that era and was known as the Collegium Insanorum, perhaps because it contained so many educated and literary patients.

Cowper experienced several additional episodes of depression and psychosis, including suffering from severe auditory hallucinations, delusions of religious persecution, and a belief that other people could hear his thoughts. In his diary he described the onset of his depression: "A strange and horrible darkness fell upon me. If it were possible that a heavy blow could light on the brain without touching the skull, such was the sensation I felt."[21]

Between such episodes, Cowper became a respected poet. Many of his best-known works were influenced by his psychotic experiences, including five stanzas entitled "Lines Written during a Period of Insanity." "The Task," written in 1785, includes "a serving maid" whose lover dies at sea:

> She heard the doleful tiding of his death—
> And never smiled again! and now she roams
> The dreary waste . . .
>
> She begs an idle pin of all she meets,
> And hoards them in her sleeve; but needful food,
> Though pressed with hunger oft, or comlier clothes,
> Though pinched with cold, asks never.—Kate is crazed.

According to Philip Martin, Cowper's description of Kate "was responsible for the massive popularity enjoyed by poems depicting madwomen in the magazines and miscellanies of the 1790s." Cowper's Crazy Kate was also the inspiration for numerous paintings, most notably Henry Fuseli's 1807 painting by that name, which was widely imitated. As Helen Small recently noted: "Between 1770 and about 1810, stories about bereaved or deserted women fallen into insanity were the subject of an extraordinary vogue in sentimental prose, poetry, drama, and painting."[22]

In "The Castaway," written one year before he died, Cowper again expressed the despair that had punctuated his adult life, as he compared his fate with that of a sailor washed overboard during a storm. Though the man shouts to his friends, they are unable to rescue him because of the wind's "furious blast," and he watches as the ship sails away. The poem's closing lines make clear the depths of Cowper's own sense of hopelessness:

> *No voice divine the storm allay'd,*
> *No light propitious shone;*
> *When, snatch'd from all effectual aid,*
> *We perish'd, each alone:*
> *But I beneath a rougher sea,*
> *And whelm'd in deeper gulfs than he.*

Cowper was widely read in the nineteenth century, and his insanity was commented upon by psychiatrists. Indeed, in 1858 the *American Journal of Insanity* noted that "in the entire annals of mental disease there is no case so widely known, or which has excited so deep an interest, as the insanity of Cowper."[23]

Thomas Chatterton, born in 1752, is generally regarded as one of England's most brilliant young poets. He published his first work at age eleven and at fifteen began writing poetry that he attributed to one Thomas Rowley, a fictitious fifteenth-century monk. The poems were well received, and Chatterton's hoax did not come to light until after his death by suicide at age seventeen. According to Kay Jamison, Chatterton was "subject to severe melancholia as well as periods of frenzied energies, occasionally incoherent enthusiasms, and extreme grandiosity." Chatterton's sister was also later hospitalized for insanity.[24]

Charles Lamb, born in 1775, was a widely read essayist whose whimsical creations included "A Dissertation upon Roast Pig" and "A Chapter on Ears." At age twenty he had an episode of mania and was hospitalized for six weeks at a private madhouse in Hoxton. During this episode he had grandiose delusions that he later described to his former schoolmate and close friend, Samuel Taylor Coleridge: "But mad I was—and many a vagary my imagination played with me, enough to make a volume if all told. . . . For while it lasted I had many many hours of pure happiness. Dream not, Coleridge, of having tasted all the grandeur and wildness of Fancy, till you have gone mad. All now seems to me vapid; comparatively so."[25]

In September 1796, eight months after Charles Lamb had recovered from his insanity, his older sister, Mary, killed their invalid mother with a carving knife as the family prepared to eat dinner in their London home. Mary "had been once before, in her earlier years, deranged," and "for the few days prior to this [murder] the family had observed some symptoms of insanity in her." Charles "was at hand only time enough to snatch the knife out of her grasp," and Mary was immediately taken to a local madhouse.[26]

Within a few weeks Mary had recovered. Charles petitioned the court to become her guardian and removed her from the madhouse. For the remainder of his life he cared for his sister despite her continuing, and increasingly prolonged, episodes of violent mania followed by "a succeeding dreadful depression," during which she required rehospitalization. Lamb's devotion to her was legendary among his friends, who often referred to him as "Saint Charles"; one friend observed that "his sister was but another portion of himself." Between episodes of insanity, Mary Lamb was able to function and in 1807, with Charles, published *Tales Founded on the Plays of Shakespeare* for children (she wrote the comedies, he wrote the tragedies), and in the following year she published *Poetry for Children.*[27]

"The Uncertain Continuance of Reason"

The madness of some of England's best-known writers contributed to the increasingly widespread belief as the eighteenth century progressed that insanity was becoming more common. As early as 1735 a letter to the Royal College of Physicians referred to madness as "epidemical" and noted: "Our nation has been observed by foreigners to abound in *maniacs,* more than any other upon the face of the earth.... I find it has of late increased so much among us, that there is scarce a family in the nation entirely free from it."[28]

In 1758 William Battie, whose patients included Christopher Smart and who was later the president of the Royal College of Physicians, opened his *Treatise on Madness* with this observation: "Madness, though a terrible and at present a very frequent calamity, is perhaps as little understood as any that ever afflicted mankind." This book was the first psychiatric textbook written for students and was also the first to adopt John Locke's 1690 suggestion by making delusional thinking the defining symptom for insanity. Battie defined delusions as follows: "Deluded imagination, which is not only an indisputable but an essential character of Madness, . . . precisely discriminates this from all other animal disorders: or that man and that man alone is properly mad, who is fully and unalterably persuaded of the existence or of the appearance of any thing, which either does not exist or does not actually appear to him, and who behaves according to such erroneous persuasion. . . . Madness, or false perception, being then a praeternatural state or disorder of Sensation."[29]

Poet, critic, and man of letters Samuel Johnson was another who believed that the incidence of insanity was increasing. In his didactic novel *Rasselas,* published in 1759, he included a fictional case history of an astronomer who developed a delusion that he could make the sun and rain obey his commands. Johnson's description of the formation of delusions has never been surpassed: "In time, some particular train of ideas fixes the attention, all other intellectual gratifications are rejected, the mind, in weariness or leisure, recurs constantly to the favourite conception, and feasts on the luscious falsehood, whenever she is offended with the bitterness of truth. By degrees the reign of fancy is confirmed; she grows first imperious, and in time despotick. Then fictions begin to operate as realities, false opinions fasten upon the mind, and life passes in dreams of rapture or of anguish."[30] In *Rasselas* Johnson also noted that "disorders of intellect happen much more often than superficial observers will easily believe. . . . Of the uncertainties of our present state, the most dreadful and alarming is the uncertain continuance of reason." Four years later, Johnson told James Boswell, his friend and later his biographer, that "insanity had grown more frequent since smoking had gone out of fashion," believing that smoking tranquilized the mind.[31]

For Samuel Johnson the issue of madness was an intensely personal one. He suffered from what is now called obsessive-compulsive disorder; he regularly touched every post along the street as he walked, avoided stepping in the paving stones, and according to Boswell, exited doorways "by a certain number of steps from a certain point, or at least so that either his right or his left foot . . . should constantly make the first actual movement when he came close to the door or passage." Johnson was intensely troubled by his obsessions and compulsions, believing they were a sign of impending madness. Such was his fear of going completely mad that, according to Roy Porter, "as a precautionary measure, [Johnson] apparently entrusted his great friend, Mrs. Hester Thrale, with a chain and padlock, for emergency use."[32]

Johnson's belief that he himself was afflicted with a form of impending madness made him sympathetic to literary colleagues who had become insane. Poet Christopher Smart, for example, "would drop to his knees in the middle of busy streets and require everyone to join him" in praying, yet Johnson denied that such behavior was necessarily a sign of insanity, saying, "I'd as lief pray with Kit Smart as anyone else."[33]

James Boswell, Johnson's biographer, noted that his friend confused insanity with other mental disorders such as simple depression: "Dr. Johnson and I had a serious conversation by ourselves on melancholy and madness: which he was, I always thought, enormously inclined to confound together. Melancholy, like 'great wit,' may be near allied to madness; but there is, in my opinion, a distinct separation between them."[34] Boswell himself knew the difference, since "one of his own children, Euphenia, was mentally deranged," and his brother, John, was intermittently insane and confined in private asylums. On one occasion Boswell reflected on his brother's illness: "It was a curious sensation when I saw my brother, with whom I had been brought up, in such a state. Madness of every degree is inexplicable."[35]

"The Hideous Malady Which So Amazingly Prevails"

Thomas Arnold, one of the best-known English "mad-doctors" during the second half of the eighteenth century, was much admired by

Boswell. He ran a private madhouse in Leicestershire and in 1782 published his widely read *Observations on the Nature, Kinds, Causes, and Prevention of Insanity, Lunacy, or Madness*. In a section entitled "Whether Insanity Prevails More in England Than in Other Countries," Arnold wrote: "Insanity, especially of the melancholy kind, has been commonly supposed to prevail so much more in this island than in any other part of Europe, that it has acquired among foreigners the denomination of the *English disease*. . . . There is, I believe, some foundation for the supposition; though, perhaps, much less than is generally imagined. . . . This, at least is certain—that instances of Insanity are, at this day, amazingly numerous in this kingdom;—probably more so than they ever were in any former period."[36] Arnold was probably responding to foreign observers, such as French scholar Pierre J. Grosley, who in 1765 had been so impressed by the large number of "Madmen and Lunatics" in England "that he devoted whole chapters" of his book to them.[37]

Arnold's response to Grosley was a classic display of Francophobia. He explained that France had less insanity than England because the causes of insanity—religious sentiment, love, and acquiring riches—were lacking in that nation. According to Arnold, under French Catholicism, "whose chief characteristic is superstition," the "pardon for sins of all sorts and sizes is so easily obtained [as] in every popish country, that few true believers . . . can be supposed to be much troubled with religious melancholy." Similarly, "Love, with them, is almost wholly an affair of art;—it has more of fancy than passion; and is rather an amusement of the imagination, than a serious business of the heart." Regarding "the desire, and prospect, of acquiring riches . . . there can be but little hope of attaining riches in a land of slaves, where the bulk and strength of a nation is depressed and impoverished . . . being subject to the will of an absolute monarch," in contrast to England's "happy land of liberty." Arnold thus concluded: "All these circumstances being taken into the account, it seems not improbable that this disorder is not only much more prevalent in England than in France, but more peculiar to this than to any other country. For even waiving the other considerations just enumerated, an *excess of wealth and luxury*, in which perhaps no nation upon earth can vie with this, seems to entitle us to an abundant share of the curse which appears too plainly to be entailed upon their possessors."[38]

It is surely a peculiar form of patriotism to view insanity as evidence of a superior civilization, but that is what Arnold was arguing. Not only was insanity increasingly prevalent in England, he argued, but the English should regard that fact with pride. In promoting this view, Arnold was expanding on the 1733 publication of George Cheyne's *The English Malady; or, A Treatise of Nervous Diseases of All Kinds, as Spleen, Vapours, Lowness of Spirits, Hypochondriacal, and Hysterical Distempers, etc.,* which Arnold referenced. Cheyne, however, who himself suffered from depression, emphasized depression and suicide as "the English malady," whereas Arnold emphasized insanity. Arnold's views of insanity as a badge of civilization were destined to resurface periodically over the next two hundred years.

In addition to Thomas Arnold, other notable English physicians expressed the strong belief in the closing years of the eighteenth century that the incidence of insanity was increasing. William Perfect, owner of a private madhouse in Kent, in 1778 published his *Select Cases in the Different Species of Insanity,* a book that would eventually be published in seven editions with slightly different titles. Perfect claimed that "instances of insanity are at this day more numerous in this kingdom than they were at any former period." A majority of Perfect's sixty-one cases appear to have had a medical origin (e.g., syphilis, mercury poisoning, encephalitis), but others appear to be consistent with a modern diagnosis of schizophrenia or manic-depressive illness.[39]

In 1788, six years after Thomas Arnold published his influential book, William Rowley published *A Treatise of Female Nervous, Hysterical, Hypochondriacal, Bilious, Convulsive Diseases.* Rowley believed that "England, according to its size and number of inhabitants, produces and contains more insane than any other country in Europe." The reason, Rowley claimed, was that "in those kingdoms where the greatest luxuries, refinements, wealth, and unrestrained liberty abound, are the most numerous instances of madness." The following year Benjamin Faulkner published *Observations on the General and Improper Treatment of Insanity,* in which he echoed both Arnold and Rowley: "The rapidity with which the disorder has spread over this country, within the last fifty years, may be attributed, in a great measure, to the encrease of luxury, . . . Inordinate desires, and the indulgence of inordinate passions, not unfrequently subjugate reason, and produce insanity."[40]

William Pargeter, a London physician who in 1792 published his *Observations on Maniacal Disorders,* was also impressed by the rising incidence of insanity. He referred to it as "the hideous malady which so amazingly prevails at this day" and said that "the frequency of this disease renders it truly alarming. . . . [It] has arrived at the height of its dominion." Like Arnold, Rowley, and Faulkner, Pargeter believed that at least some cases of insanity were associated with the increasing luxury being experienced in England. His eloquent description of the consequences of insanity is worth quoting: "It would be almost too shocking to portray the real features of this terrible complaint . . . the situation of a fellow creature destitute of the guidance of that governing principle, reason—which chiefly distinguishes us from the inferior animals around us. . . . View man deprived of that noble endowment, and see in how melancholy a posture he appears. He retains indeed the outward figure of the human species, but like the ruins of a once magnificent edifice, it only serves to remind us of his former dignity, and fills us with gloomy reflections of the loss of it."[41]

Among the best-known English physicians in the closing years of the eighteenth century was Bethlem Hospital's John Haslam, labeled by British psychiatrist Denis Leigh as "by far the most original and discerning writer on psychiatry in the period 1798 to 1828." In 1798 Haslam published his *Observations on Insanity,* which was widely circulated throughout Europe and issued in a second edition in 1809, at which time it was also praised in the popular *Quarterly Review.* Haslam noted that "the alarming increase of insanity, as might naturally be expected, has incited many persons to an investigation of this disease. . . . In our own country more books on insanity have been published than in any other."[42]

Haslam was especially impressed by the increasing number of individuals who were becoming insane at a young age. In 1789 Andrew Harper, in *The Economy of Health: A Treatise on the Real Cause and Cure of Insanity,* had written that "young people are hardly ever liable to insanity and that the attack of this malady seldom happens before an advanced period of life." Yet Haslam described cases of this new form of insanity as if they were something comparatively new:

"There is a form of insanity which occurs in young persons. . . . This disorder commences about, or shortly after, the period of menstruation." Haslam proceeded to provide the first unequivocal English description of what we now label schizophrenia, and in 1810 published an entire book on another case, *Illustrations of Madness: Exhibiting a Singular Case of Insanity.*[43]

In addition to describing schizophrenia, Haslam also provided remarkably clear descriptions of manic-depressive illness (including the rapid-cycling kind), postpartum psychosis, postvaccinal encephalitis presenting with psychosis, alcoholic psychosis, and psychosis secondary to syphilis. His *Observations on Insanity* was judged by Denis Leigh to be "a most outstanding piece of work, surpassing in merit any pervious publication both in England or on the continent."[44]

The published texts of Arnold, Perfect, Rowley, Faulkner, Pargeter, and Haslam in the closing years of the eighteenth century were part of a growing literature on psychiatry in general and insanity in particular. Denis Leigh, in *The Historical Development of British Psychiatry,* compiled a list entitled "Books Dealing with Psychiatric Illness Published in English during the Eighteenth Century." Of 112 books listed, only 9 were published from 1700 to 1725; 22 from 1726 to 1750; 29 from 1751 to 1775; and 52 were published between 1776 and 1800. Thirty-one books were published in the first fifty years of the century, and the same number in the last twelve years.[45]

The King Is Mad, Long Live the King

The insanity of King George III permanently altered the way madness was viewed in England. As noted by British psychiatric historians Ida Macalpine and Richard Hunter: "No longer could insanity be equated with ignorance or sin or superstition. If it was possible for the highest in the land to be struck down after an utterly blameless life of devotion to duty . . . surely such an illness could not be anything but natural, demanding of sympathy and amenable to medicine as any other?" Even before the king's illness, the question of increasing insanity was being debated in the wings of England's public stage; after his illness the question moved to front and center.[46]

The king's illness, diagnosed by Macalpine and Hunter with reasonable certainty as acute intermittent porphyria, first manifested itself in 1765, five years after he had ascended the throne. At that time he had gastrointestinal symptoms, abdominal cramps, and neurological pains in his arms and legs, which are characteristic of the disease, but he did not have any psychiatric manifestations. However, in 1788, during his second attack, he became insane with mania, delusions, hallucinations, and violent outbursts that required restraints.

The question of whether or not the king would recover led to the regency crisis. His enemies insisted that his son, a Whig sympathizer, take command of the throne, while his supporters sought to delay this succession, hoping for the king's recovery. Physicians on both sides were brought into the bitter debate, and hearings were held before special committees in the House of Commons and House of Lords. It was insanity "played out in a blaze of publicity such as has probably never before or since been accorded the illness even of a monarch."[47]

The effect of the king's 1788 illness on the public was dramatic. In the early years of his reign he had not been especially popular, but in later years he became more so. His devotion to his wife and fifteen children, his interest in the problems of farmers (he was often referred to as "Farmer George"), and his honesty and serious attention to the affairs of state all provided him with a common touch with which the people identified. Most had supported him in his recent confrontation with the American colonies, believing that the Americans were ungrateful children unwilling to pay their due to Mother England.

King George's insanity, therefore, was widely and passionately discussed in the streets of London. One of his ministers was "stopped in his carriage by the mob, to give an account of the King; and when he said it was a bad one, they had furiously exclaimed 'the more shame for you.'" Another minister expressed the belief that "none of their own lives would be safe if the King did not recover." When a false rumor spread that the king had died, "an universal consternation prevailed throughout the metropolis." The *Morning Chronicle* reported that "among other objects peculiarly affected by the state of his Majesty's indisposition, is the theatre which is prevented by a laudable delicacy from performing *King Lear, The Regent,* and several other dramas, on account of their striking applicability to the present juncture of affairs."[48]

King George did recover from his initial bout of insanity after five months, and the Archbishop of Canterbury composed a prayer of thanksgiving for "delivering our most Gracious Sovereign from the severe Illness with which he hath been afflicted." But the king had additional attacks in 1801, 1804, and 1810, each lasting several months. Following his final illness in 1810, when he was seventy-two years old, he lapsed into increasing senility, blindness, and deafness. When he finally died in 1820, one journal characterized it as "indeed but the passing of a shadow."[49]

It was the shadow of regal insanity which had hung over England for more than thirty years. The illness appeared to alter those afflicted, often permanently. During one of the king's prolonged episodes, Edmund Burke had written: "The King is *insane*—that is, he is dead to every civil Function. A certain animal is alive; the man is dead; the King is gone." King George had a rare form of insanity, caused by porphyria, but the more common forms of insanity loomed as specters, destined to grow and grow, and haunt England for the next two centuries.[50]

CHAPTER 4

"The Clap of Tortured Hands"

England 1800–1850

Oh! the fever of the mind! Nothing, indeed, can weigh in the smallest degree against mental sickness,—against that state in which the imagination is only active as the agent of cruelty— in which conscience, always alive to guilt, is now furnished with the tormenting implements of fancy and fear;—when there are no distinct impressions upon the brain but those of misery;—when all besides this is indistinctness, tumult, hurry, distraction!

—DAVID UWINS, "Insanity and Madhouses," 1816

For now it was indeed a dismal time, and for about a Month together, not taking any Notice of the Bills of Mortality, I believe there did not die less than 1500 or 1700 a-Day, one Day with another.

—DANIEL DEFOE, *A Journal of the Plague Year*, 1722

Nineteenth-century England was marked with increasing glory and increasing insanity. The people of Shakespeare's "scepter'd isle," en route to their coronation as God's elite, were increasingly delayed by masses of madmen in their path. It was a cruel counterpoint to England's global eminence, as if a madhouse had been built at the entrance to their castle.

The century dawned brightly on the rapidly expanding British Empire. Between 1795 and 1800, England was taking possession of Malta, Trinidad, Honduras, the Cape of Good Hope, Ceylon, and ever larger areas of India. In 1797 Lord Nelson had defeated the Spanish fleet at Cape St. Vincent, and the following year he had humiliated a French fleet at Abukir. By 1800 Britannia ruled the seas and was emerging as the century's economic and political superpower.

On May 15, 1800, James Hadfield, a former soldier in the king's army, fired a pistol at King George III as he entered the royal box at Drury Lane Theatre. The ball narrowly missed the king's head, and Hadfield was immediately apprehended. At his trial six weeks later, it was reported that Hadfield had suffered a penetrating head wound while serving in the army, after which he had shown "manifest symptoms of derangement." Hadfield's attack on the king was said to have been in response to God's command as a means for bringing about the Second Coming. Hadfield's residual head wound was so obvious that during his trial his counsel "was able to invite the jury to inspect the membrane of the brain itself," after which the jury members rendered a verdict of "Not Guilty, being under the influence of Insanity at the time the act was committed."[1]

Until Hadfield's trial in 1800, there had been no provision under English law for the continued detainment of individuals found not guilty by reason of insanity. Indeed, prior to 1780 the use of an insanity defense had been rare. Joel Eigen, in *Witnessing Insanity: Madness and Mad-Doctors in the English Court,* analyzed all trials in London's Old Bailey court at which a medical witness testified about the mental condition of the accused. He found only one case between 1760 and 1779, while for the period 1780 to 1799 he found fifteen. Nigel Walker and Sarah McCabe, in *Crime and Insanity in England,* also noted "an increase in the relative frequency with which lunatics and idiots appeared in the dock at Old Bailey" during the late eighteenth century.[2]

The irony of a madman attacking King George III, who had himself been severely deranged, was widely discussed in 1800. In 1786, two years prior to his initial episode of insanity, the king had been attacked by an insane woman, Margaret Nicholson, who had lunged at him with a butter knife as he was getting out of his carriage. Later that year, another insane woman, after escaping from Bethlem Hospital, had entered the home of Attorney General Lord George Gordon, where she was apprehended. As reported in the *Times*: "This circumstance having transpired, a report was instantly spread through the neighborhood that Lord George Gordon had assisted Margaret Nicholson in her escape from Bedlam. . . . A great crowd gathered around the house to know the truth of the circumstance. . . . When this was over [and the identity of the woman clarified] the woman was accordingly returned to her keeper, with an injunction to keep her more strictly confined in [the] future."[3]

Episodes of insane persons approaching members of the royal family had been reported with increasing regularity in newspapers in the closing years of the eighteenth century. In 1787 Thomas Stone, who had been "observed to behave in a very strange manner . . . by his landlord," was arrested "for sending various letters to the Princess Royal" because he had "conceived an attachment for her Royal Highness; also that she had conceived the same for him." The following year a Mr. Spang was arrested for trying to enter the palace. "When asked what brought him to the Queen's Palace, he said God. . . . His general demeanor was evidently marked with strong indications of insanity." In 1790 the *Times* reported that "another maniac was yesterday conveyed to the custody of the keeper of Tothillfields Bridewell [jail], he having applied at the Queen's Palace for admission to their Majesties, in a wild romantic style, saying his letter was from the Deity and must not be refused."[4]

Most such insane individuals were considered harmless and were released after a brief confinement. James Hadfield, however, clearly posed a threat to the king's life. In 1800, therefore, Parliament hurriedly passed a Criminal Lunatics Act with retrospective provisions to keep Hadfield "in strict custody." He was incarcerated in Bethlem Hospital for the remainder of his life, during which time he demonstrated his capacity for dangerousness by murdering another patient.

The idea of insanity as "the English malady" was becoming increasingly widespread. In 1804 Joseph Cox, a mad-doctor (as those who specialized in psychiatric cases were usually called) who invented the swinging chair for the treatment of insanity and whose influential *Practical Observations on Insanity* was translated into French and German, claimed that "insanity is unfortunately not only frequent but said to be peculiarly endemical to England." In 1807 William Stark, in his *Remarks on the Construction of Public Hospitals for the Cure of Mental Derangement*, noted that loss of reason is "the heaviest calamity incident to our race." And in 1808 John Reid, a London physician, wrote in the *Monthly Magazine* that "the English malady, by its visible and rapid progression, renders itself every day more deserving of the title. . . . Madness strides like a Colossus over this island."[5]

In 1807, as concern about insanity was becoming widespread, a Select Committee was appointed by Parliament "to inquire into the State of Lunatics" and hold hearings. Historians have speculated why such hearings should have taken place at this time, with proposed reasons ranging from "a coming together of the concerns of Benthamite Radicals and Evangelical Tories" to the hearings being an extension of the simultaneously developing Poor Law reform or prison reform.[6] The simplest reason is that the 1807 hearings reflected increasingly widespread concern about insanity.

Testimony at the hearings described increasing numbers of insane persons in workhouses, where they were "generally confined in some out-house or cell, or other place in which their noise gives least disturbance." Such reports contrasted with previous observations of workhouses; the *Account of Workhouses*, a 1732 survey of all major workhouses in England, "mentions them [insane persons] in only two instances, and then in passing," and in one workhouse "only two out of 62 inmates were lunatics." The 1807 Select Committee also heard testimony suggesting that increasing numbers of the insane were being held in jails. In the 1770s, prison reformer John Howard had found only "a sprinkling of the mad" in jails. By 1807 this practice had become more common, including the incarceration of an insane man who was sent to jail for having committed a murder, and three weeks later, when "allowed . . . out of the jailer's sight, . . . murdered one of his fellow prisoners." Jails, it was said, were "places highly improper for the custody, and inconsistent with the cure, of lunatics."[7]

The 1807 Select Committee also attempted, for the first time, to ascertain the total number of insane persons in England by asking county authorities to count them. The returns were highly variable, with seven of the fifty-four counties claiming that they had none. The official total was 1,765 insane persons "in poorhouses and houses of industry" and an additional 483 "in private custody." On behalf of the Select Committee, Sir Andrew Halliday visited two counties to verify the returns and reported that one county had undercounted by 24 percent and the other by 500 percent. Given such undercounts and considering the total population of counties claiming no insane persons, a reasonable estimate of their total number in England in 1807 would be between 5,000 and 6,000, or approximately 0.61 insane persons per 1,000 total population. If this estimate is correct, then the prevalence of insanity in England at that time slightly exceeded the baseline rate of insanity expected from medical conditions alone.

The outcome of the Select Committee report was the passage of "An Act for the Better Care and Maintenance of Lunatics," better known as the County Asylum Act of 1808, by which counties were encouraged to build public insane asylums, to be paid for with local taxes. According to Leonard Smith, "The Act was remarkable in a number of ways, not least because it signified, whether by design or by accident, an unusually direct intervention by the state in health and welfare provision." This was, it should be noted, the first of twenty parliamentary acts and amendments concerning insane persons, idiots, and insane asylums that would be passed during the nineteenth century. As John L. Crammer observed, "An astonishing amount of Parliamentary time was spent on this subject in the 19th century." Similarly, Vieda Skultans noted that "the number of Bills, reports of select committees and inquiries relating to lunacy rose from a mere handful in the eighteenth century to seventy-one between the years 1801 and 1844."[8]

The first of the new county asylums opened in Nottinghamshire in 1812, followed by others in Bedfordshire, Norfolk, and Lancashire. By 1824 the number of county asylums had increased only to eight, ranging in size from 40 beds in Bedfordshire to 250 beds in Lancashire. The total number of beds in these county asylums was 932, serving an eight-county total population of 3.4 million, suggesting that authorities expected utilization of the asylums to be low. And in some counties, it initially was; the Gloucestershire Asylum, which opened in 1823 with 110 beds, still had only thirty-one patients six months later.[9]

In many counties, there was considerable resistance to building an asylum, both because of costs and because of doubts regarding need. The Gloucestershire Asylum, for example, had first been proposed in the 1790s but, because of local resistance, did not become a reality until 1823. In Middlesex, "Several parishes lodged objections on grounds of cost," and those in the vicinity of the proposed asylum objected that the "cries and noises of the unhappy inmates" would be unsettling to them. In Suffolk there were "concerted local campaigns of petitions and protests" that delayed the asylum's opening.[10]

Private asylums also increased in the early years of the nineteenth century. In 1798 there had been forty-two provincial and metropolitan "licensed houses," but by 1815 this number had increased to seventy-two. Most of them were very small, and the annual admissions for all of them together averaged less than five hundred a year until 1810–1815, when these admissions doubled. The best-known private asylum continued to be the Quakers' York Retreat, which was visited by many foreign observers, including "no less than three parties sent over by the Russian royal family." Probably the most unusual visitors were "seven Red Indian braves who had been brought over to England [from America] to appear in a London theatre. After they had seen all that was to be seen [at the York Retreat], their Chief offered up a short prayer of thanks."[11]

The expansion of private asylums brought problems. According to Parry-Jones, "Many of the critics of the madhouse system asserted that proprietors bribed medical men to patronize their houses." Patient abuses were increasingly reported, including a widely publicized case of a violent inmate of Bethlem Hospital who had been held for nine years by "a chain around his neck, the other end of which was attached to a stone wall." Public criticism of such practices led to the establishment of another parliamentary committee, convened to investigate madhouse practices; this committee met intermittently for almost two years in 1815 and 1816 and heard testimony from forty-one witnesses. Its report noted, "There are not in the country a set of beings more immediately requiring the protection of the legislature than the persons in this state [of lunacy]," and it recommended more government control of private madhouses.[12]

During these years, several observers noted the continuing rise of insanity. The most influential of these was Richard Powell, secretary of the commissioners of the Royal College of Physicians, the group charged with keeping a register of all insane persons admitted to private asylums in England and Wales. Dividing 1775 to 1809 into five-year periods, Powell used graphs to show an increase in admissions of approximately 25 percent for the entire country and a much sharper increase for London, especially during the years 1790–1794. Powell said that he had undertaken his study to ascertain the verity of "the popular opinion respecting the rapid increase of that most difficult, delicate, and important disease." He concluded: "The facts also which present themselves . . . supply us, as I am led to think, with sufficient proof that the increase must actually have been very considerable, though we cannot ascertain its exact proportion."[13]

Others echoed Powell's conclusions. Bryan Crowther, in *Practical Remarks,* published in 1811, called insanity "an affection so rapidly becoming prevalent among all orders of society." George Hill, in *An Essay on the Prevention and Cure of Insanity,* published in 1814, said that insanity "is certainly not to be rated among our declining diseases" and noted the contemporary outpouring of publications on the subject. Louis Simond, an American who made a two-year tour of England in 1810 and 1811, published his observations in 1815, noting that "madness appears to be fatally common in Great Britain" and that this high incidence existed despite the fact that "the qualifications required for acknowledged insanity, are by no means easily attained in England, where a greater latitude is granted for whims, fancies, and eccentricities, than in other countries." Simond also claimed that "the higher ranks" and "the rich particularly are most exposed to this calamity."[14]

Andrew Scull also noted that "from about 1815 onwards, a veritable spate of books and articles purporting to be medical treatises on the treatment of insanity began to appear." Thomas Bakewell, a madhouse proprietor, claimed in 1815: "It is a prevailing opinion . . . that this national opprobrium [insanity] is alarmingly upon the increase." And in 1816 David Uwins wrote in the *Quarterly Review* that "nervous and mental affections of every kind are, in the present day, proverbially prevalent." The reason, added Uwins, was civilization: "In proportion as man emerges from his primaeval state, do the Furies of disease advance upon him and would seem to scourge him back into the paths of nature and simplicity."[15] It was an argument that would be repeated many times as the century progressed.

Insanity and the Romantic Writers

It was inevitable that mounting madness in nineteenth-century England would be reflected by its writers. As Ann Colley aptly observed, madness was not chosen randomly by these writers but rather was incorporated "because the nation's consciousness pushed it there . . . [as] extensions of the nineteenth-century sensitivity to madness."[16]

The English Romantic writers nicely illustrate this point. Their movement was marked by an idealization of nature, the utilization of medieval subject matter, and a revolt against classicism's restraint and rationality in favor of free expression and irrationality. Within this context, insanity played an impressive role, both as subject matter for the Romantic writers and as an affliction of the writers themselves and their family members. As early as 1806, Philippe Pinel in Paris noted: "Certain professions conduce more than others to insanity. . . . In consulting the registers of Bicêtre, we find many priests and monks . . . many artists, painters, sculptors and musicians: some poets extatized by their own productions." This claim was widely repeated in England and disseminated in leading publications, such as William A. F. Browne's influential 1837 textbook, where it was noted: "Among the educated classes of patients admitted to Bicêtre, no instances of insane geometricians, physicians, naturalists, or chemists are to be found, while priests, poets, painters, and musicians occur in great number."[17]

George Crabbe was a transitional writer between classicism and romanticism. After some early medical training, Crabbe became a successful poet. Samuel Johnson praised his work, and Jane Austen was so fond of his poetry that "she was known among her family as 'Mrs. Crabbe.' "[18]

In 1796 Crabbe's wife became insane following the birth of their third child, and thereafter insanity became a major theme in his work. Among his many portrayals of insanity was "Sir Eustace Grey"; published in 1807, it was set in a madhouse and included extended descriptions of a madman's hallucinations. The poem was "well received in its day," and a reviewer noted: "Mr. Crabbe has, perhaps, been driven to the melancholy contemplation on insanity in all its wild variety of mood, and so, alas! to our misfortune, have we." "Tales," published in 1812, was another portrait of insanity:

Friends now appear'd, but in the Man was seen
The angry maniac, with vindictive mien;
Too late their pity gave to care and skill
The hurried mind and ever-wandering will;
Unnotic'd pass'd all time, and not a ray
Of reason broke on his benighted way;
But now he spurn'd the straw in pure disdain
And now laugh'd loudly at the clinking chain.

Then as its wrath subsided, by degrees
The mind sank slowly to infantine ease;
To playful folly, and to causeless joy,
Speech without aim, and without end, employ;
He drew fantastic figures on the wall,
And gave some wild relation of them all;
With brutal shape he join'd the human face,
And idiot smiles approv'd the motley race.[19]

William Wordsworth (1770–1850), one of the leading figures of the Romantic period, eulogized Thomas Chatterton in "Resolution and Independence":

. . . I thought of Chatterton, the marvellous Boy,
The sleepless Soul that perished in his pride;
Of Him who walked in glory and in joy
Following his plough, along the mountain-side:
By our own spirits are we deified:
We Poets in our youth begin in gladness;
But thereof come in the end despondency and madness.

Wordsworth was himself subject to periods of depression and was drawn to the subject of insanity. According to Michael Shimer: "During the mental crisis in his own life (roughly between the spring of 1795 and the fall of 1797), Wordsworth wrote a group of poems that explicitly deal with the theme of madness."[20] Many of them utilized an image of a madwoman, reminiscent of Cowper's Crazy Kate. Such poems included "The Thorn":

> *She was with child, and she was mad,*
> *Yet often she was sober sad. . . .*
> *Sad case for such a brain to hold*
> *Communion with a stirring child!*
> *Sad case, as you may think, for one*
> *Who had a brain so wild!*

Another was entitled "The Mad Mother":

> *Sweet babe! they say that I am mad,*
> *But nay, my heart is far too glad;*
> *And I am happy when I sing*
> *Full many a sad and doleful thing:*
> *Then, lovely baby, do not fear!*
> *I pray thee have no fear of me,*
> *But, safe as in a cradle, here*
> *My lovely baby! thou shalt be,*
> *To thee I know too much I owe;*
> *I cannot work thee any woe.*
>
> *A fire was once within my brain;*
> *And in my head a dull, dull pain;*
> *And fiendish faces one, two, three,*
> *Hung at my breasts, and pulled at me.*

Robert Southey (1774–1843) was poet laureate of England for thirty years. Like his friend Wordsworth, Southey was drawn to the image of the madwoman. In his "Mary, the Maid of the Inn," the heroine is driven insane after being deserted by her lover and discovering that he is a murderer. This popular poem, originally entitled "Mary the Maniac," was reprinted at least eight times in contemporary magazines. Ironically, Southey's wife was later committed to an insane asylum, where she remained for three years.

Southey's wife's sister was married to Samuel Taylor Coleridge (1772–1834), a friend of Southey's since their youth. Coleridge suffered from recurrent periods of depression, was discharged from the army as insane, and is thought by some to have had manic-depressive illness even prior to his addiction to opium. His "Kubla Khan" and "The Rime of the Ancient Mariner" are both said to be about madness. As early as 1813, George Crabbe said of "The Ancient Mariner": "It does not describe Madness by its Effects but by Imitation, as if a painter to give a picture of Lunacy should make his Canvas crazy, and fill it with wild unconnected Limbs and Distortions of features." And Michael Shimer has written: "The Mariner as a mad figure need hardly be argued. So strange is his appearance, behavior, and power that little or no doubt is left to his marked abnormality. . . . The theme of madness originates, of course, in the Mariner's killing of the albatross. . . . It is a manifestation of human irrationality." In his correspondence, Coleridge likened madness to "a fiery hell": "Why need we talk of a fiery hell? If the will, which is the law of our nature, were withdrawn from our memory, fancy, understanding, and reason, no other hell could equal, for a spiritual being, what we should then feel, from the anarchy of our powers. It would be conscious madness—a horrid thought!"[21]

The poetic master of visions of hell was William Blake (1757–1827). Charles Lamb referred to Blake as "the mad Wordsworth," and Southey, after meeting Blake, said: "You could not have delighted in him—his madness was too evident." Whether or not Blake was truly insane has been debated endlessly by his biographers; what is clear is that he regularly experienced visions and communed with spirits. Paul Youngquist argued that Blake "was a poet for whom madness became a major subject. . . . Blake made poetry out of pathology. . . . Madness emerges in his poetry as a thematic preoccupation." "The Four Zoas" has been described as "a mythological investigation of madness" with "contemporary clinical parallels in the symptomology of schizophrenia."[22]

Sir Walter Scott (1771–1832) was one of the most widely read poets and novelists of the Romantic period. Although he suffered from the "black dog" of melancholy, Scott was never insane. However, he "made mental maladies a special study" and immortalized insane women, most prominently Madge Wildfire in *The Heart of Midlothian* (1818) and Lucy Ashton in *The Bride of Lammermoor* (1819). In the former, Madge is referred to as "Madge of Bedlam" and sings of her time spent there:

> *In the bonny cells of Bedlam*
> *Ere I was ane and twenty,*
> *I had hempen bracelets strong,*
> *And merry whips, ding-dong,*
> *And prayer and fasting plenty.*

One scholar has labeled this scene "one of the most poignant scenes in all of Scott's fiction, here is insanity on display . . . the face of madness grimacing at the sane world."[23]

Another of Sir Walter Scott's mad heroines, Lucy Ashton, was subsequently the heroine of eight different operas, most notably Gaetano Donizetti's *Lucia di Lammermoor* (1835), in which Lucia suffers from visual and auditory hallucinations. In the "mad scene," Lucia, overtly insane, kills the man she has just been forced to marry:

> *Alas! What a terrible calamity!*
> *Arturo, lying sprawled on the floor,*
> *Was mute and cold and covered with gore!*
> *And Lucia was tightly hugging the sword*
> *That had been the murdered man's heretofore.*
> *She fixed her eyes on me—*
> *"My husband, where is he?" she said to me,*
> *and on her ashen face*
> *a smile flashed suddenly!*
> *Unhappy girl! She had completely*
> *Lost her sanity!*

Scott's close friend, George Gordon, Lord Byron (1788–1824), was probably the most influential of the English Romantic writers.

Scott wrote of him: "There is something dreadful in reflecting that one gifted so much above his fellow-creatures should thus labour under some strange mental malady that destroys his peace of mind and happiness." Byron's "strange mental malady" was manic-depressive illness; throughout his life he suffered from recurrent periods of mania and severe depression, and he ultimately was divorced by his wife on grounds that he was insane. The fear of impending insanity haunted Byron, as he wrote to a friend: "I don't know that I shan't end with insanity, for I find a want of method in arranging my thoughts that perplexes me strangely." This preoccupation with madness was reflected in his poetry, as in his description of an insane woman in "The Dream":

> oh! she was changed,
> As by the sickness of the soul; her mind
> Had wander'd from its dwelling, and her eyes,
> They had not their own lustre, but the look
> Which is not of the earth; she was become
> The queen of a fantastic realm; her thoughts
> Were combinations of disjointed things;
> And forms impalpable and unperceiv'd
> Of others' sight familiar were to hers.
> And this the world calls phrenzy.[24]

In 1816, while working on *Childe Harold,* Byron met Percy Bysshe Shelley (1792–1822). Shelley found Byron "exceedingly interesting" but "mad as the winds." Shelley, in fact, had his own psychiatric problems, including recurrent episodes of depression and apparent hallucinations. Kay Jamison, in *Touched with Fire,* argued that Shelley, like Byron, had manic-depressive illness, although some Shelley scholars disagree.[25] Shelley and Byron spent much time together between 1816 and 1821, during which time Shelley wrote "Julian and Maddalo," a poem about two men (thought to be Shelley and Byron themselves) who visit a friend who has become insane and is incarcerated in a madhouse:

. . . The clap of tortured hands,
Fierce yells and howlings and lamentings keen,
And laughter where complaint had merrier been,
Moans, shrieks, and curses, and blaspheming prayers,
Accosted us . . .

       'Let us now visit him; after this strain
He ever communes with himself again,
And sees nor hears not any.'

         Having said
These words, we called the keeper, and he led
To an apartment opening on the sea.
There the poor wretch was sitting mournfully
Near a piano, his pale fingers twined
One with the other, and the ooze and wind
Rushed through an open casement, and did sway
His hair, and starred it with the brackish spray;
His head was leaning on a music-book,
And he was muttering, and his lean limbs shook;
His lips were pressed against a folded leaf,
In hue too beautiful for health, and grief
Smiled in their motions as they lay apart.
As one who wrought from his own fervid heart
The eloquence of passion, soon he raised
His sad meek face, and eyes lustrous and glazed,
And spoke—sometimes as one who wrote, and thought
His words might move some heart that heeded not,
If sent to distant lands; and then as one
Reproaching deeds never to be undone
With wondering self-compassion; then his speech
Was lost in grief, and then his words came each
Unmodulated, cold, expressionless,
But that from one jarred accent you might guess
It was despair made them so uniform.

Insanity "Is Not an Increasing Malady"

Even as the Romantic writers were immortalizing madness, England's light burned ever more brightly around the world. St. Lucia, Tobago, Dutch Guiana, Martinique, Guadaloupe, Sierra Leone, Gambia, Mauritius, and Java all came within the British sphere between 1800 and 1815. In 1816, at the same time as the parliamentary committee was hearing testimony regarding madhouse practices, Thomas Bruce, the seventh Earl of Elgin, presented to the British Museum the Greek marble statues he had taken from the Parthenon. It was a symbolic transfer of the glory that had been Greece to England, and John Keats marked the event by writing "On Seeing the Elgin Marbles." In 1819 the British founded Singapore and five years later took Rangoon. There appeared to be no limit to the British Empire, or to its religious and commercial influence. Many said this was ordained to be so by God, as William Blake suggested in his 1804 poem "Milton: A Poem in Two Books," later set to music and widely sung:

> *And did those Feet in ancient time*
> *Walk upon England's mountains green?*
> *And was the holy Lamb of God*
> *In England's pleasant pastures seen?*
> *And did the Countenance Divine*
> *Shine down upon those clouded hills;*
> *And was Jerusalem builded here*
> *Among those dark Satanic mills?*[26]

During the Romantic period, there also emerged the first strong voice denying that insanity was increasing in England. It was the voice of George Man Burrows, described by Andrew Scull as "one of the most well-known private madhouse keepers of the early nineteenth century." Burrows was an influential physician who had "played a major role in securing passage of the Apothecaries Act of 1815," which regularized the qualifications of physicians and helped to solidify insanity as their legal province.[27] He thus had both a professional and a financial interest in the successful treatment of insanity.

Burrows was not the first person to publicly doubt that insanity was increasing. As early as 1801 Robert Willan, in *Reports on the Diseases in London,* had claimed that there was "no sufficient ground" for believing that insanity was increasing because "the number of patients in Bethlem, St. Luke's and other hospitals is nearly uniform." Thomas Bateman, eighteen years later, repeated Willan's claim and reasoning: "Insanity does not seem to have greatly increased within the last half century. The number of patients in the public hospitals for the reception of lunatics continues nearly uniform." Both Willan and Bateman ignored the fact that Bethlem and St. Luke's had long waiting lists for admission (in 1807 there were 640 persons on St. Luke's list),[28] and since their beds were always full, the number was, by definition, "nearly uniform."

George Man Burrows, in his 1820 book entitled *An Inquiry into Certain Errors Relative to Insanity* and in *Commentaries,* published eight years later, reviewed available data on the number of insane persons in England and Ireland and concluded that the total number was approximately six thousand, similar to the estimate derived for England from the Select Committee survey of 1807. He acknowledged that "foreigners of all countries pronounce insanity as the opprobrium of England" and that "the popular opinion is that insanity is alarmingly prevalent." He argued strongly, however, that insanity was "not an increasing malady,"[29] and later, in 1828, even argued that it was decreasing in incidence.

Burrows offered two reasons for his belief that insanity was not increasing. The first was the fact that insane asylums, presumably including the one he owned, were effective in treating this condition and therefore, ipso facto, insanity had to be decreasing. He explained it as follows: "I have, therefore, no other ground for my conviction of the general diminution in the number of lunatics, than the pleasing and incontrovertible fact, that wherever asylums for insane persons have been established, from the superior mode of treatment, both medical and moral, the number who recover is much greater than heretofore; and, consequently, that the aggregate number of the insane must be lessened."[30] Burrows's second reason for denying any increase in insanity—and even arguing for a decrease—was that increasing insanity would be a national scandal and therefore it *should* not be true: "Hence, as the respective exciting causes vary, so likewise must everywhere the number of lunatics. But does it thence follow that insanity must be increasing? A conclusion so humiliating cannot be entertained without the most painful reflections; nor, if it be really so, can the consequences be indifferent, even in a national point of view?"[31]

Burrows's conclusions were widely quoted by contemporary psychiatrists and others who did not believe, or did not want to believe, that insanity was increasing. More than 150 years later, psychiatric historians Ida Macalpine and Richard Hunter, in *George III and the Mad Business*, would cite Burrows as having definitively proven that insanity had not increased in the early nineteenth century: "The question whether insanity was on the increase Dr. Burrows therefore answered with a definite no. . . . This particular ghost had at last been laid to rest and was not heard from again."[32] This declaration was a surprising error for Macalpine and Hunter, whose scholarship is generally beyond reproach; in fact, in the 1820s the ghost of increasing insanity was just beginning to walk the land.

In contrast to support he received, Burrows was also widely criticized by contemporary reviewers who did not agree with him. An anonymous reviewer in an 1821 *Quarterly Review,* for example, criticized Burrows's equating of suicide with insanity: "We question too the propriety of making the number of suicides an indication of the number of the insane, since we are not disciples of that creed which indiscriminately puts down every case of self-destruction to the score of deranged intellect." Burrows's second book on insanity was subjected to a scathing review in the same journal, where it was dismissed as "a mass of trash" and "a wretched compilation of scraps, gathered from all sorts of sources, and full of inaccuracies. . . . The author, in truth, undertook a task to which his mind was totally unequal."[33]

Even as Burrows was being praised and pilloried, Anthony Ashley Cooper was moving to the front to lead the battle against increasing insanity. Better known as Lord Ashley and later as Lord Shaftesbury, Cooper's agitation would become the single most important reason why the British psychiatric establishment never acknowledged that insanity was increasing. Adopting and adapting Burrows's arguments, he repeated them incessantly for almost sixty years, until his death in 1885.

Lord Ashley was introduced to insanity in 1827, when he was appointed to the Select Committee to consider the state of "Pauper

Lunatics in the County of Middlesex and on Lunatic Asylums." He was at the time a newly elected member of Parliament with an impeccable upper-class lineage, an education at Harrow and Oxford, and a social circle that included members of the royal family.

Lord Ashley's interest in the plight of the insane arose in part from his own problems. Suffering from periodic bouts of depression punctuated by brief bursts of elation in what would today be termed a "cyclothymic personality," he described himself as follows: "How curious and uncertain is my character. Sometimes for a while in my wildest and most jovial of spirits; at others for a longer period in cruel . . . despondency." One friend wrote of him: "Ashley's character seems to me quite unintelligible and can only be accounted for by a dash of madness." And Florence Nightingale, describing him later in his life, wrote: "Had [Lord Ashley] not devoted himself to reforming lunatic asylums, he would have been in one himself."[34]

It was not Lord Ashley's mood swings for which he was best known, however, but rather his deep religiosity and moralistic demeanor. He was a devout Evangelical Christian who prayed twice daily and studied the Bible as the literal Word of God. He was also aloof, humorless, and puritanical. A biographer characterized his outlook as consisting "of a series of negatives [which] thus removed much of the pleasure and color from life." One contemporary described him as follows: "The whole countenance has the coldness as well as the grace of a chiselled one, and expresses precision, prudence, and determination in no common degree. To judge from the set form of the lips, you would say, not only that he never acts from impulse, but that he seldom, if ever, felt an impulse in his life."[35]

One cannot fully understand Lord Ashley's approach to issues regarding insanity without understanding the importance of his religious beliefs. Evangelicalism was at the time very important in England and said to be "the religion of the vast majority of serious Englishmen." Lord Ashley was considered to be one of its leaders. As a devout Evangelical Christian, he believed that the Second Coming was imminent and that it was his job to prepare the world for it. When, in an 1845 speech to the House of Commons, he said, "Here we are sitting in deliberation today and tomorrow we may be subject to it," he meant it literally. The primary task for which he assumed responsibility was to improve the treatment of insane persons, whom he referred to as "the most helpless, if not the most afflicted, portion of the human race."[36] Any suggestion that their treatment was not improving or, even worse, that their number was increasing meant that he was failing in his self-appointed task to hasten the Second Coming. For Lord Ashley, then, improving the plight of insane persons was not merely noblesse oblige, the patrician's duty to the less fortunate, but rather a religious duty with imminent divine consequences.

Lord Ashley also believed that English Protestants were God's chosen people. He was "firmly convinced that, on several occasions in her history, Britain had been specifically favored by God.... He was not afraid or ashamed to advance British interests if he felt that they did accord with God's purpose." Catholics, in Lord Ashley's opinion, did not qualify as true Christians because of popery's "train of spiritual, moral and physical evils," and on several occasions he noted "the greater prevalence of insanity in Roman Catholic countries" as proof of their divine disfavor.[37] Given this belief, for Lord Ashley to have acknowledged that insanity was increasing in England would have been tantamount to saying that the English might *not* be God's chosen.

The 1828 Madhouse and County Asylum Act, which resulted from the report of the 1827 Select Committee, provided Lord Ashley with a vehicle for improving the treatment of the insane. He was appointed as one of the Metropolitan Commissioners to inspect madhouses, a post he would hold until 1845, when this body would be replaced by the national Commissioners in Lunacy, with responsibility for all of England and Wales. He then served as chairman of this latter group until 1885 and so effectively provided leadership on the insanity problem for fifty-seven years. Although he also became involved in efforts to protect miners, factory workers, and children being used as chimney sweeps, insanity continued to be his paramount task.

Lord Ashley's attempts to prove that insanity was not increasing would prove to be difficult since statistics to the contrary kept appearing. Foremost among these was Sir Andrew Halliday's "Report of the Number of Lunatics and Idiots in England and Wales," published in 1829, one year after the Madhouse and County Asylums Act went into effect. Halliday had participated in the 1807 census of the insane and had continued to collect data in the intervening years, during which time he also served as a personal physician to William, Duke of Clarence, who would become King William IV in 1830.

Halliday was probably the most knowledgeable person in England regarding the numbers of the insane, and his connection to King William conferred even greater authority. He divided the insane into "lunatics" (developed insanity after childhood) and "idiots" (insane since birth) and counted separately those in asylums, those in workhouses, and those kept at home. His preliminary count was 6,806 lunatics and 5,741 idiots, or 12,547 total, but he acknowledged that this was an undercount and estimated the true total at 16,500. Assuming the same proportion of lunatics to idiots in the uncounted portion of the total, the total number of lunatics in Halliday's estimate would have been 8,941, or approximately 0.79 per 1,000 total population. This figure showed, Halliday concluded, that "insanity, in all its forms, prevails to a most alarming extent in England. . . . The numbers of the afflicted have become more than tripled during the last twenty years!" He added that it was no longer possible to dispute these "melancholy facts" and that it would be "a consciousness of criminal negligence were one to attempt longer to conceal them."[38]

Halliday also thought he knew why insanity was increasing. The cause, he said, was "over exertion of the mind, in overworking its instruments so as to weaken them . . . the derangement of the vital functions, that re-act upon the brain, and derange its operation." He contrasted the large number of lunatics in England with their paucity among "the savage tribes of men; not one of our African travellers remark having seen a single madman."[39]

The idea of insanity as a badge of civilization had been suggested prior to Halliday and would be put forth many times again. As early as 1802 Thomas Beddoes had written about nations "civilized enough to be capable of insanity." Sir Alexander Morison, in his 1826 *Outlines of Lectures on Mental Diseases,* had said that insanity was increasing because "the number of insane increases with civilization." James Prichard, in his 1835 *A Treatise on Insanity,* would note that "cases of insanity are far more numerous than formerly" because insanity was caused by "the activity of the cerebral functions": "In England, indeed, this cause is very powerful. Here all the faculties of the mind act with great energy." And William A. F. Browne, whose 1837 *What Asylums Were, Are, and Ought to Be* "was to prove enormously influential," according to Andrew Scull, would claim that insanity was increasing because "as we recede, step by step, from the simple, that is, the savage manners of our ancestors, and advance in industry and knowledge and happiness, this malignant persecutor [insanity] strides onward, signalizing every era in the social progress by an increase, a new hecatomb, of victims."[40]

A Madman's Manuscript

The question of increasing insanity was being widely discussed in England in the 1830s. In 1832 the *Times* reviewed Sir Andrew Halliday's publication; in 1837 the *Penny Magazine* carried the article "Statistics on Lunacy and Crime"; and in 1839 the *New Monthly Magazine* published an extensive analysis of all the reasons why insanity was apparently increasing (e.g., "education . . . the overstraining of the intellectual powers by their premature exercise)."[41] From America, Johann Gaspar Spurzheim asked, "Why is insanity so frequent in England?" and answered that it was because the causes of insanity were more common there.

Thus, it was not surprising to readers of the *Old Monthly Magazine* when, in 1837, Charles Dickens published "A Madman's Manuscript" as one of the monthly installments of *The Pickwick Papers*. According to one scholar, Dickens was fascinated by madmen and criminals: "Wherever he traveled, he made it a point to attend executions, to visit madhouses, prisons, and morgues." In his 1993 dissertation, David Oberhelman claimed that Dickens was "reacting to the Victorian obsession with the rise in insanity and with the inadequacies of the institutions built to hold the growing population of lunatics. . . . The fear of a renewed outbreak of madness . . . lingers throughout Dickens's work." Dickens himself is said to have had a "general mood of elation, associated with hyperactivity and broken by short recurrent periods of depression," leading some to label him as having had manic-depressive illness.[42]

Dickens was remarkably knowledgeable about insanity. His personal library included Robert Burton's *Anatomy of Melancholy*, John Conolly's *On Some Forms of Insanity*, Forbes Winslow's *The Incubation of Insanity*, and W. C. Hood's *Suggestions for the Future Provision of Criminal Lunatics*.[43] The two journals Dickens edited, *Household*

Words and *All the Year Round,* regularly included articles on mad-houses and asylum reform. Most importantly, Dickens was close friends with John Conolly, one of the foremost psychiatrists of the mid–nineteenth century, and with two of the Lunacy Commissioners, Bryan Proctor and John Forster, whose full-time job was to inspect madhouses. Forster, in fact, became Dickens's first biographer when he published his *Life of Charles Dickens* in 1872. It is likely that the ideas for many of Dickens's mad characters were derived from conversations with these men.

"A Madman's Manuscript" is a strange tale, told in the first person by a madhouse inmate who is being laughed at by visitors peering into his cell. Rather than feeling humiliated, the madman delights in his status and in his ability to terrify others: "Show me the monarch whose angry frown was ever feared like the glare of a madman's eye. . . . Ho! Ho! It's a grand thing to be mad!"[44] He then recounts the onset of his illness, "watching the progress of the fever that was to consume [his] brain," the voices screaming in his ears, his attempted murder of his young wife, and then his successful murder of his brother-in-law and subsequent incarceration.

In *Barnaby Rudge,* published four years later, Dickens continued this theme. According to Oberhelman, "Madness is loosed upon the text from the onset. . . . The novel is, in that sense, a meditation on the perils of growing insanity, insanity always threatening to erupt in violence, and the impotence of traditional asylums such as Bethlem Hospital to cope with that growth." In the novel a rumor is spread that a mob, led by Lord George Gordon, who himself is depicted in the book as having the symptoms of insanity, "meant to throw the gates of Bedlam open, and let all the madmen loose. This suggested such dreadful images to people's minds, and was indeed an act so fraught with new and unimaginable horrors in the contemplation, that it beset them more than any loss or cruelty of which they could foresee the worst, and drove many sane men nearly mad themselves." Oberhelman added: "With the riots the madness does defy all forms of control and now becomes an infection, a plague—a communicable disease that can be transmitted even to those who do not harbor the propensity."[45]

Charles Dickens continued to depict mad characters in his

novels throughout his career. One of the best known is *David Copperfield*'s Mr. Dick, who believes he has things in his head that came from the head of King Charles I and were transferred to him when the king was beheaded in 1649. Such beliefs, called thought insertion, are a common symptom of the form of insanity now called schizophrenia.

Dickens also continued to visit insane asylums throughout his career. In 1842, during his first visit to America, he visited two asylums (see chapter 10). In 1851 he visited St. Luke's Asylum in London shortly after Christmas, later publishing a description of the holiday dance held for patients as "A Curious Dance Round a Curious Tree," in which he praised the non-use of restraints as part of the increasingly popular moral treatment. And in 1857, in "The Lazy Tour of Two Idle Apprentices," published with Wilkie Collins, Dickens described a fictional visit to an insane asylum, including a poignant description of patients standing idly on the wards of the asylum: "Long groves of blighted men-and-women trees; interminable avenues of hopeless faces; numbers, without the slightest power of really combining for any earthly purpose; a society of human creatures who have nothing in common but that they have all lost the power of being humanly social with one another."[46]

In 1837, in the same year that Dickens's "A Madman's Manuscript" was published, John Clare (1793–1864) was committed to Matthew Allen's insane asylum near High Beech in Essex. Clare had established himself as a leading poet in the early 1830s with works such as *The Shepherd's Calendar* and *Rural Muse*. However, he suffered from periods of depression that became increasingly severe and were accompanied by auditory hallucinations and grandiose delusions in which he believed himself to be Lord Byron, Lord Nelson, or other famous persons. He told one visitor, "They have cut off my head and picked out all the letters of the alphabet—all the vowels and consonants—and brought them out through my ears." Clare spent four years at Dr. Allen's asylum and then twenty-three more years at the Northamptonshire Lunatic Asylum, which he characterized as "the land of Sodom where all the people's brains are turned the wrong way." During his extended stay in these asylums, Clare continued writing poems, some of which reflected his despair at being confined and forgotten.

I am! Yet what I am who cares, or knows?

    My friends forsake me like a memory lost,

I am the self-consumer of my woes;

    They rise and vanish, an oblivious host,

Shadows of life, whose very soul is lost,

And yet I am—I live—though I am toss'd

Into the nothingness of scorn and noise,

    Into the living sea of waking dream

Where there is neither sense of life, nor joys,

    But the huge shipwreck of my own esteem

And all that's dear. Even those I loved the best

Are strange—nay, they are stranger than the rest.[47]

During the four years John Clare was institutionalized in Dr. Allen's asylum, Alfred, Lord Tennyson (1809–1892), whose house was a mile away, was a frequent visitor. There is no record of discussions between the two poets, though it is quite likely they met. Tennyson's motivation for visiting Dr. Allen was both personal and professional. Tennyson's father, alcoholic and paranoid, had died six years earlier, and one brother, Edgar, was confined to an insane asylum, where he remained for fifty-seven years. Another brother, Septimus, was showing mental symptoms for which Tennyson sought help, and Septimus later entered Dr. Allen's asylum as a voluntary patient.

Professionally, Tennyson was intrigued by madness and also visited the asylum in order to "study the ravings of the demented at first-hand." He used mad figures in several of his poems, including "The Sister, Rizpah," and "The Lover's Tale." But it was "Maud" that was the primary beneficiary of Tennyson's visits to Dr. Allen's asylum. It was Tennyson's "favorite poem and one which he loved to recite."[48]

"Maud," originally titled "Maud; or, The Madness," was described in a contemporary review as "the history of a madman depicted by the hand of a master." In the poem the hero becomes insane and is committed to an asylum. There he experiences visual hallucinations of his dead lover:

Is it gone? My pulses beat—
What was it? A lying trick of the brain?
Yet I thought I saw her stand,
A shadow there at my feet,
High over the shadowy land.[49]

Later, Tennyson refers to such hallucinations as "the blot upon the brain / That *will* show itself without." The poem's hero also experiences auditory hallucinations and delusions that he has died and been buried:

Dead, long dead,
Long dead!
And my heart is a handful of dust,
And the wheels go over my head,
And my bones are shaken with pain,
For into a shallow grave they are thrust,
Only a yard beneath the street,
And the hoofs of the horses beat, beat,
The hoofs of the horses beat,
Beat into my scalp and my brain,
With never an end to the stream of passing feet,
Driving, hurrying, marrying, burying,
Clamour and rumble, and ringing and clatter,
And here beneath it is all as bad,
For I thought the dead had peace, but it is not so;
To have no peace in the grave, is that not sad?
But up and down and to and fro,
Ever about me the dead men go;
And then to hear a dead man chatter
Is enough to drive one mad.[50]

Tennyson also describes other patients in the asylum:

> *See, there is one of us sobbing,*
> *No limit to his distress;*
> *And another, a lord of all things, praying*
> *To his own great self, as I guess;*
> *And another, a statesman there, betraying*
> *His party-secret, fool, to the press;*
> *And yonder a vile physician, blabbing*
> *The case of his patient—all for what?*
> *To tickle the maggot born in an empty head,*
> *And wheedle a world that loves him not,*
> *For it is but a world of the dead.*[51]

At the end of "Maud," the hero recovers his sanity, at least in part:

> *My life has crept so long on a broken wing*
> *Thro' cells of madness, haunts of horror and fear,*
> *That I come to be grateful at last for a little thing.*[52]

The Madness of Mrs. Rochester

During the second quarter of the nineteenth century, insanity appeared to be spreading rapidly. In 1827 Dugald Steward suggested that insanity could be "caught" merely by observing madmen, "the incoherent ravings and frantic gestures of a madman having a singularly painful effect in unsettling and deranging the thoughts of others." Of this period, Ann Colley, in *Tennyson and Madness*, says: "It would be safe to say that a majority feared that madness was spreading in epidemic proportions from man to man, from generation to generation, and from region to region. Many saw madness as a monster lying beneath the surface, waiting to be given an opportunity to rise and consume their England."[53]

One measure of the increasing prevalence of insanity was the overcrowding of asylums. The first eight county asylums, opened by 1823, had an average of 116 beds, "but almost at once it became clear that the number of beds needed had been seriously underestimated in most areas, and the asylums grew rapidly in size."[54] For example, the asylum at Lancashire was built in 1816 for 250 patients, but by 1844 it held 600. The Nottinghamshire Asylum increased from 80 to 206 beds, and the Bedfordshire Asylum nearly quadrupled in size from 40 to 139 beds between 1812 and 1844. Additional asylums were built, including the Middlesex Asylum at Hanwell, with 1,000 beds to serve London, but they were filled as soon as the doors were opened.

It should be noted that the increase in asylum population in the second quarter of the nineteenth century occurred despite high death rates in the asylums. At the Lancashire Asylum, cholera killed ninety-four patients in 1832, and influenza killed forty-six more in 1837. At the Wakefield Asylum, influenza killed thirty in 1837, and cholera killed over one hundred in 1849. The death rate for new admissions to the Hanwell Asylum was 18 percent for the first year, reflecting the fact that many admissions also had serious medical, as well as psychiatric, problems.[55]

A census of "lunatics" in England was carried out in 1843 and reported a total of 14,792 in public and private asylums, workhouses, and private dwellings.[56] The rate of insanity was thus 0.93 per 1,000 total population, an increase of 18 percent since 1829.

When the results of the 1843 census are examined by county, it becomes clear that the distribution of insane persons, as reported in the 1843 census, was geographically uneven. Nine counties of southern England and the Midlands (Gloucestershire, Oxfordshire, Berkshire, Wiltshire, Hampshire, Dorset, Somerset, Devonshire, and Cornwall) had a rate of insane persons per 1,000 total population of 0.46 to 0.89, with an average of 0.65. Three of these counties (Wiltshire, 0.89; Hampshire, 0.84; and Dorset, 0.76) were among the four English counties with the highest rates of insanity and are contiguous. The eight northernmost counties, by contrast, had a rate of insane persons per 1,000 total population of 0.29 to 0.52, with an average of 0.42. These include the four counties with the lowest rates (Lancashire, 0.38; Cheshire, 0.33; Staffordshire, 0.39; and Derbyshire, 0.29) and are also contiguous.[57] Thus, insanity in England in 1843 appeared to be most prevalent in the south and the Midlands and to become less prevalent as one moved north. It was a pattern that would be seen repeatedly later in the century.

The results of the 1843 census confirmed some people's fears that insanity was increasing. The previous year, an article in the *Monthly*

Review had observed that "the inhabitants of Great Britain are more liable to insanity than those of any other country in Europe, except Norway."[58] One result of such fears was passage by Parliament of the Lunatics Act of 1845, which was widely referred to as "Ashley's Act" after its sponsor. With passage of this act, each county was not merely encouraged, but mandated, to build a county insane asylum, and the Lunacy Commission was established as a national, not merely metropolitan, body. Lord Ashley was named chairman, and six full-time, paid inspectors were appointed to inspect all asylums, both public and private.

There was at this time widespread concern about conditions in many of the private asylums, which were also growing rapidly in number and size. Between 1815 and 1849 the number of private asylums doubled from 72 to 149. They were also admitting many more patients. For example, Hook Norton and Witney, the two private asylums in Oxfordshire, each admitted between eleven and fourteen patients per year in 1829 and 1830, but in 1846 Hook Norton admitted sixty-four and the following year Witney admitted fifty.[59]

Most private asylums catered to wealthy clients. For example, Eastgate House in Lincolnshire advertised itself as the "residence of a limited number of Ladies and Gentlemen of the Upper and Middle Classes," and the owner of Dunnington House in Yorkshire boasted, "I only admit a certain number of patients into my establishment and these are persons of distinction." As the public asylums became increasingly overcrowded, however, some of the private asylums opened separate units for pauper (i.e., nonprivate) patients, with the cost being borne by the county. The best-known such private asylum was Haydock Lodge in Lancashire, which opened in 1844 with accommodations for 450 insane paupers. Two years after opening, Haydock Lodge was the subject of a widely publicized parliamentary inquiry because of allegations of filthy conditions, physical abuse of patients, and a remarkably high death rate.[60]

Insane persons who could not be accommodated in public or private asylums usually ended up in the county workhouses. Although counties were mandated by law to transfer the insane from the workhouse to county asylums as the latter were opened, many counties ignored the edict because the daily cost of asylum care was approximately three times more than that in the workhouses. Consequently, workhouses continued to house large numbers of insane persons and idiots, with many workhouses even having separate wards for them. "In Oldham, Nottingham and Blackburn [workhouses], lunatic inmates even had their own matron and staff, who were separated from the remaining workhouse officers." Conditions in the workhouses were often atrocious, as was described in 1834 in a Bristol workhouse:

> In one corner of the building I discovered the most filthy, dismal looking room, which altogether presented such a sombre, wretched appearance, that curiosity prompted me to explore it. I entered it, and the scene which I witnessed, it is impossible to forget. . . . It reminded me of a coal cellar, or of any place rather than the residence of a human being. The sole tenant of this abode was a poor distressed lunatic. His appearance was pitiable in the extreme; his clothing was extremely ragged; his flesh literally as dirty as the floor; his head and face were much bruised, apparently from repeated falls. . . . He sat listless and alone, without any human being to attend upon or take care of him, staring vacantly around, insensible even to the calls of nature.[61]

Except for Lord Ashley and a small number of other social reformers, there was less public outcry about such conditions for insane persons than might have been expected. One probable reason for this was a continuing series of highly publicized reminders that some insane persons could be dangerous. In 1812, for example, John Bellingham, paranoid and insane, had shot Prime Minister Spencer Percival in the lobby of the House of Commons. In 1829 an insane Jonathan Martin set fire to the York Cathedral. In 1840 Edward Oxford shot at Queen Victoria's carriage and was subsequently declared insane. Three years later, Daniel M'Naghten shot Edward Drummond, mistaking him for Prime Minister Robert Peel. Later that same year, Richard Dadd, one of the most promising Victorian painters, murdered his father and spent the remainder of his life continuing his painting while confined to insane asylums.

Such reminders confirmed widespread opinions that insane persons should be kept confined. There was, as one observer noted in 1840, a fear of "the unfortunate incurable Toms o' Bedlam who were discharged upon the world to commit murder and arson." Studies of the use of the insanity defense and the number of criminally insane persons confined during the first half of the nineteenth century confirm that violent acts by insane persons were indeed increasing. For example, in 1837, there were 138 criminal insane persons confined in England, but by 1847 the number had risen to 337.[62]

Given this increasingly widespread fear of insane persons in mid-nineteenth-century England, it is not surprising that the literature of the period reflects that fear. The best-known example is Mrs. Rochester in Charlotte Brontë's *Jane Eyre*. Hidden for ten years in the attic of Thornfield Hall by her husband, her existence is finally revealed when Mr. Rochester attempts to take a second wife. Brontë's description of Mrs. Rochester is that of a dangerous wild animal: "In the deep shade, at the farther end of the room, a figure ran backwards and forwards. What it was, whether beast or human being, one could not, at first sight, tell: it grovelled, seemingly, on all fours; it snatched and growled like some strange wild animal: but it was covered with clothing, and a quantity of dark, grizzled hair, wild as a mane, hid its head and face."[63] When Charlotte Brontë was later criticized for her brutish depiction of Mrs. Rochester, she responded that she was merely reflecting the reality of some cases of madness "in which all that is good or even human seems to disappear from the mind and a fiend-like nature replaces it." Such a description was consistent with the increasing tenor of the times. As Ann Colley notes in *Tennyson and Madness,* "Brontë's Mrs. Rochester, locked within the tower of Thornfield Hall" was not merely "a literary convention" but rather reflected that period's preoccupation with madness, "a madness that was a pressing and threatening reality."[64]

An ironic postscript to *Jane Eyre* was Charlotte Brontë's dedication of the second edition of the book to William Makepeace Thackeray, whom she greatly admired. Unknown to Brontë, Thackeray's wife, Isabella, who had become insane, tried to drown their daughter, and attempted suicide, was being quietly confined in a house in London under the care of two women attendants. Both Mrs. Rochester and Mrs. Thackeray became mad four years following their marriages, "both were given to manic bursts of laughter," and "both were at times violent and even homicidal." When Charlotte Brontë learned of Isabella Thackeray's condition, she "was torn between amazement and mortification," apologized to Thackeray, and told a friend that it proved that "fact is often stranger than fiction."[65]

CHAPTER 5

"A Mania for Madness"
England, 1850–1890

Of all the calamities to which human nature is subjected, insanity may justly be considered as the most deplorable.

—ANDREW DUNCAN, "Present State of the
Lunatic Asylum at Edinburgh," 1812

But it was the same thing abroad, for the bad News was gone over the whole World, that the City of *London* was infected with the Plague.

—DANIEL DEFOE, *A Journal of the Plague Year,* 1722

The Great Exhibition of 1851 was a wondrous event. It was held in London's Hyde Park in the Crystal Palace, designed and built especially for the occasion, an immense glass-and-iron structure covering twenty-one acres. Exhibits, including an astonishing variety of machines, were gathered from around the world and viewed by more than six million visitors. The Reverend George Clayton described the exhibition in an 1851 sermon as follows:

You will behold there a monument of national greatness.
. . . Who then can fail to discover in the themes under consideration an indubitable evidence of England's greatness
and glory? . . . And great she truly is—great in her trade and

commerce—great in her laws and constitution—great in her freedom, both civil and religious—great in the power, the character, and the virtues of her queen, nor less in those of her royal consort, to whom this Exhibition is primarily attributable—great in the resources of her wealth, in the number and extent of her colonial possessions—great in the multitude of her subjects—great in the moral and Christian bearing of a large proportion of her people . . . great in the distribution of her Bibles, in her mission to the heathen . . . great in the presence and protection of her God. God is in the midst of her.[1]

The "indubitable evidence of England's greatness" was visible not only in the Great Exhibition but also in the thriving economy. England had become the world's richest country and by 1860 had a per capita income "50 per cent higher than that of France and almost three times that of Germany." Much of the prosperity was attributable to England's continuously expanding empire; in the fifteen years prior to the Great Exhibition, South Australia, New Zealand, Hong Kong, the Straits Settlement, the Punjab, a united Upper and Lower Canada, and the Gold Coast had all hoisted the Union Jack for the first time. The English people were proud of opening commerce while simultaneously believing that they were saving souls in the world's dark recesses. When, in 1857, Scottish physician and missionary David Livingstone published *Missionary Travels* about his exploration of Africa, the book sold 70,000 copies in the first few months.[2]

There is something inherently antipodean in a nation designating its populace as God's chosen people while simultaneously experiencing a rapid rise in the number of its insane. Such was the situation in Victorian England, and it presented the authorities with a dilemma that, though they tried mightily, they never fully resolved. A census of the insane in 1854, including all public and private asylums, reported a total of 30,538, more than twice as many as had been reported ten years previously. Taking into consideration the growth in population, the number of insane had grown from 0.93 per 1,000 total population to 1.61 per 1,000, an increase of 73 percent.

The increasing number of insane persons caused alarm. Charles M. Burnett, in his 1848 *Insanity Tested by Science*, observed: "It has long been a popular opinion that insanity is a more common disease in our country than in any other, and that this opinion has of late years been strengthened by the assertion of many that the disease is on the increase." Two years later an author, identified only as "the late Medical Superintendent of an Asylum for the Insane," described insanity as "a great national evil, spreading through numerous families, in which every remedy that medical science can suggest, and law can enforce, ought immediately to be applied." In 1854 Alfred Maddox, the proprietor of an asylum in Kent, claimed that "in no other country, compared with England, do we find such numerous and formidable examples of this extensive scourge." And three years later John Hawkes, a Medical Officer in the Wiltshire County Asylum, wrote that "the fair face of England, dotted over with her many public asylums for the relief and refuge of mental disease, presents a picture of rare and painful interest. . . . I doubt if ever the history of the world, or the experience of past ages, could show a larger amount of insanity than that of the present day."[3]

It was not only medical men who were alarmed by the rising insanity, but the general public as well. Gossip and newspaper accounts of mad persons became commonplace, as one account in the *Times* describing the "Conduct of a Lunatic in a Church," in which a man "got into the pulpit just as the clergyman was coming from the vestry to read his sermon. . . . The man clung to the gas fittings and was not removed until after a desperate struggle with the sexton and his assistants." Such public accounts often included serious misdeeds, including one under a headline of "Horrible Circumstance," in which a "maniac" named Big Hector "lately visited Edderton, in the eastern portion of this county, where, having taken hold of a child (a girl), he ate the flesh off her arm, and the poor sufferer when relieved was, and still is, in a very painful and dangerous condition." By the end of the 1850s one journal lamented "such a period as the present, when lunacy and lunatic affairs claim so large an amount of attention and interest on the part of the general public."[4]

Official concern about rising insanity was further amplified in 1859, when a census of insane persons reported that the number had grown to 36,762, or 1.87 per 1,000 total population. This was an increase of over 16 percent in just five years, and in response the House of Commons appointed a Select Committee on Lunatics to investigate. Testimony before the committee included a description of the asylum at London's Colney Hatch, which had opened in 1851 with accommodations for 1,220 "lunatic poor" but which "almost immediately ... was filled with a mass of chronic patients." "And now," the testimony continued, "within a period of five years, it has again become necessary to appeal to the county to provide further accommodation for its pauper lunatics."[5]

As chairman of the Lunacy Commission, the principal witness for the 1859 Select Committee hearings was Lord Ashley, who, by the death of his father in 1851, had become Lord Shaftesbury. He was asked a total of 922 questions during three days of testimony and acknowledged that there had been a numerical increase of "somewhere about 15,000" insane persons between 1843 and 1859. When asked whether or not this increase was real, he responded: "I am almost afraid of giving an opinion, as it may be the commencement of the most awful controversy, for there is a great difference of opinion on that point." Despite his prefatory reservations, however, Lord Shaftesbury proceeded to repeatedly and emphatically state that the increase in insane persons was not real but only "apparent": "I am satisfied that it was not a positive increase in the actual number of lunatics in proportion to the population. . . . It is not by any means in the ratio of the increase of the population. . . . I repeat that I do not believe that it is by any means in proportion to the increase of the population." Instead, he said, the "apparent" increase in insane persons was the product of "a vast number of old chronic cases [which] were brought to light that nobody knew anything about. . . . The appearance [of increase] was owing to the provision having been made for them, and the greater activity of all the authorities to look them up in all directions, and to bring them to the face of day and place them in the receptacles [asylums] prepared for them."[6] Such cases, he said, then steadily accumulated in the asylums.

Lord Shaftesbury's vested interests, prejudices, and Evangelical religious beliefs were prominently in evidence during his testimony to the Select Committee. He asserted, with no supporting data, that "at least one-half of the cases of lunacy" were caused by excess use of alcohol and that "owing to the efforts made by Teetotal societies and temperance societies, . . . the progress of insanity, which would otherwise have been a most formidable ratio of increase, has been very much checked." He denied that insanity was being caused by "religious excitement" or revivals, as some alleged, and claimed that insanity was more prevalent in Roman Catholic countries than in England. In defense of his more than thirty years of leadership on the metropolitan and national lunacy commissions, Lord Shaftesbury claimed that asylums and treatment for insane individuals had improved markedly and that the newer treatments were "without any exception the greatest triumph of skill and humanity that the world ever saw." In reviewing Lord Shaftesbury's testimony, Nicholas Hervey recently characterized it as "a congeries of imperfect observations, preconceived prejudices and direct falsehoods. . . . There was indeed a self-deceptive dishonesty about the way he passed off personal opinions as the received knowledge of the commission."[7]

The question arises as to why, during the 1859 Select Committee hearings and subsequently, Lord Shaftesbury's testimony was not publicly contradicted. Available data demonstrated clearly that, whatever the cause, insanity was increasing disproportionately to the population increase. Furthermore, there was no evidence that alcohol-induced admissions to asylums had increased, and the superintendents of most of the increasingly overcrowded asylums must have found doubtful Lord Shaftesbury's assertions that treatments had markedly improved.

The answer to this question must take into consideration the fact that Lord Shaftesbury was the official government expert on issues of insanity. He also ran the Lunacy Commission as his personal fiefdom, and in fact, it was not until 1875 that "for the first time in forty-five years, his colleagues on the Lunacy Commission . . . rejected his advice on a point."[8] Perhaps most important was the fact that Lord Palmerston, England's prime minister from 1855 to 1865 except for a brief interval, was married to Lord Shaftesbury's wife's widowed mother, and the prime minister was therefore Lord Shaftesbury's father-in-law. To contradict Lord Shaftesbury was thus to contradict the government, and the government was not at all interested in hearing that insanity was increasing.

From 1859 onward, then, the official position of the British government, as represented by the Lunacy Commission, was that insanity was not increasing. The "apparent" increases were said to be due to improved case-finding and the accumulation of chronic cases in the asylums. Once established, this official position never changed. Year after year, the Lunacy Commission's annual report listed increases in the number of insane persons in England, followed immediately by annual assurances that the increases were only "apparent" due to an "accumulation" of cases.

The Psychiatric Establishment

Lord Shaftesbury's efforts to persuade the public that insanity was not increasing were helped immensely by England's psychiatric establishment. In 1841, physicians working in the asylums had organized the Association of Medical Officers of Asylums and Hospitals for the Insane, which later became the Medico-Psychological Association and eventually the Royal College of Psychiatrists. In 1853 this organization began publishing the *Journal of Mental Science,* later to become the *British Journal of Psychiatry,* regarded as the official voice of English psychiatry. From the beginning of its publication until 1895, the *Journal of Mental Science* was edited or coedited by four psychiatrists— John Bucknill, C. Lockhart Robertson, Henry Maudsley, and Hack Tuke—all of whom aggressively promoted the idea that insanity was not increasing. Thus, the official government position and the official psychiatric position reinforced and supported each other, and no matter how alarming the reported increases of insane persons, the increases were invariably labeled as being merely "apparent."

John Bucknill was superintendent of the Devonshire Asylum from 1844 to 1862. In 1853 he became the first editor of the *Journal of Mental Science* and later became president of the Medico-Psychological Association and was knighted. In an 1858 textbook written with Hack Tuke he said:

> On no subject has there been more absurd and illogical reasoning, or more hasty generalisations, than on the proportion of the insane to the population. . . . Highly important inferences are drawn with the utmost complacency, and apparently in entire ignorance of the fallacy which underlies such loose and worthless calculations. . . . In our own country there are two reasons why the proportion of

the insane to the population appears to be greater than was formerly the case. The first is, that the disease is recognised as such to a far greater extent than formerly; and the second is, that we know, to a much greater extent than heretofore, the number of the insane throughout the country. In the short period of nineteen years, the estimated proportion of the insane in England rose from 1 in 7,300 to 1 in 769; a difference which led to the belief in the frightful increase of insanity, but which by no means warranted such a conclusion. The knowledge of an evil, and the existence of that evil, are two widely different things.

Bucknill also agreed with Lord Shaftesbury that if any portion of the "apparent" increase in insanity was real, that portion was probably attributable to "intemperance" and "the over-tasking of emotions" caused by advancing civilization.[9]

In 1862 C. Lockhart Robertson and Henry Maudsley assumed coeditorship of the *Journal of Mental Science*. Robertson was Superintendent of the Sussex County Asylum from 1859 to 1870 and a president of the Medico-Psychological Association, and he labeled the increase of insanity in England as "a manifest fallacy." In 1869 he published a widely cited article entitled "The Alleged Increase of Lunacy," in which he acknowledged that there had been "an increase in the last twenty-five years in the number of registered lunatics of more than a hundred per cent," but he claimed that this was caused by better case-finding, better statistics, and the accumulation of chronic cases in the asylums. He admitted that admissions to the asylums were still continuing to rise but said that this was no cause for concern since "the rate of increase is in a yearly decreasing ratio." He concluded that "the alleged increase of lunacy is a popular fallacy, unsupported by recent statistics."[10]

Robertson used the *Journal of Mental Science* as a forum to vigorously publicize his position. Summaries of his article "The Alleged Increase of Lunacy" were also published in popular periodicals, including the *Pall Mall Gazette*, the *Saturday Review*, and the *North British Review*, and Robertson dutifully reprinted these summaries in the *Journal of Mental Science*. In an 1871 issue Robertson included a

"Report on Insanity in Wiltshire," in which the author concluded that "the supposed increased liability to insanity in England at the present time, as compared with the earlier part of the century, may to a great extent, or even altogether, be imaginary, when the increase in the general population is considered." At the same time, Robertson continually reminded readers of the great advances being made by modern psychiatric treatments. In view of these advances, an increase in insanity was, in Robertson's view, a "terrible possibility which I entirely dispute."[11]

Henry Maudsley was one of the most important figures in nineteenth-century English psychiatry. His influence came from his fourteen-year coeditorship of the *Journal of Mental Science,* his position as president of the Medico-Psychological Association, his widely read 1867 textbook *The Physiology and Pathology of the Mind,* and not least of all, from the fact that he had married a daughter of John Conolly, the best-known English psychiatrist of the early nineteenth century. Maudsley was "very much the aristocrat's alienist,"[12] consulted by rich and influential persons throughout Europe, and at his death he left £5 million (1997 equivalent) to build a psychiatric institute that still bears his name.

Like Robertson, Maudsley acknowledged in an 1872 article that, for insane persons, "the ratio to the population has doubled since 1844." However, he added, the idea "that so many more persons should be yearly going mad now than twenty-five years ago, seems to me a supposition which is, I will not say preposterous, but is certainly not probable in itself and not supported by facts." Maudsley said that the "apparent" increase in insanity was caused by better case-finding, the accumulation of chronic cases, and government regulations that provided fiscal incentives for counties to transfer insane individuals from homes and workhouses to county asylums. He concluded: "There is no satisfactory evidence of an increase in the proportion of occurring cases of insanity to the population."[13]

Five years later, in a paper titled "The Alleged Increase of Insanity," Maudsley again noted "an alarming increase" in insanity: "It is clear that if it goes on with the same ruthless speed for the next half century . . . the sane people will be in a minority at no very distant day." Nevertheless, Maudsley concluded, "There is no evidence of an increased production of insanity." Consistent with his aristocratic inclinations, Maudsley specifically exempted the upper classes from any taint of increasing insanity; if insanity was increasing, he said, it was increasing exclusively among the lower classes. In this regard, Maudsley was influenced by Charles Darwin's *Origin of the Species*, which had been published in 1859 and which he frequently quoted. Insanity, in Maudsley's view, was but another example of the survival of the fittest:

> It is necessary to bear in mind that an increase in the number of insane persons in a country does not mean the degeneracy of the people: the capability of development is the capability of degeneration, and where the general progress is going on actively the retrograde action in the elements must be going on also: the particular is sacrificed to the general, "the individual perishes, but the race is more and more." If this be so, may we not then say that an increase of insanity is after all a testimony of development, that a great apparent evil is but a phase in the working out of good.[14]

Following Maudsley, Hack Tuke edited the *Journal of Mental Science* from 1880 until his death in 1895. Tuke was the great-grandson of William Tuke, the founder of the York Retreat, and Andrew Scull has labeled him "the most unembarrassed apologist for Victorian asylumdom." William Bynum characterized Hack Tuke as "a good 'party' man, devoted to improving the status of his profession in Britain." For example, in his *Chapters in the History of the Insane in the British Isles*, Tuke claimed "remarkable progress effected in the asylum care of our lunacy population." Although early in his career Tuke had expressed uncertainty about whether insanity was increasing or not, he later concluded that "the increase of insanity is apparent rather than real, being mainly due to accumulation."[15]

Tuke wrote extensively about the alleged increase of insanity and analyzed the available statistics from the Lunacy Commission to try to prove his point. He advocated the use of first admissions, rather than the total patients hospitalized, as "the only sound test of the increase of insanity." For example, in 1882 he recorded the first admissions per 10,000 total population for twelve years as follows:

1869	4.71	1873	4.80	1877	5.28
1870	4.54	1874	5.03	1878	5.36
1871	4.62	1875	5.19	1879	5.20
1872	4.59	1876	5.30	1880	5.19

His conclusion was that "the ratio of the yearly increase of the fresh admissions to the population has been slight," when in fact the increase was 10 percent over the twelve-year period. By 1894 first admissions per population had increased another 10 percent; Tuke dismissed the figures, saying: "I have now reason to believe that the returns which have been since published [since 1880] cannot be trusted." Edward Hare, in his seminal 1983 paper "Was Insanity on the Increase?" commented on Tuke's selective use of statistics and noted that "the untrustworthy later returns had shown a very marked increase rate of first attacks."[16]

For a "good 'party' man" like Hack Tuke, increasing insanity was simply unacceptable, as it had been for Bucknill, Robertson, and Maudsley before him. Tuke labeled the idea that insanity was increasing "a melancholy theory" that "would unsettle our belief in the onward progress of mankind, it would shake the very foundation of our faith." Increasing insanity would imply not only that the asylums had failed but also that the psychiatrists themselves had failed. It was an unacceptable possibility. As Mr. Podsnap says in Dickens's *Our Mutual Friend:* "I don't want to know about it; I don't want to discuss it; I don't want to admit it!"[17]

"A Mania for Madness"

The publication of Wilkie Collins's *The Woman in White* in 1859 marked a new phase in the use of madness in English fiction. The novel was published after the 1859 census of insane persons had reported a sharp increase in numbers and while Parliament's Select Committee on Lunatics was hearing Lord Shaftesbury repeatedly reassure its members that the increase in insanity was not real. As David Oberhelman noted in his dissertation on this subject:

By the mid–nineteenth century psychological medicine was perhaps the most controversial branch of medical science. Its development occasioned prolonged debates within all segments of Victorian society about the apparent growth of lunacy in Britain and about the authority of the alienists to declare people mad and deprive them of their liberty. . . . Victorian culture accordingly exhibited an unprecedented concern with madness and asylums, and the status of psychological medicine with its manifold theories of the forms, causes, and treatment of insanity, was subjected to intense scrutiny by the clerics, philosophers, government officials, legal scholars, journalists, and literary writers, particularly novelists. The novelists' position on psychological medicine was especially troubling for the defensive psychological community.[18]

The Woman in White belongs to a genre referred to as an English sensation novel, a type of fiction that became immensely popular in the 1860s and early 1870s. Oberhelman claimed these novels exhibited "a mania for madness itself, . . . producing a veritable Bedlam of madmen and madwomen. . . . Madness and the system of private lunatic asylums . . . are almost ubiquitous plot elements in the sensation novels. . . . Wrongful confinement . . . , the corruption of 'mad-doctors,' and the threat of hereditary madness become some of the most lurid nightmares [in the works of Wilkie Collins and his contemporaries]."[19]

Collins's novels were not the first English sensation novels to attack doctors who specialized in insanity. Henry Cockton's *The Life and Adventures of Valentine Vox, the Ventriloquist*, published in 1839, was "the first instance of a Victorian novel addressing the profession of psychological medicine in its representation of madness."[20] In the novel, Walter Goodman persuades "Dr. Holden," a dishonest asylum physician, to commit Walter's brother to a private asylum so that Walter can take his brother's money. The novel was published one year after John Perceval, son of a former prime minister, published *A Narrative of the Treatment Experienced by a Gentleman, during a State of Mental Derangement,* in which he exposed the abuses to which he had been subjected while confined by his brother in a private madhouse.

The Woman in White and the sensation novels that followed were, according to Oberhelman, "among the most widely read works in the [nineteenth] century. . . . The novels were so highly popular that they created new marketing strategies, including a line of 'Woman in White' clothing and perfumes."[21] Their broad readership popularized the issues surrounding insanity, including the public's fears both of madness and of wrongful confinement.

In *The Woman in White*, the title character, based on a woman with whom Collins had apparently had an affair, first appears almost as an apparition to a young man on a lonely, moonlit road north of London. Responding to the woman's pleas for both assistance and secrecy, the young man sends her off in a carriage and then listens from the shadows when men approach, searching for her. What he overhears soon leads him to question whether he's done the right thing in helping her:

> ". . . escaped from [an] Asylum!"
>
> I cannot say with truth that the terrible inference which those words suggested flashed upon me like a new revelation. Some of the strange questions put to me by the woman in white, after my ill-considered promise to leave her free to act as she pleased, had suggested the conclusion either that she was naturally flighty and unsettled, or that some recent shock of terror had disturbed the balance of her faculties. But the idea of absolute insanity which we all associate with the very name of an Asylum, had, I can honestly declare, never occurred to me, in connection with her. . . .
>
> What had I done? Assisted the victim of the most horrible of all false imprisonments to escape; or cast loose on the wide world of London an unfortunate creature, whose actions it was my duty, and every man's duty, mercifully to control?[22]

In 1866 Collins published *Armadale*, a novel in which another unethical psychiatrist, "Dr. Downward," confines people inappropriately in his private asylum. Indeed, according to Oberhelman, "The plague spots of madness afflict much [*sic*] of the characters and dominate the prose of the text. . . . Madness so saturates the text that any debate over figurative or literal uses of the term is rendered meaningless. . . . It illustrates the true epidemic proportions of madness in the 1800s."[23]

Collins's intense interest in madness was shared with his close friend Charles Dickens. Collins and Dickens lived together in Paris in 1855 and later traveled together and jointly wrote "The Lazy Tour of Two Idle Apprentices" in 1857. In addition, Collins's younger brother married Dickens's daughter. Collins's writings on insanity are largely unknown today, and he is remembered mostly for *The Moonstone*, which was published in 1868 and earned him the title "father of the English mystery novel."

Another widely read sensation novel of the early 1860s was *Lady Audley's Secret*, written by Mary Elizabeth Braddon. Mrs. Braddon had a special interest in insanity, since she was living with, but could not marry, publisher John Maxwell, whose wife was insane and confined to an asylum. In Mrs. Braddon's book, the "secret" is that Lady Audley is insane, a fact slowly revealed in the novel through her bigamy and subsequent murder of one of her husbands. In her confession at the end of the book, Lady Audley says: "I killed him because I AM MAD! because my intellect is a little way on the wrong side of that narrow boundary-line between sanity and insanity."[24]

Lady Audley's Secret achieved wide notoriety because it was serialized in the *Sixpenny Magazine* in late 1861 and early 1862, at the same time that the trial of William Frederick Windham was being reported in daily newspapers. Windham was an eccentric young man who had inherited a large sum of money and whose family had then declared him insane in order to protect his inheritance. The trial to determine his sanity lasted thirty-three days and included over 140 witnesses; it was "the longest and most involved lunacy inquiry of the 1800s."[25] Much of the debate in the Windham trial echoed issues in *Lady Audley's Secret*, but the outcomes differed: Windham was found by the jury to be sane, while Lady Audley was said to be insane.

Of the many sensation novels of the 1860s, the one that most truly lived up to its genre was Charles Reade's *Hard Cash*, which overtly and libelously ridiculed John Conolly, the best-known psychiatrist of his era. Conolly, who had been superintendent of Hanwell, the largest asylum in England, and president of the Medico-Psychological

Association, had been sued by a man who accused Conolly of falsely imprisoning him in a private asylum at the behest of the man's wife. At his trial, Conolly admitted that he had received a fee—a kickback—from the private asylum and that, since he had had a financial interest, legally he should not have signed the man's commitment papers. In his defense Conolly claimed: "I know the [commitment] act says that a certificate should not be signed by any medical man connected with the establishment. I do not consider myself connected with the establishment, as I only send male patients to it."[26] Conolly was found guilty and fined £20,000 (1997 equivalent).

In *Hard Cash,* Conolly is thinly disguised as "Dr. Wycherly" who, at the behest of a father, illegally confines the man's son in a private asylum to prevent the young man from exposing his father's criminal behavior. Wycherly is portrayed as a hypocrite who appears to be "the very soul of humanity" but who is in fact said to be "blinded by self interest . . . a man of large reading and the tact to make it subserve his interests." During his trial at the end of the novel, Wycherly, like Conolly, is forced to acknowledge that he received kickbacks of "fifteen per cent from the asylum keepers for every patient he wrote insane and that he had an income of eight hundred pounds a year from that source alone."[27]

Hard Cash was serialized in Charles Dickens's weekly, *All the Year Round,* in 1863 and caused much discussion. A letter in the *Daily News* said: "When we read this, a thrill of terror goes through the public mind. If what Mr. Charles Reade says be possible, who is safe?" A review in the *Times* warned readers about assuming that the book was based on facts: "The incautious reader is apt to imagine mad doctors to be scientific scoundrels, lunatic asylums to be a refined sort of Tophet [Hebrew Bible place of human sacrifices], and the visiting justices to be a flock of sheep. This is the untruthful exaggeration of fact jumbled with fiction." One asylum physician publicly challenged Reade to produce a single specific example of wrongful commitment to an asylum; Reade responded with "a lengthy enumeration of several cases of perfectly sane persons confined under the Lunacy Laws,"[28] including a case in which Reade himself had testified and in which the jury found the man to be perfectly sane.

Increasingly, the English public appeared to be more inclined to believe Charles Reade and other novelists who were sensationalizing insanity, and less inclined to believe Lord Shaftesbury and other officials who were denying that any problem existed. Newspapers and periodicals regularly reported the "melancholy increase in the number of patients in the county lunatic asylum." In 1867 the *Scotsman* noted that "the increase of this class [insane persons] has baffled all calculation." In 1868 the *Times* reported that in the previous ten years insane persons had increased "45 percent while the population is estimated to have increased rather more than 11 percent." The following year the *North British Review,* examining the statistics on insanity, concluded: "If we examine the effect of this at the end of a long series of years, we have a result which cannot fail to startle." And by 1877 the *Times* quoted a magistrate as saying that "if the lunacy continued to increase as at present, the insane would be in the majority and, freeing themselves, would put the sane in the asylums."[29]

The Mad Hatter as Snark

Acquaintances of Lewis Carroll were not surprised to see allusions to madness in his writings. Carroll had been christened Charles Lutwidge Dodgson after his mother's brother, Robert Wilfred Skeffington Lutwidge. Lutwidge was a lawyer and a member of the Board of Metropolitan Commissioners in Lunacy from 1842 to 1845, secretary of the Lunacy Commission from 1845 to 1855, and a full-time inspector on the Lunacy Commission, whose chairman was Lord Shaftesbury, from 1855 until his death in 1873. Thus, from the time Lewis Carroll was ten years old, his uncle was involved in the inspection of madhouses and related issues, including the question of whether insanity was increasing. Lutwidge testified in 1859 before the House of Commons Select Committee on Lunatics, providing the committee with "an approximate estimate of the number of Lunatics in England of all classes"—37,300—including those in jails and kept at home. This was probably the most complete enumeration of the insane done to that time.

Skeffington Lutwidge and Lewis Carroll, both lifelong bachelors, were very close friends, Lutwidge being described as Carroll's "favorite uncle." According to his diaries, Carroll usually stayed with Uncle Skeffington when in London, dined frequently with him, and shared an interest in the theater. It was Uncle Skeffington who introduced Carroll to photography, and on at least one occasion Carroll accompanied his uncle to the Surrey County Asylum to discuss photography with Hugh Diamond, a staff physician who was the secretary of the London Photographic Society. Carroll also shared with his uncle a deep interest in mathematics and religious matters. Uncle Skeffington was a founding member of the London Statistical Society and a member of the National Society for Promoting Religious Education. Carroll was a lecturer in mathematics at Christ Church, Oxford, and an ordained deacon in the Church of England. For Carroll, "religion was the most important factor in his life," but he "was a moderate" and "avoided religious zealots."[30] Lewis Carroll would therefore have disliked Uncle Skeffington's supervisor, Lord Shaftesbury, who was a rigid evangelical and was widely viewed as a puritanical zealot. One can imagine the conversations Lewis Carroll and his uncle had over dinner on photography, mathematics, religion, Lord Shaftesbury, and, of course, insanity.

Given this background, it was logical that "throughout his life Carroll displayed a fascination with mental derangement. . . . The recurrent preoccupation with anarchy and madness, in *Wonderland* especially, entices us to speculate on the part they played in Carroll's thought." A well-known example is the "Mad Tea-Party" episode in *Alice's Adventures in Wonderland*, with dialogue that would have been familiar to Uncle Skeffington:

> The Hatter was the first to break the silence. "What day of the month is it?" he said, turning to Alice: he had taken his watch out of his pocket, and was looking at it uneasily, shaking it every now and then, and holding it to his ear.
>
> Alice considered a little, and then said, "The fourth."
>
> "Two days wrong!" sighed the Hatter. "I told you butter wouldn't suit the works!" he added, looking angrily at the March Hare.
>
> "It was the *best* butter," the March Hare meekly replied.
>
> "Yes, but some crumbs must have got in as well," the Hatter grumbled: "you shouldn't have put it in with the bread-knife."

> The March Hare took the watch and looked at it gloomily: then he dipped it into his cup of tea, and looked at it again: but he could think of nothing better to say than his first remark, "It was the *best* butter, you know."

Lewis Carroll also drew upon "Maud," Tennyson's poem of madness, which was said to have influenced Carroll's *The Dream of Fame* as well as passages in *Through the Looking Glass*.[31]

On May 21, 1873, Skeffington Lutwidge was attacked by a patient while making an official inspection of the Fisherton Lunatic Asylum at Salisbury. According to the *Times*, "A lunatic named M'Kave suddenly darted towards him and severely wounded him in the temple with a large rusty nail, the point of which had recently been sharpened." Upon hearing the news, Lewis Carroll immediately went to Salisbury, accompanied by Sir James Paget, a prominent London surgeon. The following day, Lutwidge appeared to be recovering, so Carroll returned to Oxford. Six days later, however, Lutwidge's condition rapidly deteriorated, and although Carroll rushed back to Salisbury, he "arrived a few minutes after [his] dear Uncle's death."[32] Lutwidge's death came following a period when Lewis Carroll had been spending increasing time with him, including having taken a week's trip together to Scotland late in 1871.

In July 1874, fourteen months after his uncle's death, Lewis Carroll claimed that a single line of verse suddenly came into his head: "For the Snark was a Boojum, you see." Starting with that line, which would become the final line, "by degrees, at odd moments during the next year or two, the rest of the poem pieced itself together." Thus was born "The Hunting of the Snark," said to be "the longest, most intricate nonsense poem in the English language." In addition to being "set to music, adapted for the stage, and performed as a musical comedy,"[33] the poem has generated Snark clubs that still meet regularly in Oxford, Cambridge, London, and New York, and provided the U.S. Air Force with a name for one of its guided missiles.

Despite the fact that, as one Carroll scholar has noted, "no poem has ever been more analysed," "The Hunting of the Snark" has defied definitive interpretation since its creation more than 120 years ago. Most exegeses have described the poem as an allegory or satire, with proposed subjects ranging from a contemporary trial (the Tichborne case) to an arctic expedition, an antivivisectionist tract, "an unsound business venture," "the craving for social advancement," and even an adaptation of Herman Melville's White Whale. Other analysts have focused on the person of the Baker, whose death at the end of the poem is caused by a Boojum, and have concluded that "The Snark" is "a poem about being and nonbeing, an existential poem, a poem of existential agony." In support of this, scholars have cited the illness and subsequent death of Lewis Carroll's godson, who was dying of tuberculosis at the time the poem was being written. A few scholars have even claimed that Lewis Carroll had nothing in mind and was writing "deliberate nonsense." A review written at the time of the poem's publication in 1876 suggested that Lewis Carroll had "merely been inspired by a wild desire to reduce to idiocy as many readers, and more especially reviewers, as possible."[34]

Lewis Carroll himself never explained "The Hunting of the Snark," although he received numerous requests to do so. When asked, he gave elliptical replies such as, "I'm very much afraid I didn't mean anything but nonsense! Still, you know, words mean more than we mean to express when we use them: so a whole book ought to mean a great deal more than the writer meant."[35] In his preface to the poem, Carroll labeled it "a brief but instructive poem" with a "strong moral purpose."

In view of the death of Lewis Carroll's uncle shortly before the poem was undertaken, it seems reasonable to hypothesize that "The Hunting of the Snark" may have been connected to this event. The ten-person Snark-hunting crew included, in fact, the same number of members as the Lunacy commission during the eighteen years Skeffington Lutwidge was a member. (The Lunacy Commission was composed, by statute, of three physicians, three lawyers, and up to five honorary commissioners, but this "honorary complement . . . was rarely filled."[36] Analysis of the commission members from 1860 to 1872 reveals that there were ten members most of the time.) The Bellman—the aristocratic, authoritarian, self-righteous leader of the crew—bears a striking resemblance to Lord Shaftesbury, the leader of the Lunacy Commission. The Baker, who has many different names and "forty-two boxes, all carefully packed," appears to be a composite of Robert Wilfred Skeffington Lutwidge and Lewis Carroll himself, who was forty-two when he began writing the poem.

A third member of the Snark-hunting crew, the Butcher, may have been inspired by John Forster, a member of the commission from 1861 to 1872. Described as "severe and blunt" but "sympathetic," Forster was a "prolific writer who moved in Dickens's circle."[37] In the poem the Butcher is described as follows:

> The Beaver brought paper, portfolio, pens,
> And ink in unfailing supplies:
> While strange creepy creatures came out of their dens,
> And watched them with wondering eyes.
>
> So engrossed was the Butcher, he heeded them not,
> As he wrote with a pen in each hand,
> And explained all the while in a popular style
> Which the Beaver could well understand.

It is possible that all the members of the Snark crew could be matched to actual members of the Lunacy Commission if enough information was available regarding them.

A key passage to understanding "The Hunting of the Snark" occurs in the third section, in which the Baker, the hero of the tale, speaks:

> "A dear uncle of mine (after whom I was named)
> Remarked, when I bade him farewell—"
> "Oh, skip your dear uncle!" the Bellman exclaimed,
> As he angrily tingled his bell.
>
> "He remarked to me then," said that mildest of men,
> "If your Snark be a Snark, that is right:
> Fetch it home by all means—you may serve it with greens,
> And it's handy for striking a light.
>
> "You may seek it with thimbles—and seek it with care;
> You may hunt it with forks and hope;

You may threaten its life with a railway-share;
You may charm it with smiles and soap—"

("That's exactly the method," the Bellman bold
In a hasty parenthesis cried,
"That's exactly the way I have always been told
That the capture of Snarks should be tried!")

"But oh, beamish nephew, beware of the day,
If your Snark be a Boojum! For then
You will softly and suddenly vanish away,
And never be met with again!"

At the end of the poem, the Baker does find a Snark, who turns out to be a Boojum, and the Baker "softly and suddenly vanishe[s] away," just as his uncle had warned him. In this context, a Snark would appear to be an insane person, and a Boojum a particular type of insane person who is dangerous. The uncle advises the use of thimbles, forks, and soap to hunt the Snark; this is consistent with the activities of the Lunacy Commissioners, whose job it was to inspect madhouses, including the clothing, food, and cleanliness of the inmates. And when the Baker is killed at the end of the poem, he is seen to "plunge into a chasm," an echo of the fact that Lutwidge was killed by a patient named M'Kave. Even the structure of the poem, subtitled "An Agony in Eight Fits," conveys the tragedy wrought by madness that Carroll was trying to express amid superficially whimsical dialogue and double entendres. "Fit," for example, is an archaic word meaning part of a poem, but it also suggests the seizures commonly observed in asylums and M'Kave's spasm of insane homicidal rage that killed Skeffington Lutwidge.

Madness, then, underlies and permeates "The Hunting of the Snark." In the Barrister's dream, the Snark not only plays the attorney for the accused but also the judge and jury in a scene reminiscent of the Mad Tea-Party. And when the Banker in "Snark" is snatched by the Bandersnatch, he, too, becomes insane:

Down he sank in a chair—ran his hands through his hair—
And chanted in mimsiest tones
Words whose utter inanity proved his insanity,
While he rattled a couple of bones.

Indeed, there is an element of insanity to the entire undertaking of "The Hunting of the Snark," which was noted in passing by the *Saturday Review* in 1876, when the poem was first published: "The story is in verse, and describes an expedition of various lunatics, conducted by a mad bellman, in search of a mysterious object."[38]

"Bluebeard's Cupboard"

Even as reviewers puzzled over the meaning of "The Hunting of the Snark," the number of insane persons continued to rise. As early as 1862, John Arlidge, the superintendent of St. Luke's Hospital in London, had publicly commented that the increasing numbers of insane persons "might well give rise to alarming apprehension of a mental degeneracy" in the country. As the *Times* observed in 1864: "Our asylums, private and public, now contain nearly twice as many patients as they did 15 years ago. . . . But this large number does not fully represent the total amount of insanity existing in the country; there are also the insane in gaols, the Chancery patients living out of asylums, and cases kept out of view for private or other reasons." When the Select Committee on Lunatics had met in 1859, there had been 36,762 insane persons in asylums; by 1879 the number reached 69,885, and in 1899 it was 105,086. As a ratio per population, the number of insane persons in asylums rose from 1.87 per 1,000 total population in 1859 to 2.76 in 1879 and 3.30 in 1899, an increase of 76 percent in forty years (fig. 5.1). These alarming numbers were further reinforced by censuses of "mentally unsound" individuals, which included those living at home, done as part of the national censuses of 1871, 1881, and 1891; these censuses reported a 41 percent increase of "mentally unsound" individuals during the twenty-year period.[39]

The effect of the steadily rising tide of insanity on public asylums was predictable. In 1824 there had been only eight asylums, and

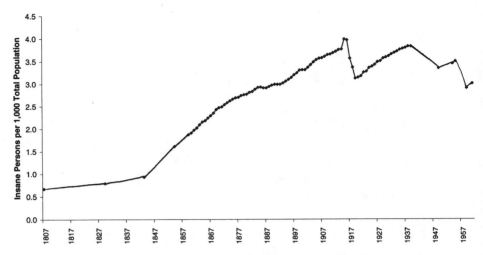

F<small>IG</small>. 5.1. England Wales: Insane Persons in Psychiatric Hospitals, Workhouses, and under Care per 1,000 Population, 1807–1961. Data on which the graph is based are taken from the annual reports of the Commissioners in Lunacy and from *Inpatient Statistics from the Mental Health Enquiry for England* reports, Department of Heath and Social Security.

their average size had been 116 beds. By 1860 there were forty-one asylums with an average of 386 beds, and by 1890, sixty-six asylums with an average of 802 beds. Each annual report of the Lunacy Commission reported new asylums under construction, new wings being added to existing asylums, and the conversion of "several houses on the estate lately occupied by attendants . . . being prepared for the reception of patients." The West Riding Asylum had opened in 1818 with 150 beds; by the end of the century, it had 1,469 beds, almost a tenfold increase. As early as 1856 John Bucknill, superintendent of the badly overcrowded Devonshire Asylum, boarded out "quiet, chronic, female patients in neighboring cottages beyond the asylum grounds" and rented "a house in the nearby seaside town of Exmouth, where he boarded forty to forty-five quiet female patients under the care of a resident medical officer . . . and two resident female nurses,"[40] harbingers of deinstitutionalization, which would come a century later.

The effect of the steadily rising number of insane persons on conditions in the asylums was also predictable and reported regularly in the newspapers:

> The barbarous means of restraint employed in some of these "dens of despair" are disgraceful to a civilized land, while the abominable filth and disregard of common decency often noticeable in others call for the instant interposition of authority. (*Times*, 1856)

> The state of Haverfordwest (South Wales) Asylum, formerly a dungeon for criminals, is a scandal to the country. . . . One specimen of the place is given in the fact that the asylum does not contain a single watercloset—the consequences are such as human decency forbids us to describe. (*The Times*, 1859)[41]

As asylum conditions worsened, it predictably became increasingly difficult to hire and retain good nursing staff. At the Kent Asylum, for example, "seven [attendants] were dismissed for leaving their patients unattended all night whilst out drinking, four for prostitution in Maidstone, three for playing cards in a corner of the suicide ward whilst a patient cut his throat, and several for sleeping whilst on night duty." The tragic consequences of inadequate staffing were inevitable: "Two attendants have recently been sentenced to seven years' penal servitude for manslaughter of a lunatic, who was found to have died from fractures of ribs and other injuries." Even as Lord Shaftesbury was telling members of Parliament in 1859 that modern psychiatric treatment was "the greatest triumph of skill and humanity that the world ever saw," the *Quarterly Review* was labeling county asylums "the Bluebeard's cupboard of the neighborhood."[42]

In recent years it has been fashionable to attribute the increase in asylum building in nineteenth-century Europe primarily to social and economic causes, best exemplified by Michel Foucault's *Madness and Civilization*. Asylums were built, argued Foucault, as part of "the great confinement" of the insane, paupers, criminals, and vagrants who were not economically productive. This thesis will be discussed at length in chapter 14, but it should be noted in opposition that there was continuing widespread resistance among the public to the building of these institutions. The financing of asylums was, until 1874, the exclusive responsibility of local governments, which meant higher local taxes each time an asylum was built; after 1874 the central government contributed approximately 40 percent of the asylum costs by paying a weekly subsidy for each pauper lunatic. The initial cost per bed for the nine public asylums operating in 1827 was £9,776 per bed (1997 equivalent), and total expenditures for insanity in England increased from £308,000 in 1840 to £11,302,000 in 1870 (1997 equivalents).[43]

Given such costs, it is not surprising that "ratepayer and taxpayer resistance to increased public expenditure was deep rooted, vituperative, and often crippling." As early as 1859, the persistent calls by public officials to build new asylums and enlarge existing ones were said to cause "terrible discouragement and complaint with the ratepayers." In Sussex "there was clearly a highly organized campaign against building a county asylum." In Buckinghamshire in 1849, "six hundred ratepayers, led by Benjamin Disraeli, renewed their opposition [to an asylum], complaining that they had already been taxed for a new jail and judges' lodging, and were now being asked to underwrite another expensive capital project." Disraeli was at the time a Member of Parliament for Buckinghamshire. An editorial in the *Westminster Review* complained of pianos and other "lavish expenditures" in public asylums: "It is no exaggeration to say that two-thirds of the permanent residents in every pauper asylum care little for the luxurious furnishings around them. A considerable proportion, indeed, could not tell the difference between a palace and a stable-yard."[44]

A large number of skirmishes in the battle over the costs of insanity took place in local workhouses. It was these institutions that had housed mentally ill individuals before the county asylums were built, and they did so at a cost of one-half to one-eighth that of asylum care. When county authorities were ordered to transfer mentally ill residents from the workhouses to the newly built asylums, they often transferred only the most disturbed and disturbing individuals and kept the rest in the workhouses. In 1828, for example, there were an estimated 9,000 "lunatics and idiots" in England's workhouses. This number decreased in the 1840s and early 1850s as more county asylums opened but then increased again by 1861 to almost 9,000, and by 1870 "workhouses held over 12,000 pauper lunatics, about 25 percent of their total number." By this time, some county asylums, faced with marked overcrowding, were quietly transferring even some chronic and nonassaultive patients back to workhouses despite laws and official psychiatric rhetoric prohibiting such transfers.[45]

In many workhouses the mentally ill were so numerous that

they were housed separately. In 1865 it was estimated that "104 out of the 688 workhouses in England and Wales had separate lunatic wards," and one, St. Luke's Workhouse, "was really to be considered as a lunatic asylum, so numerous were the cases of insanity admitted to it." A physician, examining all mentally ill individuals in London's St. Pancras Workhouse in 1865, diagnosed them as follows: mania, 76; imbecility, 44; epilepsy, 44; alcoholism, 32; melancholia, 21; and idiocy, 5. He concluded that his findings "contradict the common supposition that workhouses rarely contain any but harmless imbecile patients." The availability of care in such workhouses varied from minimal to nonexistent; at one, "The inspector found that the nurse having care of the insane females was herself decidedly of unsound mind and was rewarded with half a pint of beer daily." Charles Dickens, having visited the insane ward of a large London workhouse, described it as "a kind of purgatory or place of transition."[46]

The Causes of Insanity

As the prevalence of treated insanity appeared to rise steadily in the nineteenth century, debate about its possible causes increased proportionately. Genetics figured prominently in such debates, although estimates of the magnitude of its importance varied widely. An analysis of presumed causes of insanity for all patients admitted to English asylums from 1878 to 1887 listed 21 percent as having had a presumed hereditary origin.[47]

Intemperance was usually the second most commonly cited cause of insanity, especially by officials advocating abstinence. Lord Shaftesbury was a prominent voice in this regard, arguing that more than half of all cases of insanity were caused by alcohol abuse. Lord Shaftesbury's views were regarded increasingly skeptically as the years passed, as a 1906 *Times* article suggests: "One solemn person tells us that insanity is largely due to 'drink,' ignoring the two obvious facts that insanity is on the increase and that drinking is not, as well as the consideration that the converse of the proportion is more likely to be true. It is more likely that a tendency towards insanity finding expression in defective self-control occasions alcoholic intemperance than that alcoholic intemperance occasions insanity."[48]

Religious enthusiasts often cited moral decay as the cause, thus equating insanity with immorality. For example, Hack Tuke, a devout Quaker, said that insanity arose from "that stratum of civilized society which is squalid and drunken and sensual." John Hawkes, a psychiatrist in the Wiltshire Asylum, blamed the younger generation's being "led spell-bound by passion, the powers and resources of youth are squandered in the bed of the voluptuary; sin sinking into the heart with all its accursed stains, polluting the fountains of reason at their source, and embittering the springs of life."[49]

Another reason for the increase cited by some people was the influx of Irish immigrants. There had always been some migration to England of Irish men and women looking for work, but during the great famine at midcentury this increased sharply, especially among those unable to afford the passage to North America. According to Kerby Miller's *Emigrants and Exiles,* "between 1845 and 1855 several hundred thousand of the most destitute Irish . . . inundated British ports and settled permanently in the working-class slums and cellars of Glasgow, Liverpool, London, and other cities." Many spoke only Irish and were regarded by the English as being as backward "as the aboriginal inhabitants of Australia."[50]

Increasing numbers of Irish immigrants were noted in the English public asylums beginning in the 1850s. At the Rainhill Asylum in Lancashire, the percentage of admissions who were Irish increased from 27 percent in 1854 to 43 percent in 1866. By 1870 the *Times* noted that 45 percent of all patients at Rainhill were Irish and complained of "the enormous expenditure the county was put to in maintaining vagrant lunatics thrown on the county."[51]

In addition to genetics, intemperance, moral decay, and Irish immigrants, almost every conceivable physical, social, and psychological factor was invoked to explain rising insanity. Railway travel, which was thought to injure the brain, was frequently cited, since the development of railroads coincided temporally with the rise of insanity. The steam engine, "uterine excitement," "tight lacing," severe bee stings, constipation, "sudden change from quiet to bustle," the study of astrology, "blowing the fife all night," and "attending socialist lectures" all had adherents as causes of insanity, as did a multitude of other factors. As the *Journal of Mental Science* reminded readers in 1873, "Do not kettledrums, nips, and late hours manifestly lead to abnormal cerebration?"[52]

Underlying the debate about causes of the rising insanity lay a recurrent question of the relationship of insanity to civilization. As English explorers returned from the farthest reaches of the globe in the last half of the nineteenth century, they often reported that insanity appeared to be rare in the least civilized areas. Partially in response to such reports, the belief became widespread that insanity was an inevitable consequence of civilization. As Henry Maudsley explained in 1867: "Theoretical considerations would lead to the expectation of an increased liability to mental disorder with an increase in the complexity of the mental organization. . . . In the complex mental organization . . . which a state of civilization implies, there is plainly the favourable occasion of many derangements. . . . An increase of insanity is a penalty which an increase of our present civilization necessarily pays."[53] At other times, however, Maudsley denied that any such increase was taking place.

Amid the annual reports of the Lunacy Commission and speculation on causes of insanity in the latter half of the nineteenth century, several questions emerged that potentially offered clues to the causation of insanity. Was insanity more common among men or women? Poor people or rich people? Urban dwellers or rural folks? Northern counties or southern counties? Such questions elicited strong opinions and even occasional facts.

The question of relative liability to insanity among poor and rich had been tentatively answered in favor of the rich in the first half of the century. George Burrows had said that "hereditary insanity is most common among the highest rank of society." William A. F. Browne, one of the most influential physicians of his generation, also cited the "insane rich" as more numerous, and Andrew Scull concurred that "in the early 1840s, the best professional opinion suggested that it was the educated, the wealthy, the most cultured segments of the community . . . who had the most to fear from the spectre of madness." This was despite the fact that wealthy families often avoided using public asylums so that nobody would know their family was afflicted, and "the families of some lunatics would even send the patients abroad" to avoid disclosure.[54]

Regarding the relative liability of urban and rural dwellers to insanity, opinions in the early part of the century were mixed. In 1829 Andrew Halliday stated that insanity was more common in agricultural areas. In 1835, however, William Farr came to exactly the opposite conclusion after examining the available statistics on insanity. Two years later, William A. F. Browne also concluded that "the agricultural population . . . is to a great degree exempt from insanity." An analysis of asylum admissions in Lancashire in 1848–1850 and opinions by Maddox in 1854 and Bucknill and Tuke in 1858 all concurred with Browne, and by the latter years of the nineteenth century it was widely believed that urbanization was associated with insanity.[55]

A comparison of the growth of English cities with the rise of insanity supports this association. In 1801 there was only one city (London) with a population of more than 100,000; by 1841 there were six, and by 1901 there were thirty. Similarly, the percentage of the English population living in urban areas of more than 20,000 individuals increased from 17 percent in 1801 to 54 percent in 1891. How much of the association of urbanization with insanity was due to affected individuals moving from rural areas to the cities, as Thomas Clouston argued in 1872,[56] and how much was due to other factors such as poverty, overcrowding, and infectious diseases, all of which were proposed as explanations in the nineteenth century, is not known.

A variant of the urban-rural question is whether some geographic regions of England were more liable to insanity. This question was of increasing interest to the Lunacy Commissioners at the end of the nineteenth century, and on multiple occasions from 1871 onward they published in their annual reports insanity rates by county. The 1871 results were remarkably similar to the geographical distribution that had been reported in 1843. The counties with the highest rates of insanity were Herefordshire (3.39 per 1,000), Wiltshire (3.27), Berkshire (3.17), Oxfordshire (3.10), and Gloucestershire (3.05), all of which were in the Midlands or southern England. The counties with the lowest rates, by contrast, were Durham (1.29), Yorkshire (1.51), Cornwall (1.58), Cheshire (1.83), Derbyshire (1.84), and Lancashire (1.93), all of which, except Cornwall, were in the north.

This distribution of insanity in England remained constant through 1911, the last year for which similar county data were published. Figure 5.2 shows the insanity rates by county averaged for four of the years for which data were published: 1871, 1889, 1901, and 1911.[57] The insanity rates for the highest counties (Herefordshire, 4.7; Wiltshire, 3.8; and Oxfordshire 3.6) were approximately twice as high

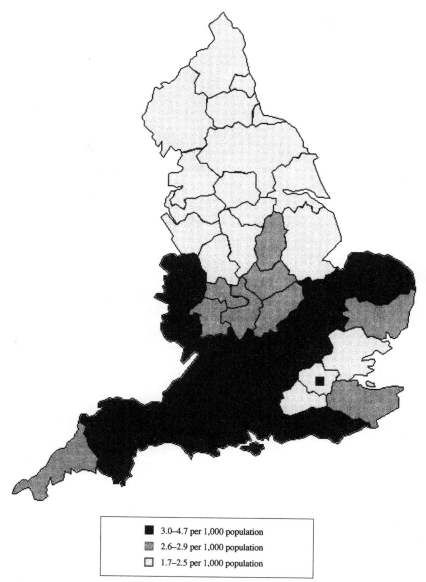

■	3.0–4.7 per 1,000 population
▨	2.6–2.9 per 1,000 population
□	1.7–2.5 per 1,000 population

FIG. 5.2. England: Insane Persons in Asylums, Workhouses, and under Care in the Community by County. Averages for Censuses of 1871, 1901, and 1911.

as the rates for the lowest counties (Durham, 1.7; Derbyshire, 1.9; and Yorkshire, 2.0) for that period.

The explanation for these regional differences was, and still is, not apparent. Since the rates were dependent on data furnished by local authorities, there may have been reporting differences, but if so, these differences were both regional and consistent from 1843 to 1911. The Lunacy Commissioners themselves considered as a possible explanation the density of population, which they measured as persons per acre. When they examined the data, however, they concluded that "there is no apparent relationship between the density of population and the ratio of insane." Thomas Clouston similarly looked for correlations between the insanity rates and recent increases in population but found it only "in some slight degree." However, when Clouston compared the insanity rates to "pauperism," as measured by the regional wages of laborers, he reported that a "parallelism shows itself in a remarkable manner": "In all the Northern Counties the rate of wages is good, and in them all, whether agricultural or manufacturing, the rate of lunacy is low . . . while the Southern and Midland Counties of Dorset, Somerset, Wilts, Gloucester, Worcester, Oxford, Hereford, and Berks, where the wages are very low, produce far above the average amount of lunacy."

Whatever the cause, Clouston concluded that "it is an astonishing fact medically that any non-infectious disease should be nearly three times as common in Berkshire as in Durham; while it is equally remarkable and interesting socially and economically."[58]

CHAPTER 6

"A Great and Progressive Evil"
England, 1890–1990

Who can think of 68,145 insane men and women—the number in the United Kingdom at the end of 1872—and endeavour in the remotest degree to realize the broken hearts, the blasted hopes, the blighted ambitions, the unfinished work, the dead affections of this great army of stricken ones, and their belongings, without feeling very sad at heart?

—ANONYMOUS, *Journal of Mental Science*, 1873

All their Predictions run upon a most dreadful Plague, which should lay the whole City, and even the Kingdom waste; and should destroy almost all the Nation, both Man and Beast.

—DANIEL DEFOE, *A Journal of the Plague Year*, 1722

By the closing years of the nineteenth century, England had become *the* dominant world power. It had assumed, in Kipling's phrase, "the white man's burden," and had overrun, annexed, or purchased one-quarter of the earth's land surface. England controlled territory from the Transvaal to Cyprus and Uganda to Fiji, had purchased the Suez Canal, and had proclaimed Queen Victoria Empress of India. By 1892, "Britain had more registered shipping tonnage than the rest of the world put together." At home, "the horsepower used in British industry increased from two million in 1870 to ten million in

1907." Benjamin Disraeli described England as having undergone a "convulsion of prosperity."[1]

Amid this economic and political splendor, reports of increasing insanity continued to appear like unbidden guests at a banquet. James Crichton-Browne, superintendent of the Yorkshire West Riding Asylum, wrote: "It is impossible for us to acquiesce in the soothing doctrine now being disseminated that the alleged increase of lunacy is only a popular fallacy"; rather, he said, it was clear that "an actual as well as an apparent augmentation in the numbers of our insane poor is rapidly in progress." In a similar vein, Martin Duncan, president of the Medico-Psychological Association, said that it was time "to admit that for once popular fallacy is supported by recent statistics. . . . There is a steady increase in the lunacy of the population of England, Wales, and Ireland. . . . Insanity remains as a dead-weight on the statistics of our social miseries." John Arlidge noted that "the increase of lunacy . . . [is] a painful and perplexing fact" and that available data "indisputably [point] to an absolutely increased production in the community." Harrington Tuke, not related to Hack Tuke, also claimed that "these figures would appear to prove that a great wave of insanity is slowly advancing, but making each year a definite progress." And Robert Jamieson of the Royal Aberdeen Hospital claimed that "the most remarkable phenomenon of our time has been the alarming increase of insanity."[2]

For the average man or woman in England, it was difficult to ignore evidence that insanity was increasing. The fiction of Charles Dickens, Walter Scott, Charlotte Brontë, Wilkie Collins, Mary Elizabeth Braddon, and Charles Reade continued to be widely read. Rumors circulated about the mental state of John Ruskin, the popular essayist and art critic who suffered from recurrent bouts of insanity from 1878 until his death in 1900 and who attributed his own hallucinations to a "state of morbid inflammation of brain." The case of wealthy Mrs. Georgiana Weldon, who "believed the spirit of her deceased mother to have entered her pet rabbit" and who sued her husband for trying to have her involuntarily hospitalized, was much in evidence in 1884; "for months, the legal columns of the *Times* were filled with accounts of Mrs. Weldon's protests and eccentricities."[3]

During these latter years of the nineteenth century, insane persons became more visible and more threatening. Newspapers articles described their presence, such as one entitled "Wandering Lunatics," about a man seen wandering on the streets: "[His] feet, arms, neck and great portions of the shoulders were bare and exposed to the piercing wind, and they had a horrible, dusky-red, mottled aspect. . . . He was moving about in a restless, indeterminate fashion, paying no heed to the lookers on, and not soliciting any charity. His lips were moving rapidly, as if he were muttering to himself. . . . It is surely a grave public scandal that such spectacles should be witnessed in the teeming thoroughfares of the metropolis." Insane persons trying to gain access to Buckingham Palace were reported with increasing frequency, such as Henry Young, age twenty-three, who "behaved in the most violent manner" when apprehended but who, "up to the time when the first symptoms of insanity were noticed, . . . had shown himself to be a steady and efficient workman."[4]

The association of insanity and violent behavior became increasingly firm at the end of the nineteenth century. Newspaper and journal articles, such as "An Insane Mother Kills Her Five Children," reported homicides caused by insane individuals. According to the *Fortnightly Review* in 1896: "Not a day passes without accounts of murder and suicide appearing in the press. . . . In many cases two, three, or more sane persons fall victims to the homicidal mania before the lunatic takes his or her own life." And despite the fact that Jack the Ripper was never actually identified, a 1902 newspaper account reported the following: "The question of the premature discharge of lunatics is a very serious one. . . . To . . . premature discharge are due many of the daily tragedies which startle the newspaper reader . . . sometimes a massacre. The homicidal maniac who shocked the world as Jack the Ripper had been once . . . in a lunatic asylum."[5]

This increasing association of insanity and violent behavior was also reflected in popular literature at the end of the century. Robert Louis Stevenson drew upon it when, in 1886, he published *The Strange Case of Dr. Jekyll and Mr. Hyde*. When the benevolent Dr. Henry Jekyll drinks his potion, he changes into a vicious Mr. Hyde who calmly tramples over a little girl and then murders an elderly gentleman by "stamping with his foot, brandishing the cane, and carrying on (as the maid described it) like a madman. . . . With ape-like fury he was trampling his victim under foot and hailing down a storm of blows, under which the bones were audibly shattered and the body jumped upon the roadway." Later, Dr. Jekyll's former schoolmate and colleague, Dr. Lanyon, is drawn into the proceedings when he receives a letter from Jekyll begging for his assistance. Lanyon is concerned about his old friend's sanity but also feels the need to protect himself: "Upon the reading of this letter, I made sure my colleague was insane; but till that was proved beyond the possibility of doubt, I felt bound to do as he requested. The less I understood of this farrago, the less I was in a position to judge of its importance; and an appeal so worded could not be set aside without a grave responsibility. . . . The more I reflected the more convinced I grew that I was dealing with a case of cerebral disease; and though I dismissed my servants to bed, I loaded an old revolver, that I might be found in some posture of self-defence."[6]

The association of insanity and violence also underlies Bram Stoker's *Dracula*, published in 1897. Adjacent to Count Dracula's English estate is "a private lunatic asylum" run by Dr. John Seward. Stoker included in his novel long descriptions of Dr. Seward's favorite patient, Renfield, who catches flies to feed to spiders, then feeds the spiders to sparrows, then asks for a cat so that he can feed the sparrows to the cat. Dr. Seward says that his patient is a "homicidal maniac" and adds:

> I shall have to invent a new classification for him, and call him a zoophagous (life-eating) maniac; what he desires is to absorb as many lives as he can, and he has laid himself out to achieve it in a cumulative way. He gave many flies to one spider and many spiders to one bird, and then wanted a cat to eat the many birds. What would have been his later steps? It would almost be worth while to complete the experiment. It might be done if there were only a sufficient cause. Men sneered at vivisection, and yet look at its results to-day! Why not advance science in its most difficult and vital aspect—the knowledge of the brain? Had I even the secret of one such mind—did I hold the key to the fancy of even one lunatic—I might advance my own branch of science to a pitch compared with which Burdon-Sanderson's physiology or Ferrier's brain-knowledge would be as nothing. If only there were a sufficient cause! I must not think too much of this, or I may be tempted; a good cause might

turn the scale with me, for may not I too be of an exceptional brain, congenitally?

Later, Renfield escapes to Count Dracula's estate, where he is seen to change into "a big bat, which was flapping its silent and ghostly way to the west." Count Dracula had inhabited the insane man's body and transformed him into a vampire.[7]

The 1897 *Special Report on the Alleged Increase of Insanity*

The status of insanity specialists in England had never been very high. Indeed, in 1829 an anonymous author in the *Monthly Review* had claimed that "the practitioner who devotes himself to the investigation and treatment of mania is considered by his brethren, in most cases, as following pursuits of doubtful respectability, and as degrading himself into the lowest ranks of the profession."[8]

By the 1890s England's psychiatric establishment had grown tired of being criticized. Lord Shaftesbury, the government's spokesperson for the psychiatric status quo, had died in 1884, after having spent his lifetime trying to prepare England for the Second Coming. A year before Lord Shaftesbury died, he had assured the House of Lords once again that insanity was decreasing "owing to the efforts of Temperance Societies" and that the improvements in psychiatric care had been "well nigh incredible." Since 1859, when Lord Shaftesbury had previously reassured Parliament that insanity was not increasing, the number of insane persons in England's censuses had increased from 36,762 to 76,765, and the rate per 1,000 total population had increased from 1.87 to 2.88. Shortly before his death, Lord Shaftesbury told a friend, "I cannot bear to leave the world with all the misery in it."[9]

The asylum superintendents were particularly unhappy that neither the press nor the public appeared to believe their reassurances that insanity was not increasing. The *Journal of Mental Science*, the official voice of the psychiatrists, carried a steady stream of plaintive remarks:

> The public press, and through it the public, leap to the conclusion that such tables take cognizance of every case of

mental affection occurring or existing in the kingdom, and alarming inferences are drawn in highly-coloured verbiage expressive of the great increase in insanity year by year. (1893)

Directly with the publication of this Report there has arisen the usual outcry in lay and even some medical papers as to the alarming increase of insanity in our midst, and our reiteration of the same series of arguments year by year, disposing of this erroneous idea, becomes somewhat wearisome. (1895)

It is somewhat refreshing for once to proceed to an examination of the annual Report of the Commissioners in Lunacy without having to encounter, at the hands of the lay and medical press, the usual yearly erroneous deductions from the statistical tables therein contained, to the effect that insanity, in its more active phases, is making rapid strides among the populace [and to have] sensation-mongers spread abroad their alarming and imaginative assumptions as to the fearful increase of insanity in our midst. (1896)

That *quoestio vexata,* the increase of insanity in our midst, has temporarily been shelved . . . and the stirring times in which we have lately been living must make us thankful for the absence this year in the lay press of those annual irritating diatribes on lunacy and its increase. It is only when other sensational matter runs short that the daily press expounds its immature and chaotic views on a subject of which its knowledge is infinitesimal. (1899)

The magnitude of the press's and the public's ignorance was illustrated, according to the *Journal,* by the fact that "an indiscreet statistician has quite recently in a popular publication computed the startling result that in A.D. 2301 we shall all be mad!"[10]

The strategy adopted by England's psychiatrists to ameliorate public alarm about possible rising insanity was to hold a "special enquiry into the alleged increase of insanity in England and Wales" under the Commissioners in Lunacy. Because the commissioners had had primary responsibility for the problem of insanity since 1845 and had also stated many times that insanity was not increasing, the outcome of the inquiry was a foregone conclusion.

The resulting *Special Report on the Alleged Increase of Insanity* was published in 1897. Large portions appear to have been adapted from an 1890 study by Noel Humphreys, a statistician, who had concluded: "Without therefore venturing to say that there has been no increase of insanity in England in recent years, many reasons have been pointed out for refusing to accept any insanity statistics that we at present possess as conclusive evidence of a real increase of the rate of occurring insanity." Humphreys's cautious conclusions were eagerly enlarged upon by England's psychiatrists. George Savage said they put to rest "one of the bugbears of the age, the idea that insanity was running like wildfire through the whole population." Hack Tuke also "rejoiced to find the conclusions at which Mr. Humphreys had arrived were so much in accordance with what might be regarded as an encouraging and satisfactory mode of viewing the great question of the alleged increase of insanity in England and Wales."[11]

The 1897 *Special Report* included data on the increase in asylum patients between 1859 and 1896. Especially damning was a table showing that first admissions had increased from 4.71 per 10,000 total population in 1869 to 5.16 in 1879, 5.29 in 1889, and 6.09 in 1895. The report acknowledged that "the upward progress . . . of first attacks out of proportion to population seems *prima facie* to indicate the increase of insanity which has been alleged, and we must now inquire if there are any circumstances which modify its apparently significant influence."[12]

The report then proceeded to propose three major reasons why the apparent increase in insanity was not real. The first claimed that there had been a large pool of unidentified insane persons residing in workhouses and with relatives, and as this finite pool had been identified and hospitalized, it had given the appearance of increasing insanity. As supporting evidence, the *Special Report* cited the general census returns for 1871, 1881, and 1891, which included insane persons living at home and in which between 11 and 18 percent more insane persons had been enumerated than had been known to the Lunacy Commissioners at the time.

This theoretically finite backlog of unidentified insane persons had been invoked by English physicians since the earliest years of the nineteenth century as the principal reason for the rising rate of insanity. It is important to point out that by 1897 most insane persons residing in workhouses were well known to the commissioners; many, in fact, had been transferred back to the workhouses from the overcrowded county asylums. There were, at the time, approximately 12,000 identified insane persons in the workhouses, the same number as had existed there in 1870. The theoretically finite backlog of unidentified insane persons living in the community never seemed to become smaller, no matter how many new asylums were opened to accommodate them. On several occasions the leaders of English psychiatry issued light-at-the-end-of-the-tunnel statements, such as this one by C. Lockhart Robertson in 1867: "Thus, I think I am justified in saying that we see the limits of our labours in providing for the care and treatment of the insane poor; and, further, that we have nearly gained the desired end. It is allowing a wide margin in our calculations for the future if we place the possible total number of pauper lunatics and idiots at 1 in 400 of the population."[13] By 1891 the total number of pauper insane persons and idiots had climbed to 1 in 298 of the population, and the unidentified pool appeared to be as large as ever. This was even acknowledged in the *Special Report*, which enumerated the unidentified pool as follows:

	1859	1896
Insane in workhouses	7,963	10,906
Insane residing with relatives	5,798	5,924

Thus, the theoretically finite pool of unidentified insane persons increasingly appeared to be infinite, since each time a person was moved to an asylum, another took his or her place in the pool. Since the argument had been made continuously for almost a hundred years, it raised the probability that the unidentified pool was not merely a backlog of cases but rather represented the production of new cases.

The second major reason cited by the 1897 *Special Report* for the apparently increasing number of insane persons was decreasing recovery and mortality rates for asylum inmates. Insofar as admissions exceeded discharges through recovery or death, the asylums inevitably became more crowded as the number of inmates increased.

There *is* evidence that recovery rates for hospitalized insane persons decreased in the second half of the nineteenth century, including studies of the asylums at Lancashire, Buckinghamshire, Colney Hatch, and Hook Norton. Such findings were cited in 1890 as evidence that "the form of insanity was worse" than it had been earlier in the century. These findings are consistent with Robert Wilkins's findings of an increasing number of young patients admitted to Bethlem with symptoms of auditory and visual hallucinations between 1830 and 1899. It is also consistent with Hack Tuke's 1892 observation that "a large number of cases of pubescent and adolescent insanity terminate more unfavorably than the mental physician, guided in his prognosis by the general truth, has been led to expect."[14]

In addition to the decreasing recovery rate, a decreasing death rate of inmates in asylums was also cited by the 1897 *Special Report* as a reason why insanity appeared to be increasing. Comparative figures did show a modest decrease in the asylum death rate, from 10.1 deaths per year per 100 patients for 1873–1877 to 9.5 per 100 for 1893–1897, and such figures were emphasized in the report. In fact, however, the asylum death rates varied widely by year and by asylum.[15] Infectious diseases such as typhus, cholera, pneumonia, tuberculosis, and syphilis were the most common causes of death in the asylums, followed by cardiovascular diseases.

What was not discussed in the 1897 *Special Report* was the possibility that institutionalizing insane persons in asylums may have effectively *decreased* their total number. As early as 1835 William Farr calculated that death rates in asylums were three to six times that of the general population at comparable age levels, and these figures were confirmed in 1879. For patients ages twenty to twenty-four, the Lunacy Commission reported in 1906 that "the insane death-rate is nearly twenty times that of the general death-rate." There are, unfortunately, no comparable statistics on mortality rates of insane persons living outside versus inside asylums. However, given the epidemics of infectious diseases that frequently devastated the overcrowded asylums (e.g., cholera in 1832–1833 killed up to 49 percent of the asylum inmates),[16] one can argue that increasing institutionalization of insane persons in the nineteenth century may have ultimately decreased their total number by killing larger numbers than would have died had they been living in the community.

The third major reason cited by the 1897 *Special Report* to explain the increasing rate of insanity was that insanity was becoming increasingly more broadly defined, with individuals being sent to asylums in the later years of the century who would not have been sent in earlier years. This possibility had been proposed by John Arlidge as early as 1859 and in the twentieth century was to become a favorite argument of Michel Foucault, Andrew Scull, and others who would claim that insanity had increased because the asylums became "a convenient place to get rid of inconvenient people."[17] This argument will be discussed in chapter 14.

Refutations of this argument were common even at the time it was first raised. In 1898, for example, the superintendent of the Staffordshire Asylum said that his admission statistics "do not lend support to the idea which one hears expressed from time to time that many people are sent to asylums who have no business there. Such is certainly not our experience; on the contrary, we find that patients are frequently not brought here until it is impossible to keep them outside." Even some members of the psychiatric establishment doubted the conclusions of their colleagues, as one psychiatrist suggested in his 1904 lecture to the Medico-Psychological Association: "Insanity is a great and progressive evil. Its progress of late has been almost phenomenal, and the expense it entails upon the public almost insupportable."[18]

Nor did the annual reports of the Lunacy Commissioners provide any support. The diagnostic breakdown for all admissions from 1895 through 1899, for example, was as follows: mania, 48 percent; melancholia, 29 percent; dementia, 16 percent; congenital insanity, 5 percent; other, 2 percent.[19]

In addition to these broad categories, insane patients who had seizures were labeled epileptic, and this group constituted a steady 11 to 12 percent of the total inmate population between 1844 and the end of the century. An additional 7 to 8 percent were said to have general paralysis of the insane, a form of brain syphilis that also remained steady from approximately 1870 until 1900. A third subset was diagnosed as having alcoholic insanity, but the magnitude of this group varied widely, depending on the belief system of the persons making the diagnoses. Finally, a subset of the patients diagnosed with dementia was said to have been "congenital idiots," later relabeled as "severe mental retardation." This group never comprised more than a small percentage of the total asylum inmates because, as C. Lockhart Robertson noted in 1867, "idiots are maintained partly at home, partly in the workhouse," and only the most "troublesome are sent to the county asylum."[20] Many asylums, in fact, refused to admit "congenital idiots" at all.

The diagnostic categories utilized in the nineteenth century, therefore, do not support the belief that the asylums were increasingly being filled with merely troublesome persons. Further evidence is provided by studies that have retrospectively rediagnosed patient case records from the late nineteenth century using modern diagnostic criteria. For example, a comparison of all admissions to Lancashire's Rainhill Asylum in 1890 and 1990, using the International Classification of Diseases (I.C.D. 9), reported the diagnostic breakdown in table 6.1. Such results lend no support to the belief that patients admitted in

TABLE 6.1 Diagnostic Breakdown of Patients at Rainhill Asylum, 1890 and 1990

	1890 Admissions	1990 Admissions
Psychoses (schizophrenia, manic-depressive illness, psychotic depression, hypomania, manic episode)	33%	40%
Depression	18%	24%
Drug-induced psychosis	0%	2%
Alcohol-related illness	8%	16%
Dementia (Alzheimer's and other)	6%	1%
Epilepsy	6%	0%
General paralysis of the insane	11%	0%
Mental subnormality	11%	0%
Acute confusional state	3%	2%
Anxiety-related illness	0%	5%
Personality disorder	0%	6%
No mental illness	4%	3%

1890 were mild cases. These findings are also consistent with retrospective diagnostic studies of patients from nineteenth-century private asylums, including Trevor Turner's study of Ticehurst Asylum, Edward Renvoize and Allan Beveridge's study of the York Retreat, Franklin Klaf and John Hamilton's study of Bethlem Hospital, and William Parry-Jones's study of Duddeston Hall and Brislington House.[21]

In conclusion, then, the 1897 *Special Report on the Alleged Increase of Insanity* provided little support for alternative explanations for the observed increasing insanity rates. The community backlog of cases of insanity never seemed to grow smaller; the declining asylum death rates would explain, at most, only a small percentage of the increasing insanity; and evidence is contrary to the thesis that insanity's definition had been broadened. The only alternative explanation for which there was evidence—that insanity was clinically becoming more severe in the nineteenth century—was hardly one that would have reassured the press or the public regarding their fears of rising insanity. The commissioners concluded their report by stating that "we have been unable to satisfy ourselves that there has been any important increase of occurring or fresh insanity." Given their own data, such a conclusion was wishful thinking.

Five months following the publication of the 1897 *Special Report,* the Commissioners in Lunacy issued their annual report for 1897, showing a total of 99,365 insane persons, an increase of 2,919 since the previous year, the increase being "the largest on record." The following year, the total increased by an additional 2,607 patients to 101,972, which the commissioners labeled "this huge mass of insane humanity."[22] The figures appeared to be an additional refutation of their 1897 report.

Nor was the English press convinced by the 1897 *Special Report.* The *Westminster Review* labeled it "ridiculous efforts to gloss over and explain away undeniable facts. . . . That there is an actual increase is indubitable, notwithstanding the dogmatic but puerile asseverations of the Commissioners in Lunacy to the contrary. . . . Were the Commissioners in Lunacy cross-examined on their own figures and the inferences they have drawn, a lamentable appearance might be predicted."[23]

The most damning criticism of the English Lunacy Commissioners, however, came from W. J. Corbet, the chief clerk of the Irish

Lunacy Department and a former member of Parliament from Ireland. He said the authors of the *Special Report* had "devoted all their energies to combating the idea that insanity is on the increase. . . . A more remarkable composition has rarely, if ever, emanated from official brain or pen." Not a man to hide his opinions, Corbet had previously accused the commissioners of "fossillized officialism" as well as "Lilliputian logic" and had compared them to "simple parents fondling their deformed offspring . . . hugging the fallacy they have themselves created, until, by constant repetition, they at length evidently believe in the soundness of their conclusions, though the figures given in their own reports are convincing to the contrary."[24]

A Temporary Solution

Following the publication of the 1897 *Special Report*, public discussion of increasing insanity in England continued for another decade, as the number of institutionalized insane increased from 101,972 (3.24 per 1,000) in 1898 to 126,084 (3.60 per 1,000) in 1908. Newspapers continued to express concern about "the grave increase of lunacy. . . . Assuming a similar increase in the future, what is the outlook for, say, 50 years hence?" And the psychiatric establishment continued to offer a multitude of reasons to explain why the increase was not real but merely apparent, as in this 1903 report: "The question that at once presents itself is whether this growing ratio means that insanity on the whole is increasing. There are several other explanations which would require to be borne in mind before admitting such an unpleasant one."[25]

From time to time, psychiatric disasters occurred, reminding the public of problems that were accompanying the rise of the patient population. For example, in 1900 one of the Lunacy Commissioners, Mr. G. H. Urmson, "was attacked and severely wounded by a male patient at the London County Asylum at Bexley with a broken knife which he [had] managed to obtain and conceal." And in 1903, fifty-one female patients burned to death when their makeshift quarters at the overcrowded Colney Hatch Asylum caught fire; newspapers recounted "the harrowing details" of "the patients locked in their dormitories shrieking with terror" and "the finding of the charred remains of the hapless victims."[26]

One final spasm of public interest in the question of increasing insanity occurred in 1906 and 1907, stimulated by a series of articles and letters in the *Times*. An anonymous "correspondent" published four long articles discussing the rise of insane persons per population, from 1 in 761 in 1844 to 1 in 272 in 1905, and prophetically predicted that, at that rate of increase, "nearly 1 per cent of the inhabitants of England and Wales" would be consigned to asylums" by 1965. The correspondent then proceeded to ridicule "the many estimable people who like to amuse themselves with hypotheses, while they close their minds firmly against unpleasant facts," and also urged "the recognition of insanity for what it is, a disease of the body differing from measles or from rheumatism chiefly in affecting a different portion of the organism."[27]

Letters of support and rebuttal continued intermittently for a full year in the *Times,* labeled by one writer as "a correspondence that like a wounded snake drags its slow length along." Thomas Clouston denied categorically that there had been any real increase in insanity and cited as one reason the fact that the Commissioners in Lunacy had said so. Other writers said the apparent increase was due to the falling death rate of asylum inmates. On the other side, Forbes Winslow stated categorically that "the increase of insanity is real and not apparent," and Clifford Allbutt, while labeling insane asylums "barracks for cerebral diseases," said that "in England and in England alone we muddle with complacency."[28]

After 1907, public interest in insanity as a national problem appeared to be waning, despite the fact that the numbers of insane persons continued to increase in the official statistics. One reason may have been a shift in public interest from the internal social issues of the Victorian era to the external international issues of the Edwardian era. Following Queen Victoria's death in 1901, her eldest son, Albert Edward, ascended the throne and ruled for nine years as King Edward VII. Edward traveled widely and focused his primary attention on relations with other European nations. In contrast to the socially responsible behavior exemplified by his mother, Edward indulged himself with horse racing and mistresses.

Another probable reason for a decreasing interest in insanity was an increasingly broad consensus that insanity was primarily genetic in origin and therefore could be controlled only by eugenic measures. Such thinking had surfaced as early as 1870 in the writings of Henry

Maudsley, who quoted Charles Darwin and later attended the lectures of Francis Galton. Maudsley compared the brains of insane and mentally deficient individuals to those of apes and chimpanzees. By 1905 psychiatrists were increasingly asking: "What can be done to grapple with the evil [of insanity] and to safeguard the sane from the contamination of the taint of insanity by inheritance." In 1906 Robert Jones, a president of the Medico-Psychological Association, argued that "in eugenics are to be found the chief remedies for the amelioration of social pathology," and the following year Thomas Clouston "called for the prevention of the marriages of those deemed 'unfit.'"[29]

In the years leading up to the First World War, the psychiatric establishment in England focused its attention more and more on eugenics as the ultimate solution to insanity. T.E.K. Stansfield pointed to the "mass of degeneracy in the lower ranks of the population which is increasing out of all proportion to the remainder of the population" and asked: "How are we as a nation to overcome the evil and stem the flow of this rising tide?" E. Faulks recommended "the compulsory sterilisation of all insane and imbecile subjects about to be discharged from our asylums." And in 1912 Geoffrey Clarke, in a paper entitled "Sterilization from the Eugenic Standpoint," said that "there is no doubt about the increase of insanity" and "it is practically universally admitted that . . . heredity is the most potent cause of insanity." Therefore, he asked: "Is it not our duty to do something for the improvement of the human race by preventing the insane, the feeble-minded and the mentally unstable from breeding?"[30]

Even as English psychiatrists were turning to eugenics to solve the problem of increasing insanity, political events were taking place in Europe that would soon focus England's attention on other problems. In Hamburg the Kaiser asserted Germany's "place in the sun" and renewed his nation's alliance with Austria and Italy. The Balkan wars had repercussions across Europe. Then on June 28, 1914, Archduke Franz Ferdinand, heir to the Austrian throne, was assassinated in Sarajevo, and within weeks Europe was at war.

The Effects of War and Influenza

World War I substantially altered the perception of insanity in England, reducing it from a growing threat to merely an ongoing inconvenience. Insanity was no longer viewed as an increasing affliction of the body politic, evoking letters in the *Times,* but instead as a chronic blemish on the human condition for which little could be done. The pervasive nineteenth-century fear that insanity was increasing was largely forgotten.

In 1914, when the war began, there were 138,055 insane persons in England's asylums. By January 1915, the number had climbed to 140,466, or a rate of 3.98 per 1,000 total population. One out of every 250 people of all ages was confined to an insane asylum, and among young adults, the rate was much higher.

World War I had a direct effect on the asylums, because hospitals were needed to treat large numbers of war casualties. Therefore, the government "took over a number of county asylums, and other asylums had to accept and house their displaced patients for the duration of the war." Insane patients who were less severely disabled were sent home, many new admissions were refused, and in the remaining asylums "extra beds were squeezed into the dormitories, the corridors [were] filled with beds, [and] other rooms were converted into bedrooms."[31] In addition, almost half of the medical and nursing staff went off to fight, and food rations for the mental hospitals were reduced.

Then, at the height of this crowding, understaffing, and reduced food rations, the influenza pandemic arrived. The death rate among patients soared, as can be seen from the deaths in the Buckinghamshire Asylum: 1910–1914; 67 average for each year; 1915, 81; 1916, 110; 1917, 129; 1918, 257.[32] In 1918, almost one-third of all the patients died in this asylum. Nationally, the total number of 1918 asylum deaths was 19,515, double the prewar rate. By 1920, then, the census of England's mental hospitals had been reduced 17 percent to 116,764. After a century of looking for a solution to the increasing insanity, one had finally emerged—war and influenza.

The number of mentally ill in England's asylums did not regain the 1915 level until 1929; the 1915 rate—3.98 per 1,000 population—was never again achieved. The asylum patient population peaked in 1939 at 158,723, fell during World War II as asylums were again taken over to serve military casualties, then climbed again to 155,000 in 1955, before beginning a progressive and continuing fall as patients were discharged with newly introduced antipsychotic medication and under the policy of deinstitutionalization.

The lack of interest in insanity in England after World War I was reflected in its literature as well. As noted by William Ober, "Nervous disorders such as neurasthenia and Freudian theories of hysteria and neurosis supplanted the Victorian notions of mania and moral insanity; the psychoanalyst replaced the alienist."[33] Whereas in the first half of the nineteenth century insanity had been a major theme among English writers, in the first half of the twentieth century its use was confined almost exclusively to writers who were themselves insane. Virginia Woolf is perhaps the best example of this.

Woolf had her first encounter with insanity at age thirteen, when for six months she experienced auditory and visual hallucinations and "was wildly excited at one time and depressed at another." She had a second breakdown at age twenty-two, at which time she made a suicide attempt; thereafter, she had intermittent but increasingly severe episodes of manic-depressive illness. In addition to periods of severe mania and depression, she also experienced paranoid delusions and hallucinations. Several of her relatives also had periods of depression, and a nephew died in an asylum, "floridly psychotic manic-depressive."[34]

As she wrote in one of her letters, insanity "was a subject that I . . . kept cooling in my mind until I felt that I could touch it without bursting into flame all over." She depicted it in *The Voyage Out* (1915), in *The Waves* (1931), and, most fully, in *Mrs. Dalloway* (1925). The novel describes a day in the life of Clarissa Dalloway, an English society matron who exhibits symptoms of mania. Septimus Warren Smith, another character, has delusions that flowers are growing through his flesh, auditory and visual hallucinations, and believes he is the founder of a new religion: "But they beckoned; leaves were alive; trees were alive. And the leaves being connected by millions of fibres with his own body, there on the seat, fanned up and down; when the branch stretched he, too, made that statement. The sparrows fluttering, rising, and falling in jagged fountains were part of the pattern; the white and blue, barred with black branches. Sounds made harmonies with premeditation; the spaces between them were as significant as the sounds. A child cried. Rightly far away a horn sounded. All taken together meant the birth of a new religion."[35]

Finally, at age fifty-nine, hearing voices and fearing that she was "going mad again," Virginia Woolf left her house, "crossed the water meadows to the river, . . . put a large stone in the pocket of her coat,"[36] and drowned herself.

After World War II

During World War II, several English psychiatric hospitals were taken over for military purposes. In the remaining hospitals, there were "acute shortages of clothing, food and heating—plus an unprecedented degree of overcrowding and understaffing."[37] When the National Health Service was implemented in 1948, half of all hospital beds in England were occupied by individuals who were mentally ill or mentally retarded. The Mental Health Act of 1959 officially encouraged community care in place of asylum care, and the process of deinstitutionalization was launched. From the 152,197 patients in asylums in 1954, the number progressively fell to less than 47,000 in 1995, or a reduction of almost 70 percent. Although this reduction is substantial, it is not as great as the 90 percent reduction in asylum beds in the United States during the same years.

Since World War II there has been no national census of mentally ill persons in England to ascertain whether insanity is increasing, decreasing, or remaining the same. However, there have been several local studies providing insanity rates that can be compared with past studies. Such comparisons are of course fraught with methodological problems, but they are nonetheless instructive insofar as they provide approximate estimates of insanity present and past.

The town of Salford is one example. Located in Lancashire, Salford has been a center for manufacturing since the middle of the nineteenth century. In 1866, an official census of "insane" persons reported 198 among Salford's population of 105,335, or 1.9 per 1,000 total population.

In 1968, a computerized case register of all treated psychiatric disorders was established in Salford and was used as the basis for subsequent prevalence surveys. In 1974, a total of 517 individuals were identified with a diagnosis of schizophrenia, paranoid psychoses, manic or mixed affective psychosis, or depressive psychosis; all borderline and questionable cases were omitted.[38] The rate (point prevalence) of insanity among the Salford population of 121,190 was 4.3 per 1,000.

In 1986, another survey using the case register reported a total of 538 individuals with insanity (418 schizophrenia, 4 schizoaffective psychosis, 52 paranoid state, 32 mania/hypomania, 20 mania with depression, and 12 psychosis not otherwise specified). Among Salford's decreasing population of 91,552, the rate (one-year prevalence) was 5.9 per 1,000. The increase over the ten-year period was thought to be at least partially due to the declining population (i.e., healthy people selectively moving away) and the longer prevalence period (one year versus point prevalence). In summary, it appears either that two-thirds of the existing cases of insanity were missed in the 1866 survey of Salford or that insanity had increased substantially during the 120-year period.

Buckinghamshire, an agricultural area in the southern Midlands close to London, is another example. As noted in chapter 2, from 1597 to 1634 Richard Napier, an astrological physician, provided medical and psychiatric consultations for the approximately 200,000 residents of what are now Buckinghamshire, Bedfordshire, and Northamptonshire. Given the existing records, it is probable that the insanity rate at that time was under 0.5 cases per 1,000 total population, even allowing for many cases having been seen by other practitioners.

The first attempt to formally count the number of insane persons in these three counties was Andrew Halliday's 1829 study. He reported a total of 478 insane persons in the population of 421,000, or a prevalence rate of 1.1 per 1,000.[39] In 1871, the Lunacy Commission reported a prevalence of insanity in these three counties of 1.5 per 1,000 (1,440 insane in a population of 566,000), but by 1911 the rate had increased to 3.2 per 1,000 (1,887 insane in a population of 587,000), thus doubling in a period of forty years.

In Buckinghamshire in another study, Professor Michael Shepherd recorded all admissions for psychoses for 1931–1933.[40] To compare this with earlier periods when life expectancy was much less, it is necessary to omit all first admissions over the age of sixty-four, most of which were diagnosed with dementia, from the 1931–1933 study. The result was an average of ninety-six new cases of treated psychoses each year in a population of 271,586, or thirty-six treated cases of psychoses per 100,000 per year. In 1631–1633, Napier had identified three treated cases of insanity per 100,000 per year, and in 1931–1933,

Shepherd identified thirty-six treated cases of psychoses per 100,000 per year in the same county.

In recent years, there have been three interesting developments that bear on the epidemiology of insanity in England. The first of these is reports that individuals who are born or raised in urban areas are more likely to develop schizophrenia or other psychoses than individuals who are born or raised in rural areas. In England, the increased urban risk factor for schizophrenia compared to the rural risk factor has been reported to be 14 percent. However, if the person was born in an urban area during the winter months, the risk factor increases to 23 percent compared to rural, nonwinter births.[41]

The fact that there is an urban risk factor for psychoses in general, or for schizophrenia in particular, has now been reported in studies in Sweden, Denmark, the Netherlands, France, and the United States, in addition to England, and is one of the most clearly established risk factors. Such studies provide a scientific basis for anecdotal observations of this phenomenon, which in England date back to 1733, when George Cheyne, in *The English Malady,* suggested that "living in great, populous, and consequently unhealthy Towns" was a major cause of the increasing amount of "nervous disorders" of his day.[42]

The second recent development bearing on England's insanity rate is the unusually high rate of insanity, including schizophrenia and manic-depressive illness, among African-Caribbean immigrants to England and even higher rates among their children who are born in England. This has been consistently demonstrated in more than twenty studies since 1988, and "its validity is beyond reasonable doubt." Other studies have suggested that Irish immigrants to England also have a high rate of schizophrenia and manic-depressive illness, but other immigrants groups, such as those from India, Pakistan, and Italy, do not have unusually high rates.[43]

The third recent development of interest regarding insanity rates in England is the possibility that insanity is no longer increasing. This possibility was initially raised by reports that the number of first admissions for schizophrenia had begun decreasing in the 1960s in Scotland as well as in England and Wales. In a spasm of optimism in the early 1990s, the *British Journal of Psychiatry* and *Lancet* both published articles titled "Is Schizophrenia Disappearing?"[44]

Additional studies have tempered this initial enthusiasm and suggested that, although schizophrenia is not disappearing, at least it appears to be no longer increasing. Changes in the diagnostic criteria for schizophrenia and in the definition of first admission have confused the issue, but in both England and Scotland the incidence of schizophrenia appears to have been stable between the 1970s and the 1990s except for the increased incidence among African-Caribbean immigrants, as noted above. Another possibility that has been suggested is that schizophrenia may be becoming clinically a more benign disease with a better outcome; if true, that would reverse the trend of the nineteenth century, when insanity apparently became a more malignant disease.[45]

In England, there is guarded optimism. After two and a half centuries of an endless litany of increase, increase, increase, a leveling-off of the incidence of insanity would be most welcome. Whether or not that truly is the case should become clearer in the near future.

CHAPTER 7

The Road to Grangegorman

Ireland, 1700–1990

We propose to show that there exists such a malady as "mental contagion"—that is to say, a disease—an actual plague—which is caught by one mind from another . . . this disease is encreasing every day to a most alarming extent.

—*Dublin Review,* 1841

So while the Plague went on raging from West to East, as it went forwards East, it abated in the West, by which means those parts of the Town, which were not seiz'd, or who were left, and where it had spent its Fury, were (as it were) spar'd to help and assist the other.

—Daniel Defoe, *A Journal of the Plague Year,* 1722

n 1731 Jonathan Swift announced his intention to leave money in his will for the establishment of an insane asylum in Dublin. In Swiftian fashion, he memorialized his bequest with these lines in his "Verses on the Death of Dr. Swift, D.S.P.D.":

> *He gave the little Wealth he had*
> *To build a House for Fools and Mad*
> *And show'd by one satyric Touch*
> *No nation needed it so much.*[1]

Swift's asylum, opened in 1757 as St. Patrick's Hospital, was the beginning of two hundred years of confinement of insane persons in Ireland on a scale unparalled in the world. Workhouse populations and prison populations ultimately declined, but Ireland's "almost extravagant expansion of asylum accommodation was unique among comparable institutions of social control."[2] Insanity was increasing everywhere in the Western world, but there was something different about *baile,* the Gaelic madness. Whatever was happening elsewhere was happening more frequently in Ireland.

The suggested increase of insanity in Ireland coincided temporally with what is called the Protestant Ascendancy. Following the victory of William of Orange in 1690 at the Battle of the Boyne, Irish Catholics were excluded from Parliament, government service, and the armed forces, from purchasing land and owning firearms, and even from owning a valuable horse. Catholic lands were confiscated and given to Protestant landlords, many Catholic churches were closed, and Catholic clergymen were required to register with the authorities. Despite such repression there is no evidence that the emerging insanity occurred disproportionately among the Catholic population. Data from the 1851 census of the insane, in fact, suggest that insanity in Ireland emerged initially in areas with more Protestants and also confirm "the opinion with respect to the more educated class being more liable to mental affections than the unenlightened."[3]

There was clear evidence of concern about insanity in Ireland by the time Swift made his bequest. As early as 1684 the keeper of the Dublin jail asked the City Assembly for financial help in providing for "madd women" under his jurisdiction. In 1708 the Dublin workhouse built six cells for "the most outrageous" of the many persons there who were "madd," "fooles," or subject to "fitts." The first proposal to build a hospital "for the reception of aged lunatics and other diseased persons" was presented to Dublin officials in 1699; it was not acted on, but in 1711 the military hospital added cells for soldiers who "happen to become lunatics."[4]

In rural areas there were also indications of increasing insanity. A well in Glennagalt, the "glen of the mad" in County Kerry, was reputed to cure insanity, and many families took their mad family members there and left them. About 1750, a writer described such individuals as being "dumb, very hairy, with dismal and ruefull looks," and said that the inhabitants of the area "feared their visitors and many had placed protective bars on the windows of their homes." For the dangerously mad in rural areas, a common solution was to put the person in a hole about five feet deep in the floor of the house and cover it with bars, "and they give this wretched being his food there, and there he generally dies."[5]

Jonathan Swift's interest in insanity originated from his own family experiences. His father had died before he was born, and Swift was partially raised by a paternal uncle who became insane and died when Swift was twenty-one. Swift was thus familiar with madness and used it in his writings. In "A Digression Concerning Madness" in *A Tale of a Tub,* (1704) Swift claimed that insanity was caused by the "Force of certain Vapours" emanating from lower regions of the body on the brain. He then satirically demonstrated how certain types of insane persons, based on their behavior while confined, would make excellent candidates as army officers, lawyers, doctors, and politicians. Swift's definition of a delusion is virtually identical to that used today: "But when a Man's Fancy gets astride on his Reason, when Imagination is at Cuffs with the Senses, and common Understanding, as well as common Sense, is Kickt out of Doors; the first Proselyte he makes, is Himself, and when that is once compass'd, the Difficulty is not so great in bringing over others; A strong Delusion always operating from without, as vigorously as from within." Swift also indicated personal fears of becoming insane: "Even I myself, the Author of these momentous Truths, am a Person, whose Imaginations are hard-mouthed, and exceedingly disposed to run away with his *Reason,* which I have observed from long experience to be a very light Rider, and easily shook off."

In his later writings Swift satirically compared the members of the Irish House of Commons to the inmates of Bethlem Hospital:

> Since the House is like to last,
>
> Let a royal Grant be pass'd,
>
> That the Club have Right to dwell
>
> Each within his proper Cell;
>
> With a Passage left to creep in,
>
> And a Hole above for peeping.

Let them, when they once get in

Sell the Nation for a Pin;

While they sit a-picking Straws

Let them rave of making Laws;

While they never hold their Tongue,

Let them dabble in their Dung; . . .

Tye them, Keeper, in a tether,

Let them stare and stink together.[6]

Swift was a governor of the Dublin workhouse and of London's Bethlem Hospital, which he visited in 1710. Once he had become well known and dean of St. Patrick's Cathedral in Dublin, Swift sought advice regarding how he might best help mentally ill individuals, and he eventually decided to build a hospital. It should be noted that, although Swift was concerned about insanity in Ireland, there was some question in his mind whether a sufficient number of insane persons could be found to fill its beds, and in his will he gave specific instructions that the hospital could be used for other conditions "if a sufficient number of ideots [*sic*] and lunatics could not be readily found."[7]

In 1742 Swift suffered a severe stroke and was declared mentally incompetent. At his death three years later, his bequest of £825,000 (1997 equivalent) went to found the hospital.

"Melancholy Spectacles of Humanity"

St. Patrick's Hospital opened in 1757 with sixteen patients. By 1762 it had forty-eight patients, and by 1789 the patient population had increased to 109, demonstrating that Swift's concern about filling its beds was not well founded. Despite the availability of the hospital, at Dublin's workhouse "lunatics and idiots soon came to form so large a portion of its inmates that in the year 1776 ten cells were set aside for their reception, and in the year 1778 this class had increased so considerably that it became necessary to fit up a house . . . capable of containing thirty patients." In Cork, a new addition to the workhouse was opened in 1792 to accommodate twenty-four insane persons; by 1822 it held three hundred. Increasing numbers of mad persons were also observed wandering at large; a French visitor in 1796 noted that "one of the most painful spectacles to be seen in nearly all the principal towns of Ireland is the number of weak-minded persons in the streets." Growing public demand "for the control of the more unruly and dangerous of those permitted to wander at large" led to passage in 1787 of "an Act . . . to establish a county system of special wards" in county hospitals, but "the new legislation was almost entirely ignored."[8]

One reason for the increasing numbers of the insane was an increasing population. Georgian Ireland was marked by economic growth and prosperity, and the population increased sharply from 2 million to 4.5 million between 1750 and 1790. Hoping to emulate the success of late-eighteenth-century rebellions in America and France, Irish nationalist forces staged an abortive uprising in 1798; the English responded by dissolving the Irish Parliament and joining Ireland with Scotland, Wales, and England by an Act of Union.

Although the increasing Irish population accounted for some of the increase in insanity, it did not appear to explain it all. In 1810 William S. Hallaran, owner of a small private insane asylum and physician to the Cork workhouse, published *An Enquiry into the Causes Producing the Extraordinary Addition to the Number of Insane,* subsequently republished as *Practical Observations on the Causes and Cure of Insanity.* Hallaran claimed it was "an incontrovertible fact that, from the year 1798 to 1809, the number of insane had advanced far beyond the extent of any former period," and he attributed this "sudden and fearful addition to the number of insane" to both psychological causes ("terror from the [1798] rebellion") and medical causes (heredity and alcohol abuse). Hallaran also predicted that "insanity, it will be shown, is, in every instance, associated with organic lesion; either entirely originating in, or ultimately combined with it."[9]

Hallaran's book and the specter of increasing insanity stimulated the English authorities to act, and in 1810 they authorized the building of a separate asylum "for the reception of lunatics from all parts of the kingdom."[10] The Richmond Lunatic Asylum, more popularly known as Grangegorman because of the street on which it was located, was built for two hundred patients, which authorities believed would allow for the transfer of all existing insane persons being housed in workhouses and jails.

The Richmond Asylum opened in 1815 with many transfers from the workhouses. Hack Tuke later noted: "To the amazement of those who had induced Parliament to make what they deemed so ample a provision, it was soon found that not only was the asylum full to overflowing, but the House of Industry [workhouse] was soon as full as before." By 1817 the governor of the Asylum noted that "applications for admission to our Institution very far exceed the means of receiving them," including an additional 370 insane persons who were still residing in workhouses.[11]

The failure of the Richmond Asylum to stem the rising tide of insanity alarmed the English authorities. An 1815 report to the House of Commons stated that "in Ireland, the necessity of making some further provision for insane persons appears to be more urgent even than in this part of the United Kingdom." Similarly, George Burrows noted in 1820 that "a conviction is entertained that insanity is very prevalent in that part [Ireland] of the United Kingdom."[12] In 1816 England's chief secretary for Ireland therefore ordered an investigation into the number of insane persons in Dublin's workhouse. Two months later, the inquiry was broadened to include the provision for insane persons in the entire country. Hearings were held the following summer, resulting in the 1817 *Report of the Select Committee on the Lunatic Poor*.

The result was the first serious attempt to assess the total number of insane persons and idiots under care in Ireland. Nineteen counties said they had no provisions for insane persons at all. Eleven others enumerated a total of 989 insane persons and idiots in asylums, workhouses, and jails, making a ratio of approximately 0.15 insane persons and idiots under care per 1,000 total population.[13] In those jurisdictions where a breakdown between insane persons and idiots was provided, insane persons constituted between 57 and 80 percent of the total.

Many individuals testifying at the 1817 hearings expressed alarm at the growing numbers of the insane. Thomas Rice, who had visited facilities in Cork, Waterford, Limerick, and Tipperary, noted "a most alarming increase of the number of the insane" since the turn of the century and cited as an example increases at Cork's asylum from 72 inmates in 1800 to 219 in 1816. Similarly, the wing of the Limerick workhouse for the insane had experienced a "vast increase of insanity" from fourteen inmates in 1804 to forty-eight in 1817.[14]

Conditions for insane persons in workhouses were described as "such as we should not appropriate for our dog-kennels." At the Limerick workhouse, according to Rice, two insane persons had frozen to death. "In one of those rooms I found four-and-twenty individuals lying, some old, some infirm, one or two dying, some insane, and in the centre of the room was left a corpse of one who [had] died a few hours before. . . . In the adjoining room I found a woman with the corpse of her child, lying upon her knees for two days; it was almost in a state of putridity." "Furious" persons were chained to their beds "for years" so that some "lost the use of their limbs" and were "utterly incapable of rising." Furthermore, "The keeper of the lunatics claimed an exclusive dominion over the females confided to his charge, and which he exercised in the most abominable manner."[15]

Given such conditions and evidence that insanity was increasing, the 1817 *Report of the Select Committee on the Lunatic Poor* recommended that four or five district asylums should be built, each containing provisions for between 120 and 150 insane persons. The expense of these asylums was to be borne by the districts. A similar recommendation had been made to a parliamentary committee in 1804 but had been rejected because of the expense, and much testimony in the 1817 hearings focused on that issue.

Four district asylums (Armagh, Belfast, Derry, and Limerick) were completed in the 1820s, and five more (Ballinasloe, Carlow, Waterford, Maryborough, and Clonmel) by 1835, with a total capacity for 1,062 patients. The cost of the asylums varied between £3.7 million and £31.9 million each (1997 equivalents), thus justifying the fears of officials about costs. Ireland therefore became the first nation with a network of government insane asylums, a fact publicly noted by Sir Andrew Halliday in 1828: "Ireland is the only portion of the British Empire where just views have been entertained of what was necessary for the comfort and cure of her insane population, and where these views have been fully carried into effect. . . . Oh that England would be wise, and would consider this, and for once take a lesson from her more humble sister!"[16]

The 1820s and 1830s in Ireland were marked politically by the emergence of the Catholic movement led by Daniel O'Connell. The anti-Catholic laws of the eighteenth century had been repealed, but the continued economic dominance of Protestants and the hated Act of Union with England were perpetual reminders of the Catholics' inferior status in their own country, in which they were a majority. The population continued to rise, reaching 8.2 million in 1841, but "close to half the population lived in one-roomed squalor of window-less mud huts."[17]

During these years the number of insane persons applying for admission to the asylums continued to increase faster than the increasing population. The district asylums were filled as soon as they were completed, and small private asylums opened for families who had money. The private asylums, like the public asylums, were under constant pressure for admission. By 1844 there were fourteen in Ireland, including the Bloomfield Retreat, started by Dublin's Quakers and modeled after the York Retreat. Jails also became increasingly crowded with the insane. An 1827 survey of the jails found that "in a few instances old jail buildings had been set aside exclusively for the insane." In some counties, insane inmates lived in conditions described as "pitiful in the greatest degree," including being chained to the wall or being confined to iron cages "like wild beasts."[18]

Censuses of insane persons under care showed a steady increase. In 1828 the total was 1,584 (0.21 per 1,000 total population), but by 1841 the total had more than doubled to 3,622 (0.44 per 1,000), and in 1844 it was reported to be 4,297 (0.53 per 1,000). Although these numbers were only a fraction of what the numbers would be later in the century, they were considered alarming at the time, and the 1841 *Dublin Review* noted that "a vast increase" in "diseases of the mind" had taken place "since the commencement of the present century."[19] Just one hundred years earlier, Jonathan Swift had expressed concern whether a sufficient number of insane persons could be found to fill the beds in his proposed asylum; by 1841, Swift's concern appeared fatuous indeed.

Despite the increasing public concern, surprisingly few Irish writers wrote about insanity during this period. An exception was novelist Sheridan Le Fanu, who in his 1840 sensation novel *The Fortunes of Sir Robert Ardagh* had the protagonist exhibit "paroxysms of apparent lunacy." Le Fanu also utilized the theme of wrongful confinement in an asylum in his 1871 novel *The Rose and the Key*. In 1845 William Makepeace Thackeray, English novelist and author of *Vanity Fair*, visited the Derry Asylum and called it "a model of neatness and comfort."[20] Thackeray's Irish wife had become insane in 1840 following childbirth and remained so for the rest of her life.

A major reason for the increasing public awareness of the insanity problem was the increasing visibility of insane persons in the community. In 1824 a visitor claimed that "on most public roads in the South of Ireland fools and idiots (melancholy spectacles of humanity!) are permitted to wander at large, and in consequence of this freedom have acquired vicious habits, to the annoyance of every passenger." Six years later, a committee on the Irish poor complained that "wandering lunatics" had been "dispersed over the country in the most disgusting and wretched state." In the early 1840s, an English visitor to County Mayo was accosted by "a wandering mad woman" who was "laughing and jabbering Irish . . . the filthiest, most ragged, most squalid of her sex, her dark hair streaming down her smoke-browned neck, her black eyes bright with partial madness."[21]

Violent episodes by mentally ill individuals also became more visible. In 1828, for example, a sea captain named Stewart sailed into Cork and was found to have murdered seven of his crew "by beating out the brains of each of them in turn as they entered his cabin"; he was diagnosed as being a "religious monomaniac."[22] In 1838 a man "who was well known to be going about deranged" and "who had been refused admission into the Richmond Asylum a short time before" shot to death a "most respectable gentlemen" in Dublin.[22] As a consequence of this act, a new law was implemented making it possible to put dangerous mentally ill individuals in jail. Five years later, a House of Lords report entitled "The State of the Lunatic Poor in Ireland" recommended "the Necessity of providing One central Establishment for Criminal Lunatics"; this recommendation was implemented in 1850 by the opening of Dundrum Asylum, an institution for the criminally insane in Dublin with accommodations for 150 patients. A similar institution would not be opened in England until 1863.

The Famine and Its Aftermath

The arrival of *Phytophthera infestans* in Ireland in 1845 had a profound effect on the nation's history. Over the next four years, approximately one million people died of starvation, typhoid, typhus, cholera, and dysentery as the potato blight decimated the major food crop of the country, and another one million emigrated. In County Galway, it was reported that "dead bodies were everywhere, lying unburied." In west Cork, the inhabitants were said to be "famished and ghastly skeletons . . . such frightful specters as no words can describe." In County Queens, families "fed on grass, seaweed and shellfish, rotten potatoes, dead animals, even human corpses." Funeral shrouds and coffins were increasingly in short supply, until in some areas the survivors simply resorted to the "reusable 'trap-coffin,' with a hinged bottom, and the mass grave became ubiquitous." As one priest lamented, "The Angel of death and desolation reigns triumphant in Ireland." Southwestern and western Ireland (Connaught and Munster) were hardest hit by both the famine and emigration, with each losing more than one-third of its inhabited dwellings between 1845 and 1861.[23]

Remarkably, the number of insane persons continued to rise steadily in Ireland during and after the famine, apparently unaffected by the potato blight and its devastating consequences. Censuses of insane persons in asylums, workhouses, and jails show that the total number per population increased approximately 10 percent per year between 1841 and 1843, prior to the famine, and by 7 percent per year between 1843 and 1851, which included the famine years. Admissions to the insane asylums increased sharply from 1846 to 1847 and then leveled off in the succeeding three years. It thus appears that the major economic and social event in Ireland's history exerted little immediate influence on its steadily rising number of hospitalized insane persons.

Famine or no famine, it had become clear to authorities in Dublin by the 1850s that the ten existing district insane asylums were overcrowded and inadequate, that many insane individuals continued to reside in workhouses and jails, and that each year the situation was becoming worse. During the 1850s and 1860s, therefore, the authorities embarked upon a second wave of asylum building as well as making additions to most of the existing asylums. During the two decades, twelve new asylums were opened in Castlebar, Cork, Downpatrick, Ennis, Enniscorthy, Kilkenny, Killarney, Letterkenny, Monaghan, Mullingar, Omagh, and Sligo, with a total of 3,482 new beds. Whereas the original ten asylums had averaged 130 beds each, the twelve new asylums averaged almost 300 beds each.

Given the postfamine depressed economy of Ireland, there was considerable resistance among landowners and local authorities to building the new asylums, especially since the population was falling because of continuing emigration. During the two decades the twelve new asylums were being built, the population of Ireland decreased 17 percent; altogether it had decreased 36 percent since the onset of the famine. As early as 1854 "a number of counties protested to the Chancellor about the high cost and imperfect work in some asylums." The cost of the new asylums varied between £2.9 million and £10.6 million (1997 equivalents). In addition, the annual maintenance costs for the asylums reached £7.7 million (1997 equivalent) by 1871, surpassing total public medical outlays for the first time and representing a major drain on the public treasury.[24]

During the postfamine period, Dublin authorities began collecting more complete census data on the number of insane persons in the country. In 1845 the local police, the Royal Irish Constabulary, had been persuaded to undertake a count of all insane persons "at large" in each of Ireland's 1,500 districts and subdistricts. Constables were instructed by their police manual to "know if possible every person in [his] subdistrict." As one report claimed: "From the general intelligence and accurate local knowledge of its members, we are satisfied that from no other source could so complete and reliable information be obtained."[25]

The police census of "at large" insane persons was repeated periodically after 1850; this, combined with the periodic general censuses of the insane in asylums, workhouses, and jails, provided authorities with an ongoing database with which to assess the number of insane persons. As might be expected, more than three-quarters of the insane persons "at large" were classified as idiots rather than insane, and more than two-thirds of them were said to be "resident with relatives" and "harmless."

In the postfamine period, authorities also undertook more complete analyses of data on insanity, looking for clues to explain the continuing rising numbers despite the declining population. For example, Frederick MacCabe, the medical superintendent of the Waterford District Asylum, claimed that in County Waterford between 1851 and 1861 "the alleged increase of lunacy is a well established fact." His reasoning was as follows:

In 1851, with a population of, in round numbers, 164,000, we have 238 insane; and this return, be it observed, includes no unknown quantity. . . . In 1861, with a population of 134,000, we have 386 insane. Here with a decrease of 30,000 in the population, we have an increase of 148 insane. These figures are very significant. I have taken one county of Ireland with which I am specially well acquainted, and if the reader will compare my results with the figures furnished by the general census of Ireland for 1851 and 1861, he will perceive that the same conclusions may be arrived at for the whole kingdom as I have reached by a more minute enquiry into the returns of one of its constituent parts.[26]

Dr. MacCabe's analysis of County Waterford was at least partially stimulated by public discussions regarding the geographical distribution of insanity within Ireland, for Waterford's rate appeared to be very high. The 1851 census had included data on insane persons (not including idiots), both confined and "at large," per total population by county. The counties with the highest rates of insane persons were concentrated in the eastern and southeastern regions, mostly in Leinster. This was the most prosperous part of Ireland; "farms were generally larger and land values higher than on the rest of the island. . . . Leinster had a higher proportion of traders, shopkeepers, and publicans than any other province."[27] The counties with the lowest rates were in Connaught (Galway, Leitrim, Mayo, and Roscommon) and Ulster (Armagh and Cavan). The difference between the counties with the highest rates of insane persons per 1,000 total population (Dublin, 1.80, and Waterford, 1.21) and lowest rates (Mayo and Roscommon, each 0.43) was threefold or greater. In the census, all insane person were registered to their county of origin ("native place"), regardless of where they were found, in order to minimize errors in county of assignment.

The 1851 census thus noted that insanity appeared to be "greatest in Leinster" and that "the province of Connaught exhibits a remarkable immunity from both Lunacy and Idiocy." Connaught was the poorest part of Ireland, consisting of "largely subsistence-oriented regions." It also observed, "It would appear that Lunatics prevail most in the cities," but speculated that this might be because many of the asylums were close to urban areas. The census also provided a breakdown by occupation and education of all insane persons and found that insanity occurred disproportionately among "the professional class, of whom 404 were affected with Insanity, a large amount considering the proportion which this class bears to the great bulk of people." The 1851 census therefore claimed to "confirm the opinion with respect to the more educated class being more liable to mental affections than the unenlightened."[28]

Increasing Numbers, Dead or Alive

The annual reports of the Irish Inspectors of Lunatics during the last half of the nineteenth century had one common and recurring theme—increasing insanity. It was "a considerable increase," "a decided increase," a "great increase," and an "appalling increase," but always it was an increase. As the *American Journal of Insanity* reported in 1861, "the increase in insanity is exciting much attention" in Ireland.[29]

The number of confined insane persons in asylums, workhouses, and jails increased from 5,345 in 1851 to 10,767 in 1871 and then to 16,688 in 1891. At the same time, the total population of Ireland was decreasing from 6.5 million to 4.7 million, so that the confined insane per 1,000 total population increased more than fourfold, from 0.82 per 1,000 total population in 1851 to 3.57 per 1,000 in 1891. Annual admissions to the district asylums increased more than threefold, from 1.5 per 10,000 population in 1851 to 5.0 per 10,000 population in 1891. An 1856 report advised that "further asylum accommodation, notwithstanding the additional institutions established within the last few years, is urgently required." An 1885 report further summarized the situation: "The struggle to obtain sufficient accommodation for the insane in Ireland seems to be a never-ending one. Year after year the Inspectors suggest the necessity of the extension of the original buildings of district asylums to meet the inevitable increasing influx of the insane. . . . But their difficulties appear insurmountable from the variety of opinion exhibited on all sides of the subject."[30]

A consequence of this increase was perpetual overcrowding of the asylums. An official commission report in 1879 observed: "From these reports year after year, and from the successive records of each asylum, there is the same complaint, the monotonous repetition of overcrowding." Another report stated, "All the district asylums throughout Ireland may be said to be more or less overcrowded," and cited the housing of 606 inmates in the Mullingar Asylum despite its theoretical maximum capacity of 430. By the 1890s it was reported, "In 19 out of the 22 asylums new works for extending accommodation and improving existing structures are either being carried out or are in contemplation."[31] The Ballinasloe Asylum, originally built for 150 patients, held 1,004; the Richmond Asylum, built for 257, held 1,398 patients, many of them sleeping on the floor.

Under such circumstances, even a minimal level of comfort and care for patients was impossible to achieve. The average number of work hours per week for attendants was 82-1/2 for the day shift and 75 for the night shift. At the Waterford Asylum, attendants "claimed in a petition that a long day's duty could run to sixteen hours; they were allowed 2-1/4 hours off duty every second evening and [were given] every third Sunday off." Merely keeping count of the increasing numbers of patients strained the system. At the Richmond Asylum, "some patients still on the hospital register were probably dead because they 'could not be found.'" And in 1898, "it was discovered that it was really Anne M____ who had died on 1 March 1866, not Mary M____, who appeared still to be alive."[32]

Given the overcrowding and understaffing, violence on the asylum wards was inevitable. The violence could be between patients, as when Thomas Hopkins choked to death John Ray in the Ballinasloe Asylum in 1873, or when Alice Chapman killed Ellen Deegan with a chamber pot in the Richmond Asylum in 1889. The violence could also be directed toward the staff, as when Margaret Kelly attacked Dr. Jacob with a stone in the Maryborough Asylum, or when John Kane injured one of the hospital governors with a knife in the Derry Asylum in 1858.[33]

Beyond the asylum walls, the effects of increasing insanity were also visible. Complaints about the number of mentally ill in jails recurred so regularly that one report of the Inspectors of Lunatics simply observed: "The general subject has been so frequently dwelt upon in our reports, that it would be mere repetition to enter further upon it here." The workhouses also continued to be filled with insane persons, especially after 1875, when the law was changed to allow the transfer of "unrecovered but harmless patients, . . . thereby relieving overcrowding in asylums." An 1879 survey found thirteen workhouses, each of which held more than forty insane persons, and forty more workhouses holding twenty insane persons or more. In the 1890s the workhouse at Ballymena housed over a hundred patients transferred from the Belfast Asylum. In an 1894 article, "The Insane in Workhouses," M. J. Nolan described "the existence of dirt, overcrowding, fleas, other disgusting vermin, filthy straw ticks, . . . [and] the absence of sanitary and lavatory accommodation. . . . One man is found who has not had a bath for five years, and a woman unwashed for ten."[34]

Also noted by the official reports was "the large number of individuals of unsound mind, or whose sanity is doubtful, wandering about in Ireland . . . not under public supervision." One such individual was a young man, "stark naked, confined to a room, and looking through the wooden bars [of a farmhouse]. . . . An English tourist happening to see this case had him removed to the Monaghan Asylum."[35] Despite some decrease in the number of "at large" insane persons reported by police censuses, there simply was not room in the overcrowded asylums for them, and many of the less disturbed cases continued to live with their families.

As the number of insane persons under care increased, the costs inevitably followed. In 1871 the annual maintenance costs for the twenty-two district asylums was £7.7 million (1997 equivalent); by 1898 this had risen to £18.9 million and was increasing much more rapidly than medical costs, poor relief, or other social expenditures.[36] The national treasury contributed approximately 40 percent of the cost, but the remainder had to be raised by local taxes. Since additions to existing asylums had to be approved by local asylum boards and grand juries, there was considerable resistance in many counties to such expenditures, and local pressure was exerted to transfer patients to workhouses, where they could be maintained at lower county costs.

At the Richmond Asylum, "Inspectors . . . sought to obtain an extension of accommodation, but [were] opposed in their attempts by the grand juries of Louth, Drogheda, and Wicklow." In Ulster there were "protests by Derry ratepayers against the new county asylum." Despite severe overcrowding and proposals to build additions to the asylum, "the County Councils of Leitrim and Sligo refused to supply the funds for carrying out the work." And in County Monaghan, "by the time the Monaghan committee agreed to carry out additions . . . the sleeping rooms had almost double their quota of beds and nearly all had patients sleeping on the floors."[37]

"This Vast Brooding Evil"

By the 1890s the issue of increasing insanity in Ireland had been labeled "a vexed question" by one Irish psychiatrist. Another psychiatrist said that "no question, I believe, is more frequently or more anxiously asked." Most laypersons and some psychiatrists believed, on the basis of their own experiences, that insanity was indeed increasing, but the Inspectors of Lunatics assured them that "lunacy at present is certainly not on the increase in Ireland." The inspectors acknowledged, however, that the possibility of such an increase called for "the consideration of all who take an interest in the welfare of the country and deserve[d] the fullest and most careful inquiry."[38] Such an inquiry took place in 1893 and consisted merely of a questionnaire sent to the medical directors of the district asylums asking whether they had observed an increase in insanity in the previous decade and, if so, what they thought was causing it. The following year the results of the inquiry were published.

The opinions of the medical directors were mixed. Some said "there is an undoubted increase in the number of the insane . . . the increase is real and not merely apparent"; others claimed that "the increase in the asylum population during the last decade is most largely due to accumulation." "Consanguineous marriages," excessive alcohol use, and dietary changes were said to be the cause of the increase; for example, William Myles of the Kilkenny Asylum wrote that "when the people lived on strong and nourishing food as meal, potatoes, eggs, etc., there was not half the madness going as there is at present."[39]

The conclusions of the *Special Report,* published by the inspectors in 1894, were contradictory. On the one hand, the inspectors concluded that "the great increase of the insane under care is mainly due to *accumulation,* and is, so far, an apparent and not a real increase." On the other hand, they concluded that "the annual increase in the face of a shrinking population of the number of first admissions, including as it does such a large proportion of first attacks, of insanity, almost irresistibly points to some increase of occurring insanity in particular districts." No statistics or data were cited to support either of these conclusions. In fact, the inspectors' own published reports for the decade in question showed a sharp increase in insane persons under care, from 2.78 per 1,000 total population in 1883 to 3.75 per 1,000 in 1893 (a 35 percent increase), and an increase in first admissions to district asylums from 4.4 per 10,000 in 1883 to 5.3 per 10,000 in 1893 (a 21 percent increase). Nor did the inspectors include any discussion of the seemingly endless supply of new cases of insanity, with jails and workhouses filling with insane persons as soon as others had been transferred to asylums; this transfer and refilling of the workhouses had in fact been going on for most of the nineteenth century.

The *1894 Special Report* on insanity was fundamentally a political document, not a scientific one. Irish nationalism was on the rise following the land reform battles of the 1880s; the Gaelic League had been founded in 1893, the Irish Republican Brotherhood was increasing its activities, and most important, British prime minister Gladstone had just introduced a Home Rule Bill. The United Irish League and Sinn Fein would follow, leading Ireland to a confrontation with its English overseers after the turn of the century.

It is, therefore, not possible to understand the issues surrounding insanity in 1894 without an appreciation of the political context. Irish psychiatrists were members of the British Medico-Psychological Association but were looked down upon by many of their English colleagues. The annual summary of Irish mental hospitals published in the *Journal of Mental Science* was routinely disdainful and, on those occasions when the Irish statistics appeared favorable, the English editors still faulted them. For example, in 1878, the Irish asylums recorded a very low number of suicides for the year. The editors of the *Journal of Mental Science* responded that "this [number] is far too good to be satisfactory for it implies too little liberty given to the patients."[40] The "right" suicide rate was apparently the English rate; more than that or fewer than that could be equally criticized.

The contempt many English psychiatrists held for their Irish colleagues was, of course, part of a general English contempt for the Irish. In 1894, for example, at the same time as the *Special Report* was being published, Thomas Clouston, coeditor of the *Journal of Mental Science,* published a paper comparing the Irish people to the indigenous Maoris of New Zealand in an attempt to explain the high Irish prevalence of insanity: "When you consider that the primitive portions of the Irish people within the last fifty years have come suddenly into intimate contact with advanced ideas in politics and with advanced people . . . it would seem surprising if some racial mental effect did not result."[41]

It was within this political context, therefore, that the Irish Lunacy Commissioners were obligated to address the questions of Ireland's insanity rate. During the 1870s and 1880s, summaries of the annual reports on insane asylums in England, Scotland, and Ireland were published seriatum in the *Journal of Mental Science,* including comparative insanity rates for the three countries. The Irish rates were invariably higher than the other two countries. It had become common knowledge in England, as well as in other countries, that insanity was peculiarly endemic to Ireland. That would not do for the new Ireland, the emerging Ireland, the Ireland that hoped to throw off its colonial English masters. Having as much insanity as England was acceptable, but having more was not. The *1894 Special Report* therefore concluded that "the seeming preponderance of insanity in Ireland as compared with England is fictitious, and depends entirely upon the greater accumulation in Ireland occasioned by the lower death-rate in that country, and (possibly) the lower rate of discharge of the unrecovered."

The related question was whether insanity was increasing in Ireland. In England the question was also very topical at the time; English psychiatrists were answering it with a resolute "no," and this became official in the English 1897 *Special Report on the Alleged Increase of Insanity.* For the Irish Lunacy Commissioners to contradict their English colleagues would have been an act of both temerity and discourtesy.

The *1894 Special Report,* therefore, concluded that the apparently increasing insanity rate was merely due to "accumulation," despite the fact that the Irish data contradicted this. The editors of the *Journal of Mental Science* thereupon commended their Irish colleagues for "the alteration which has come over their views in this very important matter" and expressed satisfaction that the views of the Irish psychiatrists have been "converted . . . to what we regard as the current view in this matter." If Irish psychiatrists had any doubt regarding the consequences of offending English sensibilities, they could be reminded by a "patient named Mahoney" in the Dundrum Asylum who "had been confined in a cell for four days for refusing to take off his hat when 'God Save the Queen' was played at a dance."[42]

There were those who objected to the conclusions of the *1894 Special Report,* none more public or more articulate than W. J. Corbet. Corbet had been the chief clerk of the Irish Lunacy Department from 1847 to 1877, with responsibility for compiling the annual asylum reports, and was therefore very knowledgeable on the problem of insanity. He had then been elected to the Irish Royal Society and had served as a Member of Parliament for twelve years, from which post he had frequently spoken out on the question of increasing insanity. As early as 1884, Corbet published an article in the *Fortnightly Review* entitled "Is Insanity on the Increase?" In it he extensively analyzed data on the "continuous and regular" increase in insanity, "as if influenced by some inscrutable law," and showed that the accumulation of chronic cases could not possibly account for most of the increase. He also pointedly noted "the morbid official anxiety manifested from time to time to explain away what people will persist in calling 'the apparent increase of insanity.' . . . How [the Inspectors] can maintain their position in the face of such an array of testimony is incomprehensible."[43]

Corbet reacted sharply to the *1894 Special Report* with a series of articles in popular journals. "It is impossible to understand," he said, "the infatuation which leads the Commissioners to a conclusion so crude and so much at variance with the statistical records to be found in their own reports." "The microbe of 'apparent increase' seemed to have taken exclusive possession of the upper cavity of officialism," Corbet claimed. The truth, he said, is that, "account for it how we may, as time progresses, the stream of insanity broadens and deepens continually. The great central fact stares us in the face, it cannot be hidden, no effort of obscurantism can conceal it. The figures given from official records indisputably prove it."[44]

Corbet's critique of the *1894 Special Report* was to prove prophetic, for in the years immediately following, insanity in Ireland increased at an even faster rate. Between 1894 and 1899 the total number of insane persons under care increased from 17,655 to 20,863, an 18 percent increase, and the first-admission rate increased from 5.3 to 6.3 per 10,000 population, a 19 percent increase. Faced with such numbers, the Inspectors of Lunatics repeatedly attempted to assure people that the increase was not real: "Such an increase in the number of insane persons brought under our official cognizance . . . would lead the general public to believe that an alarming increase of insanity is taking place in Ireland, although that is not really the case, the increase in the numbers being mainly due to accumulation."[45]

Such assurances increasingly rang hollow. In an 1896 issue of the *Fortnightly Review,* Thomas Drapes noted that "Ireland alone of all civilized countries, so far as I am aware, possesses the unique and unenviable distinction of a continuously increasing amount of insanity with a continuously decreasing population." By 1898 the *Journal of Mental Science* was comparing Ireland's insanity to a flood:

> The tide of lunacy seems ever flowing. We wait in patience, as those who have gone before us have waited, for the turn, but it does not come. Each year we scan the high-water mark, and hope, but with only a half-hearted expectancy, that the maximum limit has at last been reached, but the flood still creeps upward with a wearisome, irritating persistence, and we look in vain for the ebbing. And yet it must come. On *a priori* reasoning, if there were no other grounds for the conviction, it must come. . . . If this process were to go on indefinitely the insane must eventually outnumber the sane.

A similar theme was repeated in the *1902 Report* of the Inspectors of Lunatics, which referred to increasing insanity as "this vast brooding evil which causes so much misery": "If this rate were to continue, to follow up a no doubt somewhat fanciful idea, though one not altogether devoid of interest, computation shows that in 170 years from this, the population of Ireland would consist of exactly an equal number of sane and insane." And the following year, the inspectors asked: "How long? Can nothing be done to stay the advance of the destroyer?"[46]

Accumulation and Emigration

Given the increasing visibility of the insanity problem, it was not surprising that "the public . . . [were] constantly clamoring about the increase of insanity, and demanding an explanation."[47] The response of the Inspectors of Lunatics was to undertake another questionnaire survey of asylum medical directors in 1904 and then issue a *Special Report on the Alleged Increase of Insanity* in 1906.

By this time a clear majority of asylum medical directors believed that the increase of insane persons was real. For example, George Lawless of the Armagh Asylum wrote that "taking all the figures, they show an alarming increase in insanity in a little over one generation." To counter these opinions, the 1906 report, in contrast to the 1894 report, went beyond a mere recital of asylum directors' opinions and offered specific reasons why the increasing insanity was "largely due to the accumulation which is taking place in the public asylums."[48] These reasons included a lower asylum discharge and death rate in Ireland compared to England, greater longevity of patients, greater accessibility of the asylums because of improved roads, less stigma so families were more willing to hospitalize family members, less severely sick patients being hospitalized, the transfer of insane persons from workhouses to asylums, and the return to Ireland of emigrants who had become insane after they had left Ireland.

There was some validity for the first three of these as causes for the accumulation of patients in the asylums. The asylum discharge rates had decreased from approximately 17 percent per year in 1851 to 9 percent in 1901 as increasingly disturbed patients accumulated on the wards. On several occasions, discharged patients committed homicides shortly after leaving the hospital; "such events usually encouraged the rigidity of discharge practice." The asylum death rate had also fallen slightly, from 6.7 percent per year in the mid–nineteenth century to 6.2 percent in the early years of the twentieth century. Irish officials frequently cited the lower death rate in Irish asylums, compared with English asylums, as the reason for the higher number of hospitalized patients in Ireland; in fact, the difference in death rates was small and due almost entirely to a higher rate of general paralysis caused by syphilis in England. Irish officials therefore claimed that "the apparent excess of insanity in Ireland over that of England is due to the absence of general paralysis. . . . Strange as it may appear, the apparent preponderance of insanity in this country may be largely due to the virtue of its inhabitants."[49] Although this was undoubtedly a popular view, in fact the lower death rate accounted for only a small fraction of the increasing insanity.

The claim that insanity had become less stigmatized in Ireland, and the corollary that families were sending less severely sick patients to the asylums, are very doubtful. The insane asylums were probably as feared in 1900 as they had been in 1850 and the stigma did not significantly decrease in Ireland until recent years. Furthermore, there is no evidence that less-sick patients were being admitted in the latter years of the nineteenth century. In fact, this would have been remarkable, given the crowding of the asylums; what evidence exists points toward admissions being *sicker* in later years. For example, in 1854 only 37 percent of all admissions to district asylums were classified as "dangerous lunatics," but by 1880 this proportion had risen to 55 percent, and by 1910 to 68 percent. Similarly, Lindsay Prior, in a study of admissions to the Omagh Asylum for 1895–1905, reported that "just over 55 per cent of the case book sample were admitted by reason of violence or threatened violence to a relative or neighbour; and 25 per cent by reason of self-harm or threatened self-harm. Only the remaining 20 per cent were committed by reason of their symptoms."[50]

It was alleged by one official in 1906 that the insanity rate had increased because "the Asylum is being used to pen in imbeciles, epileptics, dements, and a large class who, with an intelligence below the ordinary level, combine a tendency to self-indulgence and impulsive irritability, and an indolent refusal to work for their support." In fact, no data supported this claim. The percentage of asylum admissions attributable to alcohol excess remained constant at approximately 8 to 10 percent over the years. The percentage of asylum admissions with mental retardation as their primary diagnosis was usually 10 percent or less, and such individuals often had violent behavior or insanity as concomitant problems. Most individuals with mental retardation who could not be kept at home were kept in the local workhouses. The workhouse was also the usual institution for elderly persons who could not be kept at home, and there was no increase in asylum admissions of individuals over age sixty-five other than as a reflection of the increasing proportion of the general population over age sixty-five (4 percent in 1851, 6 percent in 1871, and 10 percent in 1911).[51]

The claim made by the Inspectors of Lunatics in their *1906 Special Report* that Ireland's high insanity rate was partially due to transfers from the workhouses was disingenuous. The inspectors were aware that since 1875 district asylums had been legally transferring less-disturbed insane individuals *to* the workhouses, and many who returned to the asylums were the same ones who had been there before. Nor did the inspectors address the more fundamental question of the origin of the never-ending pool of insane individuals who had not been transferred to the asylums but who ended up in the workhouses.

The *1906 Special Report* also cited the return of insane emigrants as a cause of Ireland's high rate of insanity. It said that there were "1,450 insane persons known to be returned emigrants in all the district, criminal, and private lunatic asylums and workhouses in Ireland" and that insane returned emigrants constituted "slightly over 7 percent of the total number resident in these institutions."[52] In counties with especially high emigration rates, the returned emigrants made up as much as 10 percent (County Mayo) to 13 percent (County Westmeath) of the asylum population.

The *1906 Special Report* also repeated a claim that had been circulating for half a century that "the exodus of the strong and vigorous ... to other countries [leaves] behind the weak-minded and imbecile classes to form a residue of insanity out of proportion to the existing population." The high insanity rate of Ireland, therefore, was "at least to some extent due to the reduction of the population of Ireland owing to emigration." The Inspectors of Lunatics had made similar claims in their annual reports of 1890 and 1891:

> The present number of the insane in Ireland therefore properly belongs to a much larger population than now exists in the country. (1890)

> The large emigration ... tending to remove the healthy and strong, both in mind and body, and leaving the weak and infirm as a burden on the public rates, must be considered as one of the principal factors in the explanation of this large increase. (1891)[53]

Emigration as an explanation for high Irish insanity rates has some plausibility. However, there is no evidence that individuals who were "strong in mind" did emigrate selectively. Moreover, attempts to correlate Irish insanity rates and emigration rates by county have been remarkably unproductive. Six of Ireland's thirty-two counties (Cork, Kerry, Tipperary, Limerick, Galway, and Mayo) accounted for 48 percent of the total emigrants in the nineteenth century; none of them ranked among the counties with the highest insanity rates in 1851, and Galway and Mayo were among the lowest. Hack Tuke, looking for a correlation between emigration and Irish insanity in 1894, reported the link to be very weak and speculated that both insanity and emigration might be caused by a third factor, poverty. In 1911 the Inspectors of Lunatics themselves published an extensive analysis of emigration and insanity and reported that "county by county, it is found that there is no marked degree of relationship between them." "This result," they added, "is contrary to what might have been anticipated, as the steady increase in the numbers of the insane in Ireland has often been attributed in large measure to the removal by emigration of the fittest portion of the population."[54]

The most damaging evidence against emigration being the cause of increased Irish insanity is the fact that the emigrants themselves became insane at a rate at least equal to the rate of those who did not emigrate. This was noted in the *1906 Special Report* as "a curious fact . . . of grave portent to the welfare of our race. . . . Ireland furnished only 15.6 percent of all foreign-born white in the United States in 1900, but 29 percent of all foreign-born white insane in hospitals." In Massachusetts and Connecticut, Irish immigrants constituted less than 30 percent of the population but over 50 percent of the hospitalized insane. A disproportionate representation of Irish immigrants among the hospitalized insane was also reported in England, Canada, and Australia. The Inspectors of Lunatics did not comment on the fact that such data clearly contradicted their own conclusion that "the exodus of the strong and vigorous" accounted for Ireland's high insanity rate. Instead, they simply noted that "the Irish branch of the Celtic race is specially predisposed to mental breakdown."[55]

Offering additional reasons for the high insanity rates in Ireland, the Inspectors of Lunatics suggested two other explanations that had been widely cited for most of the nineteenth century and would continue to be cited throughout the twentieth—heredity and alcohol abuse. Heredity in general, and consanguineous marriages between first cousins in particular, were almost invariably cited as a primary cause of increased insanity in Ireland by both officials and laypersons. This was believed to be especially true for remote rural areas such as parts of Counties Kerry, Galway, and Donegal.

Although it is now known that genetic factors are at least predisposing factors in the causation of insanity (both schizophrenia and manic-depressive illness), there is no evidence that consanguineous marriages produce more insanity. In Ireland the areas thought to have high rates of first-cousin marriages did not have unusually high rates of insanity. Moreover, the *1894 Special Report* of the Inspectors of Lunatics described an isolated island with 348 persons where "intermarriages amongst relations are of absolute necessity," yet during forty years it had produced only one insane person.[56]

More important, four studies of consanguineous marriage rates in Ireland were carried out between 1883 and 1970; all reported that such marriages were uncommon in Ireland and occurred at approximately the same frequency as in other European countries. There have also been studies looking for a correlation between first-cousin marriages and the incidence of schizophrenia in other countries; such studies have failed to find any correlation.[57]

Finally, it should be pointed out that in Ireland more insane persons per population were kept in asylums for more of their reproductive years than in any other country. It is illogical to postulate on genetic grounds that the more insane persons are restricted from procreating, the more insane persons will be born. The reproduction rate of insane persons is low in all countries compared to the general population, but in Ireland it has been exceptionally low. As recently as the 1980s, when Kenneth Kendler and his colleagues carried out an extensive genetic study of schizophrenia in County Roscommon, the reproduction rate of individuals with schizophrenia was reported to be only one-quarter the rate of the general population.[58]

Alcohol excess as a cause of Irish insanity has also been cited by officials and laypersons for the last two centuries. W. J. Corbet, the chief clerk of the Irish Lunacy Department, was an especially strong supporter of this theory. It is well established that chronic alcohol intoxication can produce a type of dementia, but this condition is comparatively rare. In 1911 the Inspectors of Lunatics studied the issue and looked for a correlation between drunkenness and insanity rates. They found none and concluded that "alcohol possesses comparatively small importance as a cause of insanity in Ireland." Despite such data there continued to be a widespread belief in Ireland that alcohol was related to insanity, as illustrated by a traditional folk song:

> Well I went down the lea road a friend for to see,
>
> They call it the Madhouse in Cork by the Sea
>
> But when I got there sure the truth I will tell
>
> They had the poor bugger locked up in a cell
>
> So's the guard tested him, "Say these word if you can:
>
> 'Around the rugged rock the ragged rascal ran.'"
>
> "Tell them I'm not crazy, tell them I'm not mad
>
> 'Twas only the sip of the bottle I had."[59]

Insanity in Politics and Literature

The *1906 Special Report on the Alleged Increase of Insanity* was the last serious attempt to examine this problem in Ireland for over sixty years. The question of increasing insanity was overtaken by political events that pushed such questions into the background. At the Ballinasloe Asylum, for example, a junior physician who was a nationalist and an active member of the Gaelic League was appointed superintendent over a senior physician who was a Protestant. A major reason for his promotion was that the junior physician "had decided to replace the buttons on the attendants' uniforms, which bore an insignia of the crown, with ones bearing the harp and shamrock." Similarly, during a debate in Parliament in 1906, an Irish nationalist charged that "under your rule it has been the survival of the unfittest in Ireland," implying that the English were the cause of Ireland's increasing insanity.[60]

The move toward Irish independence gathered momentum. In 1905 Sinn Fein (Ourselves Alone), the political arm of the nationalist movement, was formed. Five years later the Irish Republican Brotherhood began publishing its own journal, *Irish Freedom,* and political confrontations with England increased sharply. By 1913 a series of strikes began, and an Irish Citizens Army was formed to protect strikers from the police. When World War I broke out the following year, some Irish nationalists decided that England might be vulnerable because of its war efforts, and a major rebellion was planned. This event, the Easter Rising of April 1916, was quickly suppressed by English authorities, and fifteen Irish leaders were executed. But the war for Irish freedom had begun and would continue.

It was during this period of rising nationalist fervor in the early years of the twentieth century that insanity made its first significant appearance in Irish literature. Its absence prior to this time is curious and was noted by David Healy: "This [nineteenth-century absence] is doubly surprising because in addition to apparently producing more lunatics during this period Ireland also produced more writers of genius per head of the population than any other country in the Western world. . . . Given the highest psychiatric bed usage in the world and accordingly what must have been a regular series of dramas played out in the mental health arena, one might expect some reflection of this in the national literature."[61]

It may well be that nineteenth-century Irish writers simply considered insanity an unacceptable literary subject. It was too painful, too shameful, too inviting of English ridicule. One had to consider the effect on one's sister's marriage prospects, on her children, and on her children's children.

That sentiment apparently changed with the appearance of John Synge on the literary scene. In several of his prose pieces written around the turn of the century, insanity was an explicit theme. In *Étude Morbide,* for example, the narrator's mistress goes insane and is taken to a madhouse, where she dies. The narrator himself also appears to be moving toward madness: "My nervousness is increasing. My brain by some horrible decadence is grown a register for appalling things, and my almost preternatural destiny throws such things continually about me. In the newspapers I read of men who have gone mad and slain their kindred; in reviews I find analysis of nerve decay." In Synge's "An Autumn Night in the Hills," the narrator arrives at a peasant cottage, where a woman answers the door:

> "You've come on a bad day," said the old woman, "for you won't see any of the lads or men about the place. . . . They're

after going down to Aughrim for the body of Mary Kinsella.
... She was a fine young woman with two children," she went
on, "and a year and a half ago she went wrong in the head,
and they had to send her away. And then up there in the Richmond asylum maybe they thought the sooner they were shut
of her the better, for she died two days ago this morning."[62]

Synge attributed such cases of insanity to the isolated physical
surroundings of the Irish peasants. In his essay "The Oppression of the
Hills," he noted: "This peculiar climate, acting on a population that is
already lonely and dwindling, has caused or increased a tendency to
nervous depression among the people, and every degree of sadness,
from that of the man who is merely mournful to that of the man who
has spent half his life in the madhouse, is common among these hills."
In *The People of the Glens,* written about rural areas of County Wicklow, Synge alluded to "the three shadowy countries that are never
forgotten in Wicklow—America (their El Dorado), the Union [work-
house], and the Madhouse. ... In Wicklow, as in the rest of Ireland, the
union, though it is a home of refuge for the tramps and tinkers, is
looked on with supreme horror by the peasants. The madhouse, which
they know better, is less dreaded."[63]

Apparently unaffected by political events, the number of insane
persons continued its steady rise. In 1906, when the *Special Report* was
published, there were 23,554 insane persons under care (5.36 per
1,000 total population). By 1914 the number had risen to 25,180. Over
the next five years, there was a decrease in the number of the insane
under care to 22,578 (fig. 7.1). According to the Inspectors of Lunatics,
"This reduction was not due to any lessening of admission rate in District Asylum, which actually increased in 1918, but to a heavy death
rate."[64] The excessive deaths were caused by influenza, which took the
lives of 2,243 patients in 1918 alone. Other deaths were caused by
tuberculosis and pneumonia, made worse by poor patient nutrition
during the war years. The mortality rate for all Irish asylums during
1918 was 11 percent; in the Belfast Asylum, it was 20 percent.

Irish officials kept looking for a sign—any sign—that insanity
was no longer increasing. "Shall we ever reach that happy stage of
social history when it will be possible to say there is no increase in
insanity?" they asked in 1912. In 1851 there had been 5,345 insane

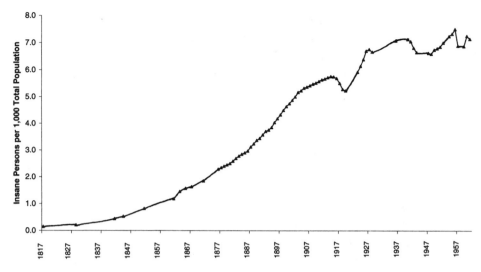

FIG. 7.1. Ireland: Insane Persons in Psychiatric Hospitals, Workhouses, and Jails per 1,000 Population, 1817–1961. Data on which the graph is based are taken from *Report of the Select Committee, 1917;* the annual reports of the Inspectors of Lunatics in Ireland; and Finnane, *Insanity and the Insane in Post-Famine Ireland.*

persons under care, 0.82 per 1,000 total population; by 1914 the number was 25,180, or 5.75 per 1,000 total population, a sevenfold increase in sixty-three years. And increasingly, officials pointed to the costs being incurred, costs that grew larger every year, reaching £19.4 million (1997 equivalent) in 1919. The *Journal of Mental Science* declared that "an eminent specialist is reported to have lately given utterance to the rather pessimistic view that it is only a matter of time until the majority of the population will consist of insane persons."[65]

During the years immediately following the *1906 Special Report,* one other study on insanity in Ireland was noteworthy. In 1911 William R. Dawson analyzed the geographic distribution of insanity and looked at possible correlations between insanity and measures of density of population, pauperism, number of emigrants, number of aged persons, land valuations, and death rates. The counties with the highest rates of insanity under care were found to have shifted modestly since 1851 away from Dublin and its surroundings (fig. 7.2). The highest rates in 1911 were found in Waterford (8.1 per 1,000 total population), Kilkenny (7.6), Meath (7.3), and Westmeath (7.1), while the lowest rates were in Antrim (3.7) and Down (3.9) in Ulster. Dawson found no correlation between insanity and any of the variables he studied except for a direct correlation between insanity and the rate of pauperism.[66] Since earlier studies had suggested that insanity in Ireland occurred more commonly among those of higher socioeconomic levels, Dawson's findings apparently represented a shift.

Politics, however, continued to dominate Irish life during these years and inevitably influenced the asylums. At the Monaghan Asylum in 1919, attendants barricaded themselves in the asylum and raised a red flag on the roof. According to one report, they were "surrounded by a force of 180 policemen and cheered on by the patients" for several days until they agreed to arbitration of their grievances. At the Clonmel Asylum later that year, attendants also went on strike, allowing several patients to escape, and attempted to burn the residence of the medical superintendent.[67]

These events were not anomalous for the times. The Irish Republican Army (IRA), led by Michael Collins, was trading atrocities with English military forces, and the war continued until a truce was called in 1921. An Irish Free State with twenty-six counties was then

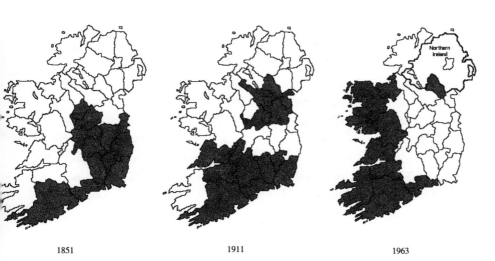

FIG. 7.2. Ireland: Counties with Highest Rates of Insane Persons. *Sources*: 1851, rate based on insane persons in asylums and in the community (*1851 Census*, 51); 1911, rate based on insane persons in asylums and workhouses (Dawson, 1911); 1963, rate based on individuals with schizophrenia and manic-depressive illness in hospitals (Walsh, 1970).

separated from Northern Ireland, which kept six counties, and Ireland became formally self-governing in 1922.

Twentieth-Century Ireland

The independence that the Republic of Ireland achieved in 1922 brought many benefits with it, but decreasing insanity was not one of them. The number of insane persons under care was 5.9 per 1,000 total population in 1923, and this increased slowly but progressively to 7.1 per 1,000 in 1940. Although they did not know it at the time, 1940 would be the crest of Ireland's epidemic of insanity. The number of beds in asylums would continue to slowly increase until 1961, but the rate of total insane persons under care never exceeded the 1940 numbers. New asylums were opened at Ardee in 1933 and at Castlerea in 1940, and there were modest additions to some of the existing asylums. The first psychiatric outpatient clinic opened in 1935, and in 1945 a new Mental Treatment Act was passed that made voluntary admissions to the asylums possible for the first time.

During the years between the world wars, insanity became more prominent in Irish literature, especially in the works of William Butler Yeats, James Joyce, Samuel Beckett, and Sean O'Casey. Yeats's work was almost certainly influenced by the insanity of his sister, Lollie. Even as a child, Lollie had been subject to "prolonged fits of gloom," and as an adult she was often "terribly depressed." Lollie's sister described her as "getting less and less sane. . . . Dr. Goff knows she is incurable." Her psychiatric state continued to deteriorate and reached a nadir in 1911, when she was said by her father to be "full of bitter delusions about everybody. It was quite crazy." The problem, as seen by other family members, including her brother, was that Lollie "had been the object of the unflagging but indecisive attentions of Louis Purser," a sometime suitor for many years, with no resolution of the relationship.[68]

Unrequited love as a cause of insanity had been a common theme in English literature for over a century, as evidenced by various depictions of "Crazy Kate." However, it became prominent in Ireland only in 1929, with Yeats's series on "Crazy Jane," originally published as "Cracked Mary," in *The Winding Stair and Other Poems*.[69] During this same period he wrote other poems dealing with madness. An example is "Tom the Lunatic," Yeats's version of the Tom o' Bedlam tradition.

According to Yeats, impetus for his Crazy Jane poems "was founded upon an old woman who lived in a little cottage near Gort," where Yeats wrote many of his poems. But according to one Yeats scholar, "Some doubts have been expressed as to whether the origin of Crazy Jane is quite so simple as this statement suggests."[70] Surely the psychiatric problems of his sister Lollie were not far from Yeats's mind as he was writing these poems.

Just as William Yeats's sister probably influenced his poems, so did James Joyce's daughter influence Joyce's prose. According to Joyce's biographer, Richard Ellmann, Lucia Joyce first "began to manifest . . . little oddities of behavior" at age twenty-two. Three years later, in 1932, "signs of mental derangement were becoming increasingly apparent,"[71] and she was hospitalized for the first time. By 1935 she had been diagnosed with schizophrenia and thereafter spent most of the rest of her life in a psychiatric hospital in England.

Joyce had a remarkably close relationship with his daughter, and "as her schizophrenia became more and more manifest, he became more and more partial to her." According to Ellmann, "Joyce had a remarkable capacity to follow her swift jumps of thought which baffled other people completely," and he consistently refused to acknowledge her increasing insanity, attributing her strange behavior instead to clairvoyance. In a letter written when her diagnosis was obvious, he said: "Whatever spark of gift I possess has been transmitted to Lucia and has kindled a fire in her brain."[72]

Carl Jung, the Swiss psychoanalyst who was the twentieth psychiatrist to examine Lucia, also noted cognitive similarities between Joyce and his daughter, likening them to "two people going to the bottom of a river, one falling and the other diving." Jung diagnosed James Joyce as having a "latent psychosis" and surmised that he was using alcohol to control his abnormal thinking. However, except for one reference to Joyce's having experienced auditory hallucinations,[73] there is nothing to support Jung's diagnosis.

What is undisputed is that Lucia's illness had an important effect on *Finnegans Wake*, which Joyce wrote between 1922 and 1939. Biographer Ellmann noted that "Joyce had had difficulty since 1931 in working out the final aspects of *Finnegans Wake* and saw Lucia's turmoil during the same period as parallel to his own. . . . Joyce cherished the secret hope that, when he got out of the dark night of *Finnegans Wake,* his daughter would escape from her own darkness."[74]

Many critics have noted neologisms, vague associations, and other psychoticlike elements in *Finnegans Wake.* Nancy Andreason, a psychiatrist and Joyce scholar, summarized these as follows: "Like his last biological child, his final literary child, *Finnegans Wake,* must ultimately be diagnosed as psychotic. . . . Although eccentric, the man never became psychotic. But his art did."[75]

Lucia Joyce may have also influenced Samuel Beckett, who was a frequent visitor to Joyce's Paris household during the years when Lucia was becoming progressively more psychotic. Lucia fell in love with the young Irish writer, and "as her self-control began to leave her, she made less effort to conceal the passion she felt for him." Beckett bluntly rejected her advances, leading James Joyce to inform Beckett "that he was no longer welcome."[76]

Beckett's later work includes the theme of insanity. In *Malone Dies,* written in 1951, the protagonist, Macmann, finds himself in St. John of God Hospital in Dublin, a private insane asylum with buildings "bulking large in spite of their remoteness and all astir with little dots or flecks forever appearing and disappearing, in reality the keepers coming and going." In one cell near Macmann is a catatonic "young man, dead young, seated in an old rocking-chair, his shirt rolled up and his hands on his thighs, [who] would have seemed asleep had not his eyes been wide open." In another cell was "a small thin man pacing up and down . . . asking himself questions in a low voice, reflecting, replying." Perhaps even more pertinent to Lucia Joyce's influence on Beckett was his 1972 play *Not I,* a madwoman's disjunctive monologue in which the protagonist described her auditory hallucinations ("the buzzing . . . dull roar . . . in the skull"), disconnected thoughts ("steady stream . . . mad stuff . . . half the vowels wrong . . . no one could follow . . . till she saw the stare she was getting"), and uncontrolled verbiage ("the whole brain begging . . . something begging in the brain . . . begging the mouth to stop . . . and the brain . . . raving away on its own").[77]

Perhaps the bleakest portrait of an Irish insane asylum was that presented by Sean O'Casey in his autobiographical *Drums under the Window,* written in 1945. In a chapter entitled "House of the Dead,"

O'Casey described the onset of general paralysis (brain syphilis) in a young man and the man's subsequent commitment to the Richmond Asylum in Dublin. The incident was based on O'Casey's 1905 rescue of his sister Ella from an attack by her husband, Nicholas Beaver, named "Benson" in the story, who was in the throes of a psychotic episode. After subduing his brother-in-law, O'Casey had personally escorted him into the asylum, which he later described as a "brotherhood of Bedlamites": "Long rows of lifeless windows mirrored long rows of lifeless faces, . . . a whole stonily grinning gallery of God's images turned to dull grey clay, the emptiness of a future age in every face. . . . Lost amid the quiet storm of lunacy distilling a sour air everywhere. . . . Only ghosts of things and men are here . . . nothing but vacancy reaching to where God has gone from." Benson, he declared, "would be dust to dust and ashes to ashes before he was dead."[78]

Elsewhere in the book, O'Casey describes the Partrane Asylum north of Dublin. Outside the asylum the narrator hears a yell, "an insensible burst of jagged laughter, turning into a savage yell, that gradually declined into a long-drawn, weary, piercing wail making him cold and making him shiver." He then reflects on what he has heard: "So behind this fair, sparkling, laughing curtain that Nature let down before him many dark and evil things were lurking, or hung entangled in the bright colours and satisfying scents like decaying flies in the iridescent and lovely-patterned web of the spider. Forgotten for the moment, he had already seen these things with his own eyes, and his hands had handled them."[79]

The Rediscovery of the Insanity Problem

Following World War II, in which Ireland remained officially neutral and Northern Ireland, as part of the United Kingdom, fought with the Allies, Ireland experienced a period of economic and political instability accompanied by a resurgence of emigration. The number of hospitalized insane increased slightly from 1940 until 1961, at which point the process of deinstitutionalization began. In fact, looking at the entire course of insanity in Ireland (fig. 7.1), it appears that its incidence leveled off slowly in the twentieth century, after climbing steeply throughout the nineteenth century.

In the postwar period, studies on insanity resumed. The immediate precipitant for the new studies was the publication in 1961 of a World Health Organization report comparing by country the number of psychiatric hospital beds. Ireland led the list with 10.8 beds per 1,000 total population, followed by Northern Ireland (7.4), Denmark (7.2), and Sweden (6.7). England and Wales (5.3) and the United States (5.7) had half as many psychiatric beds per population as Ireland, while countries such as France (3.3) and Australia (3.3) had only one-third as many.

Dermot Walsh, the acting superintendent of St. Loman's Psychiatric Hospital in Dublin, drew attention to these results in a 1968 article in the *British Journal of Psychiatry* in which he observed: "There seems little doubt from available statistics that the Republic of Ireland has the highest rate of hospitalized psychiatric morbidity in the world. . . . This author believes that these rates reflect a genuinely increased rate of morbidity in Ireland." Walsh added that the Irish rate of first admissions to psychiatric hospitals was "also one of the highest in world." Based on this first-admission data, Walsh calculated that "18 of every 100 males and 15 of every 100 females surviving to age 65 would experience at least one admission to a psychiatric hospital." Studies in 1981 on admission rates for schizophrenia to psychiatric hospitals confirmed that first-admission and readmission rates were two to three times higher in Ireland than in England.[80]

Walsh's observations rekindled interest in the Irish insanity problem and led to additional studies. Two studies in the 1970s in which the same psychiatrist diagnosed patients in both Ireland and England established the fact that diagnostic differences were not the cause of the differing insanity rates between the two countries. Further studies of hospitalized patients in Ireland also confirmed that the high rate of insanity was not due to less severely affected patients being hospitalized there.[81]

Contemporary studies also established the fact that insanity was not geographically evenly distributed in Ireland and that this uneven distribution had changed over the past hundred years. Data on rates of hospitalized psychoses (schizophrenia and manic-depressive illness) were published for 1963, prior to the widespread deinstitutionalization of psychiatric patients. Among the Irish counties, Galway (9.4 per 100,000 total population), Mayo (7.8), Sligo (7.5), Kerry (7.3), and

Clare (7.0) had the highest composite rates, while Dublin (3.6), Carlow (3.7), and Louth (4.0) had the lowest.[82] In 1851, Galway and Mayo had had the lowest rates of insane persons per population, whereas in 1963 they were among the highest. For Dublin and surrounding counties, the opposite was the case; in 1851 Dublin had had 4.1 times more insane persons per population than Galway, whereas in 1963 Galway had 2.6 times more than Dublin. As shown in figure 7.2, it is as if epidemic insanity had passed over Ireland, moving slowly from east to west during the intervening century.

In addition to this shifting geographical distribution of insanity in Ireland, there was evidence that some areas of the country had especially high rates. As early as 1896, a study of three hundred persons in County Meath reported "29 insane, 7 idiotic, 4 goitrous, 2 suicides, and over a score neurotic." More recently, in the 1990s, studies in Counties Cavan and Monaghan also demonstrated an uneven geographic distribution of schizophrenia. In one part of County Cavan, for example, nine cases of schizophrenia were diagnosed among 465 adults ages fifteen and over; two of the nine were sisters, but the others were unrelated and had no family history of schizophrenia. Similarly, in County Roscommon a study done in the 1980s found forty-eight cases of active psychosis (thirty-two of whom met formal diagnostic criteria for schizophrenia or schizoaffective disorder) among an adult population (ages fifteen and over) of 2,051 individuals (i.e., one out of every forty-seven adults was actively psychotic).[83] County Roscommon is among the poorer counties in Ireland; at the time of the study, 28 percent of houses did not have indoor plumbing and 51 percent did not have a telephone.

There was also good news for Ireland in these recent studies. In the studies of Counties Roscommon and Cavan, the individuals identified with psychosis were almost all over the age of forty, suggesting that the incidence of insanity has decreased in recent years. This decline has been confirmed by other recent incidence studies and was also suggested by the multination incidence study of schizophrenia carried out by the World Health Organization in the 1980s in which Dublin was one site.[84] Given the fact that the 1963 data had found Dublin to have the lowest prevalence of psychoses of any area in Ireland, the comparatively low incidence of schizophrenia found in Dublin in the World Health Organization study was not surprising.

It is not politically correct today to talk about high insanity rates in Ireland, either past or present. One Irish researcher attributed the reports of high rates in the past to the fact that "asylums may have been places where the confused or dependent elderly were cared for, especially in a time of famine and poverty." Other researchers have claimed that the high first-admission rates in the past were caused by patients being admitted to more than one district hospital, despite the fact that cross-county migration of patients was unusual in Ireland. They added: "The question of high rates of schizophrenia in Ireland is an old issue that originated with reported high admission rates of Irish emigrants to New York State hospitals at the turn of the century," that is, the idea that Ireland had a high incidence of insanity was an American idea.[85]

The unique history of insanity in Ireland will not disappear, however, merely by wishing it away. From the days of Jonathan Swift almost three hundred years ago, something unusual happened in Ireland to cause a sharp increase in insanity, a shifting geographical pattern, and a more recent moderation of incidence so that it is no longer unusually high. Rather than simply dismissing such patterns because they do not conform to social or political expectations, they should be studied for clues to the causation of insanity. As part of his generous legacy, Jonathan Swift would most certainly have wanted it that way.

CHAPTER 8

"A Constantly Increasing Multitude"
Atlantic Canada, 1700–1990

Of all the maladies to which the human constitution is incident, the alienation of the intellectual powers is at once the most calamitous and interesting. The possession of those powers places man in an exalted rank in the creation. . . . Deprived of them, he resembles only the ruins of a splendid edifice, or the disorganized fragments of a delicate and complicated machine.

—WILLIAM NEVILLE, *On Insanity,* 1836

But as I am now talking of the Time, when the Plague rag'd at the Eastern-most Part of the Town; how for a long Time the People of those Parts had flattered themselves that they should escape; and how they were surprised, when it came upon them as it did; for indeed, it came upon them like an armed Man, when it did come.

—DANIEL DEFOE, *A Journal of the Plague Year,* 1722

There is virtually no mention of insanity in accounts of Canadian settlement prior to the eighteenth century. Within the seventy-five volumes of the *Relations,* published annually by the seventeenth-century Jesuit missionaries, for example, there are descriptions of epilepsy and other medical conditions, but there is no account of insanity among the native population and only one case among the French settlers.[1] The Jesuits' descriptions of native Canadians who are psychiatrically disturbed are, in fact, classic descriptions of a well-studied cultural spirit-possession syndrome called *windigo,* which was common among the Algonkian-speaking Indians of northeastern Canada in the areas where the Jesuits were working.

The first attempt to provide care for insane persons in Canada was in 1714, when Monseigneur de Saint Vallier "erected a small dwelling . . . for the reception and treatment of those suffering from mental diseases" in Quebec City. This church-managed institution was eventually expanded to hold eighteen persons, and additional smaller facilities were erected by Catholic orders in Montreal and in Three Rivers later in the eighteenth century. In 1824 a special committee of the Legislative Council of Lower Canada, in what is now Quebec, was appointed to survey the problem of insanity. It reported that a total of twenty-six insane persons were confined in these facilities and twelve more were in jails. The population of Lower Canada at that time was just under half a million.[2] There were not yet any facilities for insane persons in the most eastern of the British colonies that would eventually become Atlantic Canada—New Brunswick, Prince Edward Island, Newfoundland, and Nova Scotia.

New Brunswick

In November 1835, a small cholera hospital in Saint John was converted to an insane asylum, giving New Brunswick "the honor of [being] the first of the old British North American provinces to make special provision for its insane" other than through religious organizations.[3] At the time, New Brunswick had almost 120,000 people, including the original French settlers, Tory Loyalists from the United States who had settled in the Saint John region following the American Revolution, and a recent influx of British, especially Irish, immigrants who had come to Canada to work in the burgeoning lumbering, fishing, and shipbuilding industries.

The moving force behind the asylum was George Peters, a twenty-four-year-old Saint John native who had trained in Edinburgh, where he had been exposed to new ideas regarding the treatment of the insane. Peters was the visiting medical officer for the Saint

John almshouse and jail, where he found lunatics in restraints, "some of them perfectly naked and in a state of filth." Such individuals were confined under an 1824 statute that directed "dangerous lunatics" to be "kept safely locked up in some secure place" for the safety of themselves and others.[4]

Peters received support for his asylum proposal from the justices of the peace in Saint John County, who were "alarmed at the growing number of mentally disturbed inmates in the gaols." There were also "many others [insane persons] throughout the Province whose friends were pressing their claims to have them provided for." The commissioners of New Brunswick initially estimated that "the number of insane persons in the province might amount to about fifty" but then reestimated the figure to be 130, or approximately 1 per every 1,000 total population. In their 1837 report, the commissioners also noted: "It is the decided opinion of most persons who have investigated the subject that insanity is on the increase."[5]

The first patients to be admitted to the Saint John Insane Asylum were "two dozen reputed lunatics" who had been confined in the jail and almshouse. By the end of 1836, a total of fifty-six individuals had been admitted; according to Peters, "Many of these unfortunate lunatics have been for months and a few of them for years confined in gaol, or in some dark, ill-ventilated and cold room or cell at the residence of their friends." Diagnostically, twenty-eight of the initial patients were "maniacs," including "a man who had cut his throat from ear to ear," thirteen were "imbeciles" with severe mental retardation, one was a "melancholic," one was "fatuous," and the remaining thirteen had delirium tremens, which Peters considered "not, strictly speaking, insane, nor generally considered proper subjects for a lunatic asylum."[6]

The most salient aspect of the first patients admitted to the hospital in 1836 was the disproportionate number of Irish immigrants among them. Of the first fifty-two admissions for whom place of birth was recorded, thirty-nine of them, or 75 percent, had been born in Ireland, compared with a rate of approximately 20 percent Irish-born persons among the general New Brunswick population. In 1851, by which time there were ninety-nine patients in the asylum, fifty-one of them were Irish immigrants. And this number did not, of course, include insane Irish immigrants who had died en route to New

Brunswick, such as Patrick Coughlin, who arrived in 1849 and was recorded by a port official at Saint Andrews, New Brunswick, as "insane, now dead." By 1871, Irish immigration to New Brunswick had substantially declined, so that the Irish-born constituted only 8 percent of the general population, yet they still made up 35 percent of the Saint John Insane Asylum population. In 1885, when Hack Tuke made his tour of American and Canadian insane asylums, he recorded surprise in noting that among admissions to the New Brunswick asylum since 1875, there had been 308 non-Canadian-born patients, of which "no less than 200 were of Irish extraction."[7]

Rising Numbers

The insane asylum in Saint John became overcrowded almost as soon as it opened its doors in 1835. By 1845, overcrowding had become so marked that the building of a new asylum was being widely discussed. Similar discussions were taking place in Nova Scotia and on Prince Edward Island, and on July 15, 1845, representatives of the three colonies met in Saint John to discuss the possibility of jointly building an asylum. The discussions came to naught, and on April 3, 1846, the New Brunswick House of Assembly voted 14 to 13 to build a new provincial asylum. The close vote reflected substantial opposition to the decision, with the *Saint John Morning News* labeling it "the worst example of financial mismanagement by the ruling clique." The new asylum was planned to accommodate 180 patients, approximately one for every 1,000 population, which the newspaper said "was far too large."[8]

The first wing of the new asylum opened in 1848 and was immediately overcrowded. Such conditions made patient care difficult and the recruitment of good staff almost impossible. Peters noted that those applying for attendant positions were "coarse and ignorant, their only qualification for the position being good muscular development and the absence of all proper sensibility." Instances of attendants' abuse of patients became public, including two instances of "gross misconduct," with dismissal of those involved, and in late 1849 Peters himself was forced to resign.[9]

The new superintendent of the New Brunswick Hospital for the Insane, as the new asylum was called, was John Waddell, a native of

Nova Scotia who had been trained in medicine in Glasgow and Paris. He immediately complained to the legislature regarding the overcrowding, noting that "highly excited inmates were unavoidably mixing with the better class of patients."[10] A wing was added to the asylum in 1852 and other additions were made in 1864, 1879, and 1881. They were filled to more than capacity as fast as they were completed, and by 1881 the asylum, whose official capacity was 200, held 325 patients. The decennial census of 1881 for New Brunswick counted a total of 1,017 insane persons, which meant that there were two more potential patients living in the community for every patient hospitalized.

The rising insanity was noted by the general public. As early as 1845, a Fredericton newspaper carried a fictional account about a man "who suddenly, inexplicably, went mad." Some people claimed that insanity was caused by alcohol abuse, whereas the Saint John *Daily Evening News* blamed it on the stresses of modern living: "The race for riches grows more eager daily. Speculation grows more daring.... The mental powers are subjected to sudden and heavy strains." One aspect of modern living specifically cited as a cause of insanity was railroad travel: "It is probable that to this cause more than to any other the great increase of insanity in those countries where Rail Roads and other great public works are revolutionizing the business transactions and over-stimulating the energies of the people, may be attributed." Earlier in the nineteenth century it had been speculated that insanity was more common in the agricultural areas, but by the latter years there was a consensus that it was more common in urban areas.[11]

Insanity also made its appearance in Canadian novels of this period. According to a study of "eleven novels written by Maritime authors of the 1866–1890 period, ... the lunatic appeared frequently." Typical were the novels of May Agnes Fleming, a New Brunswick native and one of the most widely read Canadian writers of the nineteenth century. Madness was part of the plot for her books such as *A Terrible Secret* (1874) and *A Mad Marriage* (1875). In the former, for example, a young woman is murdered and the event "turns the brain" of her husband to madness; in the end, it is revealed that it was the husband who himself committed the murder while suffering from "monomania."[12]

By 1881, in an effort to decrease the overcrowding, admissions to the asylum were legally restricted to "lunatics clearly dangerous and violent." Patients were being kept in the hospital cellar, and the crowding was said to be "so close that sanitary laws [were] in some measure disregarded." As noted in the Saint John *Daily Telegraph:* "The evils involved in this simple fact [overcrowding] are such as could not well be described in our columns for the details would be offensive and even shocking." In 1885 a farm annex to hold 150 chronic patients was added, but still the beds filled. Applicants for admission had to be turned away, with many ending up in jail. In 1895 the chief of police of Saint John "requested that a cell in the city jail be padded and set aside especially for insane inmates, of whom he had had thirty-five during the year."[13] The number of asylum patients per 1,000 population in New Brunswick had risen from 0.39 per 1,000 total population in 1837 to 1.77 per 1,000 in 1901, more than a fourfold increase.

There was one bright moment in this dreary nineteenth-century history of the New Brunswick asylum. In 1861, Queen Victoria's husband, Prince Albert, visited Saint John and passed by the asylum. The hospital superintendent reported the following effect on the patients:

> The interest manifested by many of the patients in reference to this event, was at once normal and beautiful; the conversation that it suggested respecting Her Majesty the Queen, eliciting expressions of loyalty and love, the desire to see His Royal Highness, the waving of handkerchiefs and other demonstrations of joyous delight, as he passed the hospital, all indicate that, for the time, the idea of the presence of Royalty, and the circumstances connected with it, possessed their thoughts to the exclusion of those subjects which at other times disturb or excite, and when he had passed, embarked, and was gone, and the crowd that followed had dispersed, our household resumed its ordinary quiet all the happier for what they had heard and seen, and probably improved in their mental health.[14]

It is not noted whether the many Irish immigrants among the patient population were similarly affected.

Prince Edward Island

The smallest of Canada's provinces, Prince Edward Island became a separate colony in 1769 with a population of less than 1,000. Until 1799 it was named Saint John Island, but, according to one historian, because Saint John in New Brunswick and Saint John's in Newfoundland were geographically proximate, the situation "gave rise to mistakes and inconveniences in postal matters,"[15] and so the island's name was changed.

By 1831 the population of Prince Edward Island surpassed 30,000. The first acknowledgment of a problem with insane persons was a resolution that year in the House of Assembly establishing "a select committee to inquire into the expediency of making legislative provision for the care of insane persons." The subsequent report recommended the building of a combination asylum and workhouse but noted "the great expense likely to be entailed on the public by providing separately for persons so situated."[16] There the matter rested for fifteen years, mired in politics and fears about the cost.

By the 1840s it was becoming increasingly difficult to ignore the problem. The census of 1841 counted seventy-eight insane and thirty deaf and dumb persons among the 47,042 population, which was increasing rapidly because of a shipbuilding boom. Finally, in 1846 a building was constructed "capable of accommodating about 20 inmates without using the basement cells," and on May 1, 1847, the first eight patients were admitted under the care of John Mackieson, "a well-connected physician" who had come from Scotland in 1821 and had married the daughter of one of the island's leading families.[17]

The settlers of Prince Edward Island were predominantly of Scottish and English in origin. Irish-born residents made up 10 percent of the total population in 1848 and 25 percent in 1861. In hospital admissions, however, Irish-born patients were disproportionately represented, constituting between 27 and 33 percent of admissions each year from 1848 through 1864.[18] These included such individuals as William Donovan, a shoemaker, diagnosed with dementia; Arthur Woods, a laborer, diagnosed with "mania mitis"; Catherine Murphy, a spinster, diagnosed with "moral insanity"; and James Conolly, a farmer, diagnosed with "melancholia tranquilla."

From the opening of the asylum, "overcrowding was the great menace," despite additions to the existing building in 1859, 1867, and 1875. In 1856, for example, the medical superintendent reported that "many applications for admission from various parts of the county . . . have been met with refusal." Admissions increased from ten in 1848, to thirty-two in 1858, and fifty-six in 1868. The following year the medical superintendent said, "We have been obliged to crowd 16 male lunatics together in one sitting room of ordinary dimensions," and in 1871 he reported that many of those unable to obtain admission to the asylum were "at present quartered in the County Jails awaiting their turn."[19]

By this time, only the most severe cases were being admitted to the asylum. In 1870, for example, only four of the fifty-three patients in the hospital at the end of the year had diagnoses other than mania, dementia, or melancholia; two had mental retardation and the other two, "dipsomania." At the time, the hospital had a quaint custom of listing each patient's "favorite pursuit or hobby" as part of the annual asylum report. For 1864 these pursuits included "marching," "talking and singing," "scrubbing, etc.," "desponding," "lying in bed," and "want[ing] to go home."

In 1874 the Prince Edward Island Lunatic Asylum came under intense public scrutiny. The grand jury made a surprise visit to ascertain conditions therein and issued a scathing report:

> The Grand Jury find it difficult to ask your Lordships to believe that an institution, so conducted, would be allowed to exist in a civilized community. In a cell below the ground, about six feet by seven feet, they found a young woman, entirely naked, beneath some broken, dirty straw. The stench was unbearable. There were pools of urine on the floor, evidently the accumulation of many days, as there were gallons of it. . . . The sufferings of these poor people, on the sultry nights of summer and in stormy weather, when the doors are necessarily closed, must far exceed all that we have been told of the Black Hole of Calcutta. . . . The beds and bedding are, with hardly any exception, so abominably filthy that, if they be not alive with vermin, it is because vermin could not exist in such an atmosphere as

surrounds them. . . . It is the feeling of every juror that he would rather see any friend of his die and be buried than to be condemned to a living death in that asylum. We know of no crime so great as to be deserving of a punishment so terrible as to be incarcerated in one of its underground cells.[20]

According to one historian, "This presentment made a profound sensation. . . . The whole province was thrown into an uproar." Dr. Mackieson, the superintendent, was indicted by the grand jury despite his social connections, but the attorney general, who happened to be Mackieson's nephew, refused to prosecute the case. Richard Gidley, the asylum keeper, was also indicted, accused of patient abuse and also of using hospital employees and patients to work on his son's farm. Ultimately, both Mackieson and Gidley were fired but not further prosecuted.[21]

The grand jury report received widespread publicity, both in the local press and in Ottawa. The Charlottetown *Examiner* called Prince Edward Island "the one community in America in which lunatics are treated in a manner unworthy [of] the civilization and Chrisitanity of the age." A new superintendent, Edward Blanchard, was appointed and a hospital addition for twenty-eight patients was approved. The following year, the provincial legislature approved the construction of a new hospital despite major resistance regarding its cost. At this time in Canada, "the public purse gave more to asylums than to any other form of social service," including general hospitals, jails, and reformatories. Advocates for the new asylum on Prince Edward Island cited an American study showing that it was less expensive to cure individuals with insanity and return them to function than to hospitalize them over many years. Therefore, they concluded, "We can lose nothing by our charities in this direction." Such arguments, combined with public embarrassment about existing asylum conditions, carried the day, and in 1877 the building of a new asylum was begun. Two years later all eighty-six patients were transferred to the new building, and Blanchard publicly praised "the great improvement in the demeanor of the patients, the wonderful diminution in the noise . . . and the overcrowding so terribly prevalent in former days."[22]

The publicity generated by the grand jury report also brought more visitors to the asylum. In his annual report for 1877, Blanchard complained of "strangers" who came to visit "out of morbid curiosity": "Many people seem to think that a man has no sooner been stricken with insanity than he forfeits all claims to the rights and privileges of humanity, and is to be regarded much in the light of a wild beast in a menagerie, when the truth is, many are rendered much more sensitive than they formerly were, and are not only annoyed, but retarded in their recovery by such visitors." This was similar to complaints in the 1840s at the Lunatic Asylum in Toronto, which was said to be "visited like zoos" by people wishing to view the inmates.[23]

The improved conditions in the asylum were not to last for long. In 1879 there were twenty-six admissions to the asylum, the following year thirty-five, and by 1882, admissions had increased to forty. In 1881 the medical superintendent complained in his annual report that "already the wards for females are fast becoming overcrowded and something will shortly have to be done to increase our accommodation for this sex. . . . These wards will comfortably provide accommodation for forty patients, while we already have in them fifty-five." By 1885 all admissions to the hospital had to be stopped after August for the duration of the year "because the house became so crowded at that time that it was found impossible to make room for more."[24]

Despite the crowding, an increasing number of insane persons continued to arrive at the asylum's door—fifty-three in 1889, fifty-five in 1895, and sixty-seven in 1901. The number of hospitalized patients per 1,000 total population had increased from 0.26 in 1855 and 0.27 in 1861, to 1.89 in 1901, a more than sevenfold increase. The decennial censuses, which counted "persons of unsound mind" living in the community, reported almost two more such persons for every one hospitalized. The 1898 annual report of the medical superintendent noted: "It needs but a glance at statistics to prove that insanity is on the increase."[25]

Newfoundland

None of the British colonies in eastern Canada was enthusiastic about joining other provinces in confederation in 1867, but Newfoundland was the least enthusiastic. Newfoundland did not, in fact, formally join with Canada until 1949, and even then the vote was close.

Newfoundland was initially colonized in the seventeenth century by fishermen from the West Country of England. The introduction of European diseases among the indigenous Beothuk Native Americans decimated the tribe, and its last member died in 1829. Because of their custom of spreading red ocher and grease on their bodies as protection against mosquitoes, the Beothuk were known as "red Indians," which gave rise to the European stereotype for all North American natives.

In the eighteenth century in Newfoundland, there was an influx of Irish settlers, especially from Counties Cork, Waterford, and Wexford, and by 1750 the Irish outnumbered the English in St. John's, the principal city. Divisions between Irish and English, Catholics and Protestants, and liberals and conservatives became the permanent staple of Newfoundland politics, exacerbated by the relative poverty of the colony as profits from the fishing industry were sent back to England. From 1815 to 1818 the island experienced famine conditions, especially during the harsh winter of 1817–1818, during which "three hundred houses of St. John's were destroyed by fires, . . . [and] a shipload of Irish immigrants left their vessel at the edge of the ice and crawled ashore on their hands and knees to beg provisions from the half-starved inhabitants."[26]

By this time, Newfoundland had a population of approximately 30,000. The few insane persons who were violent were confined to basement cells in St. John's general hospital, which had opened in 1813; "the chronic insane, including idiots, were assigned more or less permanent quarters on the second story adjoining the sick wards. During the winter the wards were unheated [and] snow entered around the windows."[27]

The first indication that insanity might be increasing was in 1834, when the hospital surgeon complained about the "rattling, scratching, jumping and other incontrollable noise" coming from the insane patients, who "usually numbered about seven" and were "chained to benches and walls with their food being passed into them in tins tied to the end of long poles." In an 1836 report, the surgeon described that "one lunatic, a man named McCabe, had lost almost all his fingers the previous winter through frostbite." The chief justice investigated and subsequently described "a scene of wretchedness and misery . . . which must be heart-rending to . . . [all] whose minds are imbued with the smallest tinge of humanity."[28] The sheriff also reported that three lunatics were being held in the local jails. There was some public discussion of the need to build a separate building for insane persons since the general population had passed 75,000, but nothing was done.

In 1838 Henry Stabb, a native of Devon in southwest England whose family had a "long-established involvement there in [Newfoundland's] fish export trade," arrived in St. John's. Stabb, who had been trained in medicine at Edinburgh, "took an immediate interest in the welfare of the mentally ill and sought to introduce the moral treatment method he had observed during his student days." He viewed the insane as "being unquestionably diseased people, and insanity [as] being invariably accompanied, if not produced, by organic or functional disease." In 1842 he offered to take responsibility for the insane patients for a modest salary and even offered to live in the hospital with them: "For Lunatics, especially, can only be treated with a reasonable hope of success, by a Medical Man residing with them, and under whose constant care they ought to sleep, awake, eat, drink and act. A system of management, now practised in all Asylums for the Insane, because, by it, the peculiar nature of the insanity of each Patient,—from simple wandering of the mind, through numerous gradations, up to furious delirium,—may be detected."[29]

The hospital board initially rejected Stabb's offer. However, by 1845, the board, having become aware of "the great increase of the Lunatic Patients" and "the great augmentation in that Asylum of the numbers of these unfortunate beings," decided to employ Stabb and to recommend the establishment of a separate institution "for the reception and cure of persons of unsound mind."[30] Stabb immediately left for France and England to gather ideas from the best asylums, including Salpêtrière, Bethlem, and Hanwell.

On his return to St. John's in 1847, Stabb was disappointed to learn that the money allocated for the building of an asylum could not be spent "owing to the poor state of the colony's finances." Undaunted, Stabb proposed the utilization of a government-owned farmhouse at the edge of town as a "Provisional Asylum for the Insane." The plan was approved, and in November 1847 eleven lunatics were transferred to the farmhouse. At the time, Stabb estimated that "there were between fifty and sixty cases of insanity on the island" among the 100,000 inhabitants, or approximately 0.5 per 1,000.[31]

The provisional asylum became overcrowded almost immediately. In his 1849 report, Stabb noted that "a great increase of the numbers of insane patients has taken place, viz.: from 23 to 42, being an increase of three-fourths." He lobbied hard for the construction of a proper asylum and was assisted by a visit to Newfoundland by Dorothea Dix in 1848. Dix, who pledged £4,200 (1997 equivalent) of her own funds to help, was viewed as a kindred spirit and was greatly admired by Stabb. In one letter to her, Stabb wrote: "There is no earthly pleasure like that of being instrumental in doing great things for the wretched, lifting a poor insane person from degradation and misery unutterable, to much comfort and hope, even to reason and health! . . . It is unquestionable that it is a privilege, and not a task—to help the miserable."[32]

Stabb's persistence ultimately paid off, and in July 1853 construction on a new asylum for seventy-five patients began. Opposition to the plan, however, continued to be significant. When Dorothea Dix returned to Newfoundland in 1853 to lend support and try to raise additional funds, she was completely unsuccessful, due, in part at least, to "the local population's resentment of Dix's puritanical piety and almost messianic zeal, which alienated both Catholics and Protestants alike." And in 1855, the local *Patriot* editorially attacked the new asylum "as altogether upon [*sic*] too extensive as well as expensive a system. . . . Treatment in the lavishly expensive Insane Hospitals here, we cannot but regard the outlay as a reckless waste of an enormous sum of money."[33] Despite such opposition, the new asylum opened in December 1854, and all fifty inmates were transferred to it from the provisional asylum.

"Apparently on the Increase"

In examining existing data on the earliest cases of insanity admitted to the Newfoundland asylum, two aspects are prominent. The first is that most patients who were admitted were severely affected by their illnesses. For example, in his 1849 report, Stabb described a woman who had been insane for five and a half years who was, when admitted, "a frightful object, in filth and rags, lower limbs contracted, knees touching the chin. . . . She spent the whole night and day in roaring and cursing, saying she was on fire for her sins. . . . The calls of nature were to her as to the brutes." Almost all admitted patients suffered from a form of mania or dementia. The few who were admitted with "amentia" (mental retardation) were either severely affected or were also insane. For example, in 1849 Stabb admitted a mother and daughter, both diagnosed with "amentia," who were described as "sent from Fortune Bay, where they lived under a large rock and lived on shell fish, etc. . . . [They are] scarcely above the condition of wild animals." As Patricia O'Brien noted in her history of the Newfoundland asylum: "One suspects that the vast majority of nineteenth-century asylum patients were either legitimately psychotic or manifested severe behavioural symptoms owing to some form of neurological or physical condition. There was far too much pressure on asylum beds for the situation to have been otherwise."[34]

The other prominent aspect of the early admissions to the Newfoundland asylum was the disproportionate representation of Irish immigrants. In 1857, most of Newfoundland's population was second- or third-generation and English or Irish in origin. The largest recent immigrant group was Irish, yet it constituted only 6 percent of the total population (7,383 out of 124,288). But in 1849, eleven out of twenty-five admissions (44 percent) to the provisional asylum were Irish born, and in 1851, the figure was eight out of nineteen (42 percent). Since most recent Irish immigrants lived in St. John's and were thus close to the asylum, this may partially explain their disproportionately high rate of admission. Included were such patients as I. L., a fisherman described as "an irritable maniac just released from chains"; T. P., a fisherman "subject to periodical fits of violent excitement"; and M. C., a woman suffering from "puerpal [postpartum] mania." Eight years later, three Irish women were added to the permanent asylum roster when they were shipwrecked off the Newfoundland coast and brought ashore. They had tried to emigrate to America but had been refused entry in New York because of their insanity and were en route back to Ireland when their boat went down.[35]

The new asylum filled up as quickly as had the provisional one. In December 1855, at the end of just one year, Stabb complained about "the crowded state of the wards and bedrooms" and, noting that "the attic, which was designed for a different purpose, has been filled with

patients," he recommended that an additional wing be built. In 1858
Stabb reported that it was necessary to refuse admission to some
applicants and that "8 persons who took away their insane relatives
received a small annual sum for their support" as one means of relieving the overcrowding.[36]

In 1859 Stabb offered the opinion that "insanity in this country
[is] apparently on the increase." The following year, he again noted
"the increase of insanity in [sic] the island" but guessed that the
patients' increased longevity partially explained their accumulation.
Stabb's reasoning was undoubtedly influenced by the fact that the
death rate among the asylum patients had been unusually low from
1858 through 1860; the rate subsequently increased, and a longitudinal analysis of asylum mortality rates from 1855 to 1889 shows no
overall decrease whatsoever.[37]

The increase in insane persons appeared to grow each year.
During the 1860s, applicants for admission were commonly turned
away, and "as beds became available, the Board of Works chairman
selected from among the waiting applicants, who were often held in
jail in the meantime." It also became common practice to transfer
some of the chronic patients from the asylum to the workhouse, thus
reversing the flow of earlier years; by 1870 Stabb reported that "the
wretched temporary wards for the insane in the Poor House are full of
patients, as well as the wards of the Asylum."[38]

The following year, both the asylum and poorhouse were so full
of insane patients that "the government began to board mental
patients in private homes at rates ranging from $1.00 to $1.20 per
week." It also converted the Signal Hill Hospital, previously used for
smallpox patients, into an ancillary asylum. "Thus, mental patients
were now scattered between the asylum, the poorhouse, the Signal Hill
Hospital, five or more boarding homes, and the St. John's Hospital to
which patients in need of serious medical or surgical attention were
referred."[39]

Despite what must have seemed like trying to reverse an incoming tide, Stabb never gave up. In 1857 his wife's sister, who had come to
live with them, became mentally ill and was sent to Philadelphia for
ongoing treatment. In 1866 an epidemic of scarlet fever killed four of
his seven children within three weeks. Despite such personal tragedies,
Stabb persisted in his efforts to improve patient care and to raise funds

to build more hospital facilities. Further additions to the hospital were built in 1863, 1873, 1877, and 1881, but they were immediately filled. In 1868 Stabb proposed a tax on all fishermen "which, assuming that there are 25,000 fishermen, at $1 each per annum, would establish an adequate fund for the purposes required." Instead, "the government dramatically reduced the per patient level of asylum expenditure," so that by 1886 Stabb claimed that "the annual expenditure for each individual inmate of the Asylum is less than any similar Institution in British America."[40]

By this time, Stabb was seventy-four years old and in failing health. He continued as superintendent until 1889, when he retired. He had been working to improve the treatment of insane persons in Newfoundland for almost half a century and must have been discouraged by what he saw. At the end of 1847, the year Stabb opened the provisional asylum, the patient population had numbered seventeen, and he had estimated that "there were between fifty and sixty cases of insanity on the island" among the 100,000 inhabitants. By the end of 1889, there were 179 patients in the asylum and others in the Signal Hill Hospital, general hospital, poorhouse, boarding homes, and jails, or living at home with their families. The population in 1889 was approximately 200,000, a doubling since 1847, while the number of insane persons appeared to have increased by more than tenfold.

Henry Stabb was succeeded in the position of asylum superintendent by Kenneth MacKenzie, a native of Prince Edward Island who had been trained in Edinburgh. MacKenzie's tenure was relatively brief after an official inquiry reported that "he had been drunk during most of his visits" and "had suffered from delirium tremens when he had wandered about at night in a dressing gown with a burning candle and had required constant supervision." Most seriously, however, "he had attempted to force his attentions on some of the women."[41] It became clear to the hospital board that the new superintendent was as much in need of help as some of the patients, and he was forced to resign after less than two years on the job.

Nova Scotia

During the second half of the eighteenth century, Nova Scotia was an ethnic potpourri that had emerged with the fortunes of war and the arrival of new immigrants. Most of the original French settlers, known as Acadians, had been deported in the mid-1750s during the final phase of the British-French struggle for control. Many of them had gone to Louisiana, where their descendants became Cajuns. After the assumption of complete British control in 1763, the population grew with Yorkshire English, Gaelic-speaking Scottish Highlanders, Ulster Irish, and a residue of Acadians. Following the American Revolution, Loyalist refugees arrived from the United States along with a group of German Protestants, many of whom had been attached to British forces during the Revolutionary War.

Halifax, the capital, was a military town, founded as a British naval base and garrison in 1749 and "infested with grog shops, brothels, boarding houses and tenement accommodations for military dependents and the civilians who preyed upon the army." In 1759, when the population of Acadia was approximately 15,000, authorities opened a combination workhouse and jail in Halifax to accommodate "all disorderly and idle persons, and such who shall be found begging, or practising any unlawful games, or pretending to fortune-telling, common drunkards, persons of lewd behaviour, vagabonds, runaways, stubborn servants and children, and persons who notoriously misspend their time to the neglect and prejudice of their own of their family's support." The only mention of insane persons at this time was in the statutes, where it was noted that "if any person or persons committed to the said House of Correction be idiots, or lunatic, or sick or weak, and unable to work, they shall be taken care of and relieved by the master or keeper of the said House."[42]

In the records of the later years of the eighteenth century, there are suggestions that insane persons were becoming more prominent. A 1774 law directed that dangerous lunatics be "kept safely locked up in some secure place" and chained if necessary, and added, moreover, that "nothing herein contained shall . . . restrain any friend or relative of such lunatics from taking them under their own care."[43]

By the turn of the century, Nova Scotia had grown to over 60,000 inhabitants, and the workhouse, now known as the Poor's Asylum, was averaging over two hundred admissions each year. Records for the years 1802 through 1811, which include a breakdown by diagnostic category for all admissions, show that individuals admitted for reasons of "physical condition" or "poverty related" constituted the vast majority each year, while admissions for "mental conditions" made up between 3 and 11 percent of the total. For example, in 1809, nineteen admissions out of the total 288 (7 percent) were admitted for "mental conditions." Among the nineteen were ten "insane," three "weak in mind," two with "mental imbicility" [*sic*], two with "irregular living," one diagnosed as "lunatic," and one with "fits."[44]

By the 1830s, the Poor's Asylum had achieved notoriety in Halifax as a dumping ground for all unfortunates. One legislative committee reported that the asylum's buildings "were originally intended for the indigent and aged only, but are now made to serve for a general hospital, a lunatic asylum, an orphans house, a sailors hospital, and a lying-in institution." Another committee noted that "the close association of lunatics and children did not create a very healthy atmosphere. . . . The need for separate accommodation for lunatics is apparent."[45]

In the 1840s, the problem of insanity in Nova Scotia became more publicly visible. The colony was undergoing rapid growth because of the thriving lumbering and shipbuilding industries, with a consequent doubling of the population between 1815 and 1840. Much of the increase was accounted for by immigrants, 43,000 of whom entered Nova Scotia between 1815 and 1838. The majority of these were Scottish and English in origin, but they also included 2,000 immigrants from Ireland who arrived in 1827 and brought with them an epidemic of typhus. That winter "more than 500 coffins were carried from the poorhouse."[46] The association of the Irish immigrants with the typhus epidemic did not improve their social standing among the local residents.

Increasingly, suggestions were made that insanity might be on the rise. The 1844 annual report from the Poor's Asylum showed that "one eighth of the total number housed therein were insane with no hope or chance of recovery," and the number appeared to be growing; by 1849 the asylum had a waiting list for beds reserved for the insane. An 1846 report to the Assembly noted that "since public attention has been turned to this subject [lunacy], the extent of this most distressing malady has been found everywhere much greater than is generally supposed." And when Lieutenant-Governor Sir John Harvey opened the 1847 session of the Assembly, he specifically noted the problem of "pauper lunatics" as "that class of unhappy beings which I grieve to believe is rapidly increasing in these colonies." Harvey had a personal interest in such things because his son had become insane and had been sent to Boston for treatment.[47]

Because of such sentiments, the House of Assembly in 1846 designated a committee "for ascertaining the most suitable Site in the Province for a Lunatic Asylum, and for ascertaining the probable expense of founding and sustaining such an Establishment."[48] In carrying out this mandate, the committee undertook a survey to ascertain the number of insane persons in Nova Scotia so that it could recommend an appropriate size for the asylum. The committee wrote to "the Members of both branches of the Legislature, also to the Sheriffs, Chief Magistrates, and principal Medical Men in the different Counties," asking each to count "the number of Lunatics" as well as "the numbers of Deaf and Dumb persons" within their jurisdictions.

The number of replies was smaller than expected but allowed the committee to estimate that among the population of 250,000 "there are not fewer than three hundred Lunatics in Nova Scotia," including forty in the Poor's Asylum and twenty-five who had been sent by their families to asylums in New Brunswick or the United States. Returns from Pictou County, which were thought to be especially complete, counted forty-six insane persons among a population of approximately 30,000, or 1.53 per 1,000 total population. The committee therefore recommended that the new insane asylum should "be constructed for only one hundred and twenty patients at first, yet so as easily to admit of future additions."[49]

During the 1840s, Hugh Bell emerged as the leading proponent for the building of an insane asylum for Nova Scotia. He had been born in Ireland but was raised in Halifax and had had a successful career as a bookkeeper, brewer, journalist, Methodist preacher, and member of the Assembly. In 1844, at age sixty-four, Bell was elected mayor of Halifax. He immediately offered to donate his annual salary of £12,750 (1997 equivalent) to a fund to build an insane asylum, and by 1845 had solicited other donations and raised the fund to almost £38,250 (1997 equivalent). He had been a commissioner for the Poor's Asylum and had been shocked by seeing "naked men and women with arms and legs chained to floors of tiny cells." In a report to the Assembly, Bell noted: "The bodily sufferings of this class of people are far greater than is imagined—and that many are now enduring hardships and cruelties in the common jails of the country, and shut up in solitary places of confinement, whose condition is worse than that of the criminal, and whose misfortunes are aggravated by the ignorance and neglect of those who have them in custody." Such outcomes were not necessary, Bell said, because "if taken in time and with proper treatment, the disease is as susceptible of cure as any other disorder."[50]

In 1845, in order to learn more about the treatment of insane persons, Bell traveled to the United States and visited asylums in Maine, New Hampshire, Massachusetts, Connecticut, New York, and Pennsylvania. Upon his return, he gave the Assembly a complete written report of his findings. "In almost every county in Europe and America, and nearly every town," he said, "asylums are now provided for their [insane persons'] especial benefit and by a system of kindness and sympathy . . . many are restored."[51]

At the same time as Hugh Bell was lobbying for an insane asylum for Nova Scotia, Dorothea Dix was doing likewise in the United States, and in September 1849 she visited Halifax. She later recalled that she "found in a department of the Halifax Poor House . . . *forty-four* insane men and women suffering under different forms of the malady which placed them in a most helpless condition."[52]

Three months after her visit, Dix sent a strongly worded petition to the Legislative Assembly concerning "that class of unhappy beings, which I grieve to believe is *rapidly increasing in these Colonies*" and "numbered now by hundreds in the Province of Nova Scotia." Such individuals are often "incarcerated in filthy, unventilated apartments, cold, comfortless huts and cabins, and in dreary cells and dungeons; not seldom fed and sheltered with less care than the brutes, and Pariah-like, cast beyond the pale of respect, affection, and sympathy." Dix claimed that "when brought under *early, efficient* treatment" insanity was "equally manageable and curable as a fever or a cold," and she presented extensive data from American asylums to demonstrate that in the long run it was less expensive to treat such individuals than not to treat them. "It is time," she added, "that people should have learnt that to be insane is not to be disgraced—that sickness is not to be ranked with crime; and that mental disability is almost invariably the result of mere bodily ailments." She finished her petition by challenging the legislators: "Shall Nova Scotia be last and least in responding to the loud calls of humanity—shall she be latest and alone in affording evidence of godliness, civilization, and the improvements and great moral works which characterize the present age!"[53]

Dorothea Dix's petition failed to move the Assembly. Discouraged, Bell wrote to her that "even you cannot thaw the frozen atmosphere that envelops the sympathies, or rather the place where the sympathies ought to be, of our legislators." As one observer noted in reviewing these events, "It was not a matter of economic restraints as money was spent on roads and the railway, it was that the asylum was not a priority in the house of assembly." Opposition to building an asylum continued to be strong, and Bell was occasionally fleered in the local press:

> Our own Hugh Bell,
>
> Our little Hugh Bell,
>
> He's busy a-building a lunatic cell.[54]

Despite the opposition, Dorothea Dix continued to support Bell's efforts, returning to Nova Scotia in September 1852 and again in June 1853. In one of her most effective approaches, she challenged the members of the Assembly to imagine themselves as insane inmates of Poor's Asylum:

> In imagination, for a short hour, place yourselves in their stead, enter the horrid noisesome cell, invest yourselves with the foul, tattered garments which scantily serve the purpose of decent protection; Cast yourselves upon the loathsome pile of filthy straw, find companionship in your own cries and groans or in the wailing and gibberings of wretches miserable like yourselves. Call for help and release, for blessed words of soothing and kind offices of care, 'til the walls are weary of sending back the echo of your moans; then, if self possession is not overwhelmed under the imaginary misery of what are actual distresses of the insane, return to consciousness of your sound intellectual health, and answer if you will longer repose or delay to make adequate appropriations for the establishment of a Provincial hospital for those who are deprived of reason

and thereby of all that can gladden life or make existence a blessing.[55]

In 1854 in Nova Scotia, there were "four murders committed within a year, all by men who were subsequently found to be insane." In one case, a soldier suddenly killed one of his comrades because he believed that "persons were putting offensive smells to his nose, and in his bed clothes. . . . His is the act of a madman." In another, a man brutally murdered a woman "in a most shocking manner. . . . Persons who have known him for some time speak of his lunacy."[56] Such highly publicized homicides committed by insane persons illustrated the need for treatment of those afflicted and encouraged the Assembly to carry through on building an asylum.

At last, on May 16, 1855, ground was broken for an insane asylum on a bluff across the harbor from Halifax. When the cornerstone for the asylum was laid at a ceremony in June 1856, "The citizens flocked—by ferry, by tugs, by sailboats and by row-boats—to witness the rites," which included two bands, the volunteer artillery, an honor guard, and Masonic groups such as "the Army Masons in scarlet" and "the African masons in ivory and black." "And to crown all, an immense fog settled upon the city . . . and the jolly old rain poured down."[57] It was not an auspicious beginning.

"This Fearful Affliction"

The first patients were admitted to the asylum, named Mount Hope, in December 1858 under the care of the superintendent, James DeWolf. A native of Nova Scotia, DeWolf had been trained in medicine in Edinburgh and had practiced in rural Nova Scotia and in Newfoundland. The initial patients included "two men [who] were brought [there] by water from a distant part of the province, confined in low rough plank boxes or coops. They were exposed on the deck of the vessel for nine days to the inclemency of the weather, and fed through a small opening." Another patient from a distant county took thirty-nine days to reach the institution.[58]

By the end of 1859 the asylum held 55 patients, and three years later there were 130. "Overcrowding was an almost constant condition," according to a history of Mount Hope, and each year DeWolf pleaded for additional buildings and more beds:

> 1864: As predicted in former reports, the hospital is now crowded "beyond its capacity to afford either comfortable or healthful accommodation." The time has arrived when admissions must necessarily be limited to correspond with the discharges. The plea for increased accommodation for the insane, is one that appeals to every class in the community. None, however exalted their position, or however humble their lot, can claim exemption from a liability to this fearful affliction.

> 1865: The reports of this hospital from year to year, bear evidence of the anxiety of your superintendent that additional rooms should be provided. The first appeal was kindly met by the erection of the South wing, and no sooner was this built, than it was filled to its utmost capacity. It appears now absolutely necessary, not merely for the sake of those who are crowded together here, but still more for the care of those unable to gain admittance, that further and adequate provision should be promptly made, by extending and completing the hospital.[59]

In 1865 the number of patients in the hospital reached 150; less than three years later the number reached 200, and by 1875 there were more than 300 patients. During these same ten years in which the patient population more than doubled, the total population of the province grew by less than 15 percent, from approximately 350,000 to 400,000. The growth in patient population occurred despite the fact that "from the beginning the Nova Scotia asylum at Mount Hope was governed by a law that allowed recent and acute cases of insanity to be given preference over more chronic cases. . . . Mental defectives and cases of long-term illness were refused admittance."[60]

The increasing numbers of insane persons in the Nova Scotia asylum were mirrored by increasing numbers of individuals of "unsound mind" being counted in the Nova Scotia general censuses.

In 1851 the number of such individuals was 465; in 1861 the comparable figure was 657, or 1.99 per 1,000 total population. By 1871 the census had increased to 1,254 individuals of "unsound mind," or 3.23 per 1,000. Such figures concerned DeWolf, and in his 1876 annual report to the Assembly he concluded: "Assuming that the returns are approximately correct we have evidence here of a marked and steadily progressive increase, and although every allowance be made for imperfect returns in 1851, the fact remains, that while the advance in the population was at the rate of forty per cent (40) in twenty years, the numbers of those of unsound mind increased one hundred and sixty-nine per cent (169) in the same period."[61]

DeWolf and many of his colleagues attributed most of the increasing insanity to reproduction by those genetically inclined toward insanity. "The prime factor among the causes of insanity," according to Alexander Reid, DeWolf's successor, was "hereditary predisposition." DeWolf reported that "there are among our inmates a mother and her two daughters, neither [sic] of whom appears at all to recognize the others," as well as several sibling pairs. DeWolf's proposed solution to the problem of increasing insanity was eugenics: "Would that it were possible, by the enactment of prohibitory laws, to prevent those with either incipient or innate insanity, as well as the habitual drunkard, from entering into the married state."[62] DeWolf did not explain why the insanity rate was continuing to increase rapidly despite the confinement of increasing numbers of insane individuals that made their reproduction virtually impossible.

In Nova Scotia, as elsewhere, there were many other theories regarding the causes of rising insanity. "The monster evil of intemperance, with its associated vices and accidental accompaniments," was always a popular target for reformers. Another Halifax physician accounted for the increasing insanity as follows: "The close and constant aggregation of the young together (in the vitiated atmosphere of a crowded mill,) has a tendency to excite the emotional and effective sensibilities of our nature, and to awaken the sexual passion before its proper time. The effect of this in the production of insanity need not be pointed out to anyone practically conversant with the subject." Blaming modern living as a cause for insanity became increasingly popular, especially among reformers: "Our cities are overcrowded with a jostling, rushing throng, amid artificial conditions of life, subjected to the exhausting effects of high pressure existence, coupled with anxiety and worry, and to which are in many cases added to the deleterious effects following the use of narcotics and alcoholic stimulants and the evil results of excessive and impure sexual indulgence. As a consequence more people are exposed to the conditions which make for insanity."[63]

It was also noted in the early years of the Nova Scotia asylum that a disproportionate number of inmates were Irish immigrants. In 1861 a provincial census included data on the asylum's ninety-seven patients and listed the place of birth for ninety-one of them. Of these, sixty-six had been born in Nova Scotia or one of the surrounding colonies, four in Scotland, one each in England, France, and Barbados, and eighteen in Ireland. Thus, Irish-born patients constituted at least 19 percent of the patient population even though they made up only 3 percent (9,313 out of 331,057) of the general population. This overrepresentation of Irish-born patients in the Nova Scotia asylum was similar to the situation in New Brunswick, Prince Edward Island, and Newfoundland. It was also reflected in traditional folk songs from Nova Scotia, such as "Riley's Courtship," in which young Willie Riley, who is courting the squire's daughter, is banished to Ireland, "Loaded with heavy irons / Confined in Sligo jail." In reaction, the young woman becomes insane:

> Three nights this lonely lady
> In grief and sorrow spent,
> Till overcome with anguish
> She quite distracted went.

> She wrung her hands and tore her hair,
> Crying, "My only dear,
> My cruel-hearted father
> Hath used you most severe."

> Unto a private madhouse
> They hurried her away,
> Where she was heard each morning
> For to weep and pray

Her chains loud she'd rattle,
And then would cry and rave,
"For me poor Willie Riley
Is treated like a slave." [64]

Given the crowded conditions in the asylum and the severity of patients' illnesses, problems were inevitable. In 1861 the asylum's steward was dismissed, apparently for having had sex with several inmates. Six years later, there was an inquiry into the death of a young male patient whose family was given a "bruised, lice-ridden corpse." In 1877 an inmate froze to death, and allegations were made that the "wards were filthy and no treatment was being carried out." [65] A commission was appointed to investigate but was controlled by politicians opposed to DeWolf. After hearing forty witnesses, the majority of whom were hospital employees who had been dismissed by DeWolf for drunkenness and abuse of patients, DeWolf was himself dismissed, along with three senior assistants.

Alexander Reid, who succeeded DeWolf, had good intentions but also faced the continuously increasing demand for admissions to an already overcrowded asylum. Reid believed that insanity's "manifestations take place through the brain and nervous system, a material organism subject to ordinary pathological conditions" and that it should therefore be treatable. However, if the patients did not receive proper treatment, Reid said, they would "gradually sink into a vegetative species of life, with total obscuration of the mind, so to remain often for many years before death opens up a new scene to the occluded and imprisoned soul." [66]

Reid realized that the Mount Hope asylum would never be large enough to provide care for the increasing numbers of insane persons in Nova Scotia, so he explored alternatives. Building a second asylum just for chronic patients, building cottages on the hospital grounds, and having each county in the province erect its own small asylums were all considered. After much public discussion regarding costs, the last option was chosen, and in 1886 the plan was implemented. By 1890 eleven county hospitals for insane persons had been built, which brought temporary relief to the crowded wards at Mount Hope.

The county hospital solution proved illusory, for these facilities were soon overcrowded as well, and pressure for Mount Hope to admit more patients increased again. In 1894 George Sinclair, who had succeeded Reid in 1892, reported that "during almost the entire year our wards for male patients have been dangerously overcrowded. . . . We have been obliged to reject many applicants for admission." Rhetorically, he asked: "Is a man less a citizen and a brother because his brain and not his liver is at fault?"[67]

By 1896, admissions to Mount Hope had increased to 130, "the largest number ever received during a period of twelve months." Only twenty-three of these were readmissions. No central statistics were kept on the county hospitals, so it was not possible to determine the total number hospitalized. In 1898, Sinclair noted that the constant overcrowding of the county asylums and Mount Hope "furnish the public with a very reasonable pretext for supposing that sufferers from mental disease must be increasing."[68] Sinclair speculated that some of the increase was being caused by patients living longer, but in fact the death rate in the Mount Hope Asylum was higher in the 1890s (6.1 percent per year) than it had been in the 1860s (5.7 per year).

As the century closed, pessimism settled over Nova Scotia like its ubiquitous fog. William Hattie, who had become superintendent in 1898, observed: "It is useless to mince matters. I am not reflecting upon any who have preceded me in office here. The treatment to-day is not very different from what it has been since the doors of the institution were first opened, and the statistics of to-day are scarcely better than were those of ten, or twenty, or thirty years ago." "Insanity," he added, "is a fearful malady; there is none other so much dreaded, none other capable of causing such suffering to patient and such distress to friends."[69]

"This Dread Malady Is Rapid Growing"

The beginning of each new century brings hope, and Canadian officials hoped for an abatement of the steadily increasing number of insane persons. As part of the censuses of Canada in 1901 and 1911, a count was made of all blind, deaf and dumb, and insane persons. The census enumerators were instructed that "the degree of infirmity should not be absolute or total, but so sufficiently marked in any one

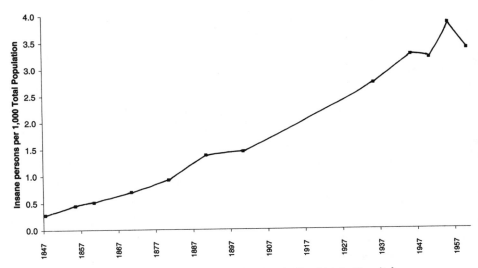

FIG. 8.1. Canada (Atlantic Provinces): Insane Persons in Psychiatric Hospitals per 1,000 Population, 1847–1960. Nineteenth-century data on which the graph is based are taken, for Nova Scotia, New Brunswick, and Prince Edward Island, from the annual reports in each province's *Journals of the House of Assembly*, and for Newfoundland, from O'Brien, *Out of Mind, Out of Sight*. Data for the twentieth century were provided by Statistics Canada.

of the classes as to have reached the stage of incapacity." Enumerators were also instructed to note whether the infirmity had existed from birth or early childhood, thus separating mentally retarded individuals from those insane.[70]

A similar "census of infirmities" had been carried out in 1891 and provided a basis for comparison. In the intervening decades between 1891 and 1911, the insanity rate for both institutionalized and noninstitutionalized persons on Prince Edward Island had increased from 3.1 to 4.2 per 1,000 total population, Nova Scotia had increased from 3.0 to 3.4 per 1,000, and only New Brunswick had remained unchanged at 2.7 per 1,000 (fig. 8.1). These censuses also indicated that approximately 55 percent of all insane persons in these provinces were in the asylums, with the remainder living in the community. Newfoundland was not included in these national censuses since it was not part of Canada at that time.

By 1905 there was a widespread realization in Canada generally that insanity was continuing to increase. Reflecting on the results of the 1901 census, Thomas Burgess, in an article in the *Montreal Medical Journal*, observed:

> In 1891 there were 13,342 insane persons in a population of 4,719,893, in 1901 there were 16,622 in a population of 5,318,606, being an increase, in ten years, of nearly twenty-five per cent, in the number of lunatics, whereas the increase in the total population was less than thirteen per cent. . . . It is the consensus of opinion that insanity is on the increase in Canada as elsewhere. . . . It has become a burning question whether something cannot be done to lessen an evil which imposes upon the community an enormous load of taxation for the maintenance of a large and constantly increasing multitude of those mentally afflicted.[71]

The main cause of the increase, said Burgess, was "hereditary taint," and a secondary cause was "our high-pressure civilization" in which "nervous systems have been laid more open to the unkind influences of material and moral forces." Throughout Canada in the early years of the twentieth century, heredity continued to be thought of as the main cause of insanity; an admission note for an insane patient to the New Brunswick hospital stated this theory most succinctly: "Wrong made from the first."[72]

In New Brunswick, overcrowding of the hospital in Saint John continued to grow worse, so a second hospital was built at Campbellton. The total number of hospitalized insane patients grew from 587 in 1900 to 2,218 in 1955, an increase of 378 percent, during which time the province's population increased 56 percent.

On Prince Edward Island, the story was similar. In 1900, there were 195 patients in the provincial mental hospital, and in 1955 there were 388, an increase of 99 percent. However, during these same years the population of the province *decreased* from 103,259 to 99,285.

Newfoundland also experienced continuing overcrowding in the hospital at Saint John's. At the turn of the century the hospital, with 170 patients, was described as having "surface sewage . . . seep[ing] into the incoming main" water supply, and "rats were [said to be] everywhere."

Waiting lists, refusals of admissions, and the transfer of patients to the workhouse or to boarding homes all became commonplace, and the situation grew worse with each passing year. In 1943 the bed capacity was 325, but the patient population of the hospital was 629: "Cots in the dormitories touched head to foot and side by side; patients took turns in the beds; and in most wards, sleeping, eating, and recreational areas were virtually indistinguishable."[73] By 1950, the hospital had 688 patients, an increase of over 300 percent since 1900, during which time Newfoundland's population had increased 64 percent.

In Nova Scotia, the county hospital plan, which had been implemented in 1886 as a means of decreasing overcrowding of the asylum in Halifax, did not solve the problem. By 1904 there were seventeen county asylums, but the asylum in Halifax, renamed the Nova Scotia Hospital, noted in its annual report that "in spite of the presence of municipal asylums in seventeen localities throughout our province, there has been a notable increase in the number of admissions to the hospital. This can scarcely be regarded in any other light than indicating a decided increase in the proportion of the insane to the general population. . . . It is painfully evident that in our province the prevalence of this dread malady is rapidly growing greater." Two years later, the superintendent reported "a greater congestion of our wards than any year in the history of the institution" due to "the extraordinarily rapid increase in the number of admissions." In 1909 the superintendent again reported continuing increases in admissions and severe overcrowding and concluded: "Our experience certainly appears to favor the view that insanity is becoming increasingly prevalent."[74]

The situation in New Brunswick, Prince Edward Island, Newfoundland, and Nova Scotia was representative of Canada as a whole. As fast as hospital additions could be completed, they were filled. Some of the newly admitted patients were elderly individuals with dementia, as was true in England, Ireland, and the United States, but the great majority were insane. In 1952, for example, among all patients in public mental hospitals in New Brunswick, Prince Edward Island, Newfoundland, and Nova Scotia, 79 percent had diagnoses of psychoses.

The continuing twentieth-century increase in insanity was of concern to Canadian authorities. In 1937 one observer noted that "mental cases" in Canada were increasing four times faster than the general population and predicted that "of all the children now going to school, a greater number will enter mental institutions than will graduate from College."[75]

By the late 1950s, the exodus of patients from Canada's public mental hospitals had begun. Saskatchewan led the way by decentralizing the care of psychiatric patients to small regional hospitals and by implementing community treatment programs, but all provinces began moving in this direction. Because of this movement toward deinstitutionalization, there were no longer any centralized statistics that could be used to ascertain whether or not insanity was continuing to increase.

There are suggestions, however, that it might have been. Data on first admissions for individuals with schizophrenia to all psychiatric inpatient facilities are available from 1950 to 1970 and show a marked increase. For all of Canada, the first admissions for schizophrenia increased from an average of 2,749 per year for 1950–1954 to an average of 5,263 per year for 1966–1970, a 92 percent increase during a period in which the general population increased 37 percent. As a rate, the first-admission increase was from 1.9 per 10,000 total population to 2.6 per 10,000. This increase in first admissions for schizophrenia per 10,000 population was observed in New Brunswick (from 1.8 to 2.6), Prince Edward Island (1.7 to 2.6), Newfoundland (1.7 to 2.2), and Nova Scotia (from 2.6 to 4.0).[76] It is possible that at least some of this increase can be explained by such factors as better reporting of data, changing diagnostic practices, and easier access to admission beds, but there are no data to support these explanations. It seems likely that some of the increase in first admissions reflected a true increase in the incidence of this disorder.

Studies of the prevalence of schizophrenia and affective psychoses in Canada also support the possibility that insanity increased significantly in the years following World War II. For example, Roger Bland analyzed the 1978 national data on mental illness in Canada and estimated the prevalence of schizophrenia to be 8.6 per 1,000 persons and the prevalence of affective psychosis to be 6.8 per 1,000 persons, both figures being relatively high by international standards.[77]

Unfortunately, however, no Canadian data exist that can be used to say with any degree of certainty whether or not insanity in Canada is continuing to increase. The available data suggest that insanity did increase slowly but steadily from approximately 1850 to 1950 and that at least schizophrenia may have increased more sharply between 1950 and 1970. Beyond 1970, it is not possible to say.

The absence of data to definitively ascertain whether insanity is increasing, remaining the same, or decreasing is inexplicable, given insanity's cost. For example, a recent study of schizophrenia alone, not including manic-depressive illness, estimated that 221,000 Canadians were affected, or approximately 7.4 per 1,000 total population. The total annual cost for these individuals was estimated to be $1.12 billion (Canadian dollars) in direct costs and $1.23 billion more in lost productivity and premature mortality. These figures were, according to the authors of the study, "a conservative estimate of the financial burden of schizophrenia in Canada," which did not include "the financial costs to families" or "attach a dollar value to the obvious pain and suffering or impact on quality of life for persons with schizophrenia or their families and friends."[78]

In 1824 a Special Committee Report to the Legislative Council of Lower Canada recommended improved services for insane persons based on "the best feelings of our nature, as no human being can be considered exempt from insanity, that awful visitation of the Almighty."[79] Almost two centuries later, the number of insane persons in Canada is at least ten times greater, as a proportion of the population, than it was in 1824, and the need for improved services is still outstanding.

CHAPTER 9

"The Disease Whose Frequency Has Become Alarming"

The United States, 1700–1840

And, once more, we may say, that we have reason to plead for this class, because they cannot plead for themselves. It is one of the evils of insanity, that it cannot gain a fair hearing, or make known its wants. It laughs in horrid mirth, while coals of fire are on its head. It shrinks and shudders before the phantoms of its own creation. It sits in morbid silence while disease is gnawing upon its life. The insane plead not for themselves, but will not every generous heart feel yet more for them, in remembrance of their forlorn condition?

—ROBERT WATERSTON, 1843

In a Word, people began to give themselves to their Fears, and to think that all regulations and Methods were in vain, and that there was nothing to be hoped for, but an universal Desolation.

—DANIEL DEFOE, *A Journal of the Plague Year,* 1722

As in Mother England, insanity in the American colonies existed but did not appear to be common in the seventeenth century. "It is unlikely," Richard Shryock notes, "that the settlers of the English colonies brought with them many who, in contemporary thought, were mentally abnormal. Those who were obviously 'of unsound mind' were presumably left behind during the Atlantic passage."[1]

Larry Eldridge made an extensive search for cases of mental abnormality, including insanity, depression, and mental retardation, in the official records of the British American and Caribbean colonies from 1607 to 1700. For that period, he identified eighty-two cases among a total population that reached approximately 300,000 by the end of the century. An example of insanity was an Albany man whom neighbors asked to be removed "because of the danger of houses taking fire because of his craziness." Eldridge concluded that "mentally disturbed persons appear but rarely in the records. . . . Mental illness seems not to have been widespread in the early colonies." Henry Viets made a similar search of the seventeenth-century archives of Massachusetts, whose records were the best preserved of any of the original colonies, and similarly concluded that "mental diseases seem to have been rare, although occasional accounts are found of hysteria."[2]

Those persons who were insane were cared for by their families whenever possible. When that was not feasible, other families were asked to help. For example, in Rhode Island in 1655, Puritan minister Roger Williams asked the people in his congregation to take turns providing care for a "distracted" woman who had fallen into "a former distempure of Weakness and distraction of mind . . . lest by her Distemp and Bitterness of ye Season she should perish amongst us." Other insane persons were boarded out to families or, if they were considered to be dangerous, confined. In 1689, for example, the town of Braintree, Massachusetts, authorized payment to the brother of Goodwife Witty to build "a house seven feet long and five feet wide near his own house for his insane sister's habitation."[3]

One of the first American statutes specifically referring to insane persons was enacted in Massachusetts in 1676. Apparently concerned about the increasing numbers of "distracted persons in some tounes that are unruly," it ordered town authorities "to take care of all such persons, that they doe not damnify others; and also to take care and order the management of their estates in the times of their distemperature."[4] In 1699, Connecticut passed a similar "Act for relieving Idiots and Distracted Persons," and other colonies followed thereafter.

The best-known examples of possible insanity in colonial America were those associated with the Salem witchcraft trials of 1691–1692. During these trials, nineteen persons were executed, two died in prison, and one died from torture. According to one observer at that time, "Some of these are known to be distracted, crazed women." Mary Glover, for example, was described as a "wild Irish woman" who, during her trial, offered "absurd and incoherent statements" and "readily confessed to being in league with the devil," who apparently spoke to her.[5] She was almost certainly insane. How many other victims of the Salem trials were also insane, and how many were suffering from hysteria, is difficult to ascertain from the existing records.

Cotton Mather, a prominent Puritan minister, played a central role in the Salem witch trials and also wrote about insanity. In his "Magnalia Christi Americana" (1702), "Insanabilia" (1714), and "The Angel of Bethesda" (1724), Mather emphatically stated that insanity was caused by sin and that mentally ill individuals were therefore agents of the devil. Mather's own wife, Lydia, was said to be subject to "violent outbursts," which Mather attributed to "Satanic Possessions."[6]

Cotton Mather was also among the first Americans to suggest that insanity might be increasing. In 1702, he warned about the growing number of colonists who "have contracted these melancholy indispositions which have unhinged them from all service or comfort."[7] One wonders whether Mather's concern about rising insanity might have contributed to his willingness, and the willingness of other officials, to accept the satanic stories of young Salem women, which in retrospect seem quite fantastical.

The eighteenth century dawned on England's American colonies, with 275,000 people scattered widely. The largest city was Boston, with 7,000 inhabitants. Late in 1699, William Penn returned from England to his Pennsylvania colony. While in England, Penn had proposed the creation of a congress to be composed of delegates from each American colony and presided over by a president to be named by the king. It was an idea whose time would come.

Colonial officials had to adjudicate occasional cases involving insanity. In 1711 in Connecticut a law was passed "To Provide in Case of Sickness, Including Insanity, Feeble-mindedness, and Similar Conditions," and four years later another law specified the fiscal responsibility of relatives for insane persons. By 1727 "the number of disorderly persons in the colony became so great that it was decided to build a colony workhouse" whose residents would include "persons under distraction and unfit to go at large whose friends do not take care for their safe confinement." In 1750 the population of Connecticut passed 100,000, and occasional descriptions of individuals with insanity can be found in the public records, such as Susannah Roberts of Wallingford, "Who is so disordered in her reason and understanding that she passeth from place to place naked," and Roger Humphry of Simsbury, who "became delirious and distracted and in his distraction killed his mother."[8]

Two years after Connecticut built its first workhouse to include insane persons, Massachusetts officials requested a separate facility at the Boston almshouse to keep "Distracted Persons Separate from the Poor."[9] In 1746, Boston town overseers suggested that the old jail be converted into a "mad house," but the suggestion was not acted upon. Five years later, the overseers complained about the increasing number of "distracted helpless and infirm people" in the workhouse.

In 1763, Thomas Hancock, a wealthy merchant and the uncle of John Hancock, left a £36,000 (1997 equivalent) bequest to Boston for the building of "a convenient House for the reception and more comfortable keeping of such unhappy persons as it shall please God in his Providence to deprive of their reason." Town officials rejected the plan, arguing that "there were not enough insane persons in the province to call for the erection of such a house."[10] Massachusetts had a population of over 200,000 at this time, with 15,500 living in Boston.

Historian Mary Ann Jimenez, who undertook an exhaustive search of Massachusetts records for cases of insanity from 1700 to 1840, identified twenty-seven "insane almshouse residents from 1757 to 1779" in Boston. She concluded that although occasional cases could be identified, "it is very difficult to find evidence about an issue that was (for whatever reason) not perceived to be a significant issue." Among the cases of insanity identified by Jimenez was a woman who hanged herself after going "some weeks" during which "she never slept a wink"; a man who wandered around in "filthy clothes, deranged," laughing in a "wild, insane manner" and doing bizarre things, such as "throwing the Bible into the fire after cutting it in two"; and a minister who "wept almost continually, even when in the pulpit." Another minister "began wearing a handkerchief over his face in 1738 because he felt himself unfit for the company of others. . . . While leading his congregation in prayer, . . . he stood with his back turned to them."[11] After three years of such behavior, the church council removed him from his post; a hundred years later, Nathaniel Hawthorne immortalized him in a short story, "The Minister's Black Veil."

In reviewing the cases of insanity in eighteenth-century Massachusetts and Connecticut, two aspects stand out. The first is the large number of cases in which the person's insanity was intermittent in character. An example is James Otis, who had several periods of "incessant talking" and bizarre behavior but who between episodes practiced law and was elected to the Massachusetts provincial assembly. The second is the large number of insane persons who were from an educated (e.g., Harvard College) and/or an upper socioeconomic (e.g., clergyman) background. This may be due to a selection bias among researchers, although Jimenez, who has probably done the most thorough search of eighteenth-century records for cases of insanity, says that she found very few cases from lower socioeconomic backgrounds despite looking for them. That the skewed socioeconomic distribution of insanity may have been real at this time is also suggested by an 1817 lecturer who told his Boston audience that insanity was indeed "more frequent among the upper classes," and an 1843 observation that "this malady oftenest comes to the most richly endowed minds."[12]

Hospitals for the Insane

At the same time as the citizens of Boston were discussing, but doing nothing about, creating a separate facility for insane persons, the citizens of Philadelphia were acting. In 1748, Thomas Bond returned to Philadelphia after having visited hospitals in London, including the Bethlem Asylum. He enlisted the help of his friend Benjamin Franklin in petitioning the Pennsylvania Assembly for funds to build a hospital for insane and other sick persons. Their petition noted that "the Number of Lunaticks . . . hath greatly increased in this Province" and that "some of them going at large are a Terror to their Neighbors who are daily apprehensive of the Violences they may commit."[13] It is unclear whether the observed increase in "lunaticks" was due to an increasing incidence or whether it simply reflected the increasing population of Pennsylvania, which had more than doubled to over 100,000 since 1730, Philadelphia alone having about 17,000 residents.

The Assembly approved the petition and allocated £150,000 (1997 equivalent) toward the building of a "hospital for the reception and relief of lunatics and other distempered and sick poor," and in 1751 the hospital was opened. Four of its first six patients were insane, and by the 1780s insane patients constituted one-quarter of all admissions and occupied half of the hospital beds because many remained. The wife of a wealthy Philadelphia merchant, for example, stayed for almost twenty-five years.[14]

Most of the beds in the Pennsylvania Hospital were reserved for "the most dangerous and disruptive lunatics," such as a woman who had murdered her infant and a farmer who had burned down his barn to rid it of rats. A notebook with patient histories, as recorded by the hospital manager, detailed cases of severe depression with psychotic features ("I am the Devil, I am the wickedest man upon the Earth") and probable manic-depressive illness ("she had lived seven thousand years in the moon . . . directs the tracks of the whale and every fish in the sea . . . one day I found her eating boiled mice"). However, according to Rajendra Persaud, who has studied the notebook, "there is only one account in the whole notebook of anything approaching schizophrenic symptoms," a young man who became insane with auditory hallucinations at age twenty-one and never recovered. The author of the notebook labeled this case as "novel and curious," which Persaud interpreted as meaning that "schizophrenic symptomatology was rare during this period."[15]

Almost from the opening day of the Pennsylvania Hospital, the insane persons hospitalized there were regarded as great curiosities by the public. In 1762 it was noted that "the great crowds that invade the Hospital give trouble and create so much disturbance" that special security precautions were instituted. According to hospital records, "the insane wing was such an object of public curiosity that the managers decided to charge an admission fee." Five years later, the fee was increased to four pence to try to restrict "the Throng of people who are led by Curiosity to frequent the House on the first day of the week, to the great disturbance of the Patients."[16] Additional restrictions were instituted in 1784 and 1791.

Largely because of the Pennsylvania Hospital, Philadelphia became "the medical center of late eighteenth-century colonial North America." The Quaker tradition of helping the less fortunate was partially responsible for this; two-thirds of the men who signed the original hospital petition and most of the hospital's managers were Quakers. Pennsylvania was also among the wealthiest of the colonies; "manufactured furniture, clocks, crystal, silver plate, fine china, lace, and such luxury utensils as forks appeared in the inventories of their estates with a frequency unmatched in other regions."[17]

Among the leaders of American medicine to emerge from Philadelphia during the late eighteenth century was Benjamin Rush, often called the father of American psychiatry. He had been a member of the Continental Congress and a signer of the Declaration of Independence when, in 1783, he joined the staff of the Pennsylvania Hospital, where he treated patients for thirty years. Rush believed that many cases of insanity were caused by an abnormal flow of blood in the brain, and in 1812 he published the first American textbook of psychiatry, *Medical Inquiries and Observations upon the Diseases of the Mind.*

Rush claimed that "in the United States, madness has increased since 1790," and he attributed this to "an increase in the number and magnitude of the objects of avarice and ambition." Rush was especially opposed to the new banking system: "The funding system and speculation in bank script, and new lands have been fruitful sources of madness in our country." He believed that wealthy individuals were more likely to become insane because the "poor do not have time to worry about the things that make the rich insane." George Hayward, in an 1818 review of Rush's work, also expressed concern about "the alarming increase of insanity within a few years, and the uncommon attention which it has lately excited in this vicinity." Rush's belief was undoubtedly strengthened by the increasingly overcrowded wards of the Pennsylvania Hospital, necessitating in 1796 the building of a new wing with eighty beds exclusively for insane patients.[18] In the forty-five years since the hospital had opened, the population of Philadelphia had more than tripled, but the increase in insane patients was occurring at an even faster rate.

At the time Pennsylvania opened its hospital in 1751, Virginia, which had a population of 231,000, almost twice that of Pennsylvania, had made no provision for its insane citizens. In 1766 the English governor, Francis Fauquier, aware of the new hospital in Philadelphia as well as developments in England, recommended that a hospital be built. "Every civilized Country has an Hospital for these People" who "are deprived of their senses and wander about the Country, terrifying the Rest of their Fellow Creatures," he said. There was apparently little support for Fauquier's idea until three years later, when the *Virginia Gazette* reported "a murder committed by a lunatic previously considered harmless" and editorialized about "the number of miserable people who have lost the use of their reason, that are daily wandering about."[19]

The hospital, the first American facility dedicated exclusively to the insane, opened at Williamsburg in 1773 with thirty beds. It was surprisingly little used in its early years, being only half full as late as 1796. When it reached its full capacity of thirty patients for the first time in 1799, the population of Virginia had grown to over 800,000. If there had been the same proportion of individuals with severe mental illness in Virginia in the 1780s as was reported in the United States in the 1980s, there would have been approximately 17,000 insane individuals in Virginia at that time.

South Carolina was also influenced by the opening of the Pennsylvania Hospital and immediately began planning its own facility. Among its plantation owners there was much wealth, and "in Charleston they enjoyed lives of luxury and cultivation, attending plays, balls, and galas, consuming fine foods and wines, purchasing English books, furniture, luxuries, and sending their children to English schools." In 1754 local officials discussed building a separate building for insane residents of the workhouse; the following year the Assembly debated a proposal to build a hospital "for confining Persons disordered in their Senses."[20]

Nothing came of these proposals, so in 1762 a group of prosperous citizens founded "The Fellowship Society of Charles Town" for the purpose of erecting a hospital "for the reception of lunatics and other distempered persons in the province." Six years later, the Assembly finally allocated funds for building a separate building for insane persons behind the poorhouse. The building was unfortunately located next to the city arsenal, which, during the Revolutionary War, blew up; the madhouse was destroyed and most of its inmates were killed.[21]

New York was also influenced by the developments in Philadelphia. At the time, New York was only the seventh most populous colony, but New York City had 17,000 inhabitants and was growing rapidly. In 1769, Samuel Bard, the son of a man who had helped found the Pennsylvania Hospital, proposed a similar hospital for New York to accommodate both insane and otherwise sick people. At the time, the only accommodation for insane persons was a dungeon in the "Publick Workhouse and House of Correction." The proposal was accepted by the governor, and funds were allocated to help build a hospital that would include "cells for the reception of Lunatics."[22] In 1775, as the hospital was nearing completion, it was destroyed by fire. Reconstruction was interrupted by the outbreak of the Revolutionary War, and the hospital was not finally opened until 1791.

In the forty years between 1750 and 1790, then, Americans for the first time began perceiving insanity as a problem. Before 1750, there had been virtually no provision made for the insane except by families or local officials. In the four decades following 1750, Connecticut, Massachusetts, New York, Pennsylvania, Virginia, and South Carolina all began publicly debating the problem and making proposals regarding what should be done. During this time, the population of the thirteen colonies increased more than threefold, from 1.2 to 3.9 million. It was also during this time that people began congregating in larger towns, changing the character of what had been almost exclusively rural living.

Is there any evidence that insanity was actually increasing in America during those years? As the population increased and as people began congregating in larger towns, existing cases of insanity certainly would have become more visible. However, based on the population of 1790, if there had been the same number of cases of insanity per population as exist today, then one would have expected approximately 86,000 insane persons in the thirteen states. The records of the hospitals, poorhouses, and other institutions of that period account for only a tiny fraction of these. Therefore, if this number existed, they must have remained at home or wandered the countryside. An alternative explanation is that there were not 86,000 insane persons at that time but rather far fewer.

"The Father of the American Novel"

Benjamin Rush was not the only American in the 1790s who believed that insanity was increasing. Edward Cutbush, one of Rush's students, published *An Inaugural Dissertation on Insanity* in 1794 in which he argued that "the rapid accumulation of the value of bank script, in the year 1791, by which many of our citizens became wealthy, produced Insanity in many instances." The increasing insanity was noted most frequently in "males and females from the age of fifteen to forty-five."[23]

Another student of Benjamin Rush's, Elihu Hubbard Smith was a close personal friend of and "literary adviser" to Charles Brockden Brown. Brown has been called "the father of the American novel," and he was "the first American fiction writer who founded his fiction upon American facts and localized his stories on American soil." He was also "the first American writer to develop an international reputation" and is said to have "made a powerful impression" on Percy Bysshe Shelley in England. Brown influenced the work of James Fenimore Cooper, Edgar Allan Poe, and Nathaniel Hawthorne, the last of whom told Brown that "no American writer enjoys a more classic reputation."[24]

Insanity is the central theme of Brown's work. "In three of Brown's greatest novels—*Wieland, Edgar Huntley, and Ormond*—the depiction of madness takes center stage; and, indeed, the depiction of madness in one form or another can be found in almost everything Brown wrote." According to one critic, "Madness, as depicted in Brown's fiction, is almost imminent—it is always impending or close at hand. . . . Madness is latently within all men, submerged within and held precariously in check by reason and self-control."[25]

Brown's interest in insanity arose in part from his close friendship with Elihu Hubbard Smith and other students working under Benjamin Rush. Brown had also been brought up as a Quaker in Philadelphia and was therefore acquainted with the Pennsylvania Hospital. In one of his novels, the insane character is taken to the Pennsylvania Hospital from New York because the latter "does not afford a place of confinement for lunatics." Brown also had an interest in science and in emerging theories regarding insanity. In 1798, with two friends, he founded the *Medical Repository,* "the first periodical in the United States devoted entirely to scientific research."[26] And he read and referenced scientific works such as *Zoonomia,* by Erasmus Darwin, grandfather of Charles; published in 1796, it contained an extensive discussion of insanity, delusions, and hallucinations.

According to Charles Pridgeon's *Insanity in American Fiction from Charles Brockden Brown to Oliver Wendell Holmes,* "The medical profession's increasing concern for the pathology of mental disorders represents the single most important reason for Brown's choice of madness as a major topic for his fiction." Insanity was becoming widely discussed in the 1790s, a subject of both curiosity and concern. "Indeed, one would be justified in noting that Brown established himself as the first major serious novelist in the United States largely because he shared this growing concern for mental disorders."[27]

In *Wieland,* his most popular novel, published in 1798, Brown took the plot from a well-known 1781 murder in New York in which an insane man had killed his wife and four children. In the novel, Theodore Wieland, who has a family history of insanity, hears the voice of God telling him to kill his wife and five children, which he does. The novel dramatizes the transformative aspects of Wieland's insanity, as when Wieland's wife realizes her husband's intent: "Surely, surely, Wieland, thou dost not mean it. Am I not thy wife? And wouldst thou kill me? Thou wilt not; and yet—I see—thou art Wieland no longer! A fury resistless and horrible possesses thee."[28]

Wieland's sister, Clara, is "terrified by the irresistibility and imminence of the madness that [has] struck her brother, by the fear that she too might be likewise transformed 'into a creature of nameless and fearful attributes.' "[29] In the end, she does become temporarily insane, and Theodore commits suicide.

Perhaps of greatest interest is Brown's introduction, or "advertisement," for his novel. He tells the reader that "the incidents related are extraordinary and rare. . . . The power which the principal person is said to possess can scarcely be denied to be real. It must be acknowledged to be extremely rare; but no fact, equally uncommon, is supported by the same strength of historical evidence." Brown is telling the reader that what he is describing really can and did happen, despite the fact that "some readers may think the conduct of the younger Wieland impossible." His explanation clearly suggests that insanity, or at least the murder of children by an insane parent, was not a familiar idea to Brown's readers.

Charles Brockden Brown was, in fact, merely the first in a series of early American writers who used insanity as a common theme. In the opinion of Charles Pridgeon, "Through 1861 only one major American writer of fiction, Washington Irving, had not significantly treated the subject of mental derangement." This interest in insanity "to a large extent represent[s] the response of writers to a national interest in the origins, nature, and treatment of insanity." Pridgeon adds that "the deranged characters in fiction were peculiar products of an era during which America—consciously in search of moral progress—initially confronted the threat of insanity."[30]

Increasing Concern

In the early years of the nineteenth century, the United States was too busy getting itself established to worry about problems such as insanity. The population had tripled between the end of the Revolutionary War and 1815, and the Louisiana Purchase had extended the nation's borders to the Rocky Mountains. Its capital had been moved from cosmopolitan Philadelphia, with a population of more than 50,000, to Washington, a town of 2,464 free inhabitants and 623 slaves. The British registered their opinion of the new capital during the War of 1812 by burning it.

There were, however, suggestions that insanity might be a growing problem for the nascent nation. In New York, the small hospital that had opened in 1791 had averaged twenty-two admissions of insane patients per year, and in 1806 the state legislature authorized the erection of a separate building for up to eighty patients. At this time there were estimated to be two hundred "pauper insane in the state, confined . . . to jails and alms-houses"[31] among its total population of approximately 900,000, or 0.2 per 1,000 total population. In 1816 it was decided to build a new hospital for two hundred insane persons outside the city limits, and this opened in 1821 as the Bloomingdale Asylum. The cost of construction was borne both by the state and by private subscription, and the state guaranteed an annual subsidy to the hospital for the next fifty years.

The New York legislature continued to monitor the situation and in 1825 ordered a census of insane persons. A total of 819 were found in the state, or approximately 0.5 per 1,000 total population; in addition 1,421 "idiots" were identified. Of the insane persons, it was said that three-quarters were "either confined in private families, poorhouses or jails, or roaming at large." Alarmed by these findings, in 1827 the legislature passed "An Act Concerning Lunatics," which specified that "no lunatic shall be confined in any prison, gaol or house of correction."[32]

The findings from the 1825 census and continuing reports of insane persons being confined in county jails despite the 1827 legislation led Governor Enos Throop to action. In his 1830 message to the legislature, he called attention "to the deplorable condition of the insane poor" and appointed a committee to explore building a new public asylum. The committee recommended building hospitals "to accommodate all our insane . . . to correct the evils and disastrous consequences of the existing system as to pauper lunatics." In view of the increasingly widespread suspicion that insanity was increasing, the committee added: "Let these hospitals be enlarged or multiplied as the malady increases, so as to accommodate at least all the insane poor."[33]

In Pennsylvania also there were suggestions in the early years of the nineteenth century that insanity was becoming a more common problem. The new wing of the Pennsylvania Hospital that had been built in 1796 was soon overcrowded, and the Society of Friends approved the building of a new hospital at Frankford, six miles from the city. Opened in 1817, admissions were initially restricted to members of the Friends "as may be deprived of their reason,"[34] but the hospital was later opened to all.

An extension for females was added to the Pennsylvania Hospital in 1825, but "by the late 1820s overcrowding again strained the . . . Hospital's resources." In 1828 the hospital manager, William Malin, advised that a new and larger hospital was needed. Discussion on this continued for ten years until a committee of the Pennsylvania legislature approved the plan, noting that the incidence of insanity had been sharply underestimated and adding: "To have the mind diseased, distracted and tormented; and to endure, beyond all this neglect, abuse and cruelty . . . presents a picture of human woe which few can contemplate without a tear of pity."[35]

Although the Pennsylvania Hospital had been open for over half a century, it continued to be a magnet for visitors. In 1822 a hospital report noted that "in order to further check the curious visitation of the insane patients, the rule was adopted to increase the fee for admission to the house from twelve and a half to twenty five cents." Six years later, in his 1828 report, William Malin observed: "The great publicity of the Hospital is also an evil of no small magnitude. The morbid curiosity displayed by a majority of the visitors to the Hospital is astonishing, and their pertinacity in attempting, and fertility in pretexts and expedients, to gain admission to the 'mad people' is not less so.... Even females who have tears to bestow on tales of imaginary distress, are importunate to see a raving madman."[36]

The visitors, Malin said, ignored signs to stay out and even pried open doors to get a look at the insane patients. If, as some historians have maintained, insanity was widespread in the community before cases began to be hospitalized in the early nineteenth century, it seems odd that so many people would find insane individuals of such great interest and flock to see them.

Concern about the increasing numbers of insane persons was not restricted to rapidly growing states, such as New York and Pennsylvania, but was also exhibited in Connecticut, whose population had increased just 25 percent over forty years, the lowest growth rate of any of the original thirteen states. In 1812 the Connecticut Medical Society instigated a census of insane persons and estimated that there were between five hundred and seven hundred in the state.[37]

Nine years later, another census was undertaken on "the disease whose frequency has become alarming." It reported that "the entire number will scarcely fall short of a thousand," but might, in fact, be twice that. Many cases of "moody melancholy" were found living at home, "enslaved by the phantoms of their own imagination—phantoms which hover around their dwellings and pursue them in their customary rambles." Such individuals were a terrible burden for their families, whose "peace is interrupted, their cares are multiplied, their time is engrossed, and their fortunes reduced or entirely dissipated in attempting to restore to reason one unfortunate member." The census also found a clustering of cases of insanity, with "six towns adjoining each other on the banks of the Connecticut River" having a total of 172 cases, while "six other towns, also contiguous to each other" had only two cases. The 1821 census concluded that "from the little attention which it [insanity] has hitherto excited among medical men, we are induced to believe that here, as in other countries, as the community has risen on the scale of refinement, it has been more and more exposed to the disease in question."[38]

The outcome of the 1821 Connecticut census of the insane was an agreement to use both state and private funds to build an asylum, which opened in 1824 as the Hartford Retreat. In arguing for the building of the asylum, officials stated explicitly that it would "diminish the number of the insane" because "many whose cases are now deemed hopeless would regain their reason."[39] The asylum, officials argued, would "also diminish the expense of their maintenance" by treating cases of insanity early in their course and thus preventing their evolution to chronic cases. These arguments, widely used by officials in other states to persuade state legislators to appropriate funds needed for asylum construction, would appear increasingly naïve as the century progressed.

Massachusetts, meanwhile, had also finally recognized the necessity for an insane asylum. In 1801 the Reverend Jedidiah Moore had called for the building of a "hospital for lunatics" because such individuals, roaming freely, were often "a terror to female delicacy." Nine years later a committee of prominent citizens urged the creation of a "hospital for the reception of Lunatics and other sick persons."[40] This led directly to the building of the Massachusetts General Hospital, which opened in 1818 with a separate section for insane patients; this section was later renamed the McLean Asylum after a generous benefactor.

During the 1820s it became increasingly apparent that the McLean Asylum had not solved Massachusetts's insanity problem. In 1827 the Boston Prison Discipline Society published a report detailing the living conditions for more than thirty insane individuals confined to local jails: "One was found in [an] apartment in which he had been nine years. He had a wreath of rags round his body, and another round his neck. This was all his clothing. He had no bed, chair or bench. . . . A heap of filthy straw, like the nest of swine, was in the corner."[41]

An investigation of state prisons the same year reported similarly abysmal conditions for the insane prisoners: "Many of them have never been accused or charged with any crime, and have remained many years in the most wretched condition. Less attention is paid to their cleanliness and comfort than to the wild beasts in their cages, which are kept for show. Some of these miserable beings have been confined for twenty years or more, and seem to have been left to wallow in their own filth."[42]

These reports circulated widely among Boston's leading citizens. One result was an 1829 inquiry by the state legislature to ascertain the number of "lunatics and furiously mad," the most seriously disturbed insane persons in the state. Reports from 114 of the state's 310 towns enumerated 289 "lunatic persons," of whom 161 were confined, 38 of them in chains. Significantly, two-thirds of the insane persons in confinement had been confined for less than two years, suggesting a relatively recent onset of their problems.[43] An additional 60 patients were confined to the McLean Asylum.

The results of the 1829 inquiry were referred to a legislative committee chaired by thirty-four-year-old Horace Mann, who was just embarking on his career as a reformer. Mann's committee recommended the immediate construction of a new asylum in Worcester for 120 patients: "While *we* delay, they *suffer.*—Another year not only gives an accession to their numbers, but removes, perhaps to a returnless distance, the chance of their recovery. Whatever they endure, which we can prevent, is virtually inflicted by our own hands."[44]

When the new hospital opened as the Worcester State Lunatic Hospital in 1833, it gave preference to "lunatics furiously mad, and dangerous to the peace and safety of the community." Over half of the admissions the first year came from jails and almshouses, and eight of the first forty admissions had committed homicides. According to Gerald Grob's *The State and the Mentally Ill,* which details the development of the hospital, "almost from the very day that the first patient was admitted, the hospital proved incapable of meeting the demands placed upon its facilities."[45]

In the latter part of 1834, half of all applications for admission to the Worcester Hospital had to be rejected because of overcrowding. In 1835, the hospital began *returning* chronic patients to local jails, exactly the opposite of its intended purpose, and "by the end of the decade, the hospital was returning incurables to local facilities at a rapid rate." New wings were added in 1836 and 1837, raising the hospital capacity to 229, and two more wings in 1842 increased the capacity to 450, a threefold increase in just nine years. In 1837, officials in Boston, seeing patients returned as quickly as they were being sent to the Worcester Hospital, decided to open their own asylum to provide care for the increasing numbers of insane persons in the workhouse; in 1832 a report had described fifty of them as "more or less insane and about half may be described as 'furiously mad' requiring almost constant confinement."[46] The hospital was opened in 1839 as the Boston Lunatic Hospital.

The rapid rise in the number of insane individuals was puzzling to state and hospital officials. There is no indication in the clinical records that diagnostic categories were being broadened; Grob noted that during the 1830s and 1840s, all the patients "were clearly . . . psychotic."[47] The population of Massachusetts was increasing but more slowly than most other states; from 1820 to 1840 it increased from 523,000 to 738,000, a rate of increase that was only half that of the nation as a whole. It should also be noted that overcrowding was occurring despite considerable resistance by towns to sending individuals to the Worcester Hospital, since the towns had to pay for the cost of each person's care. This fiscal arrangement continued until 1904, with the consequence that towns sent only their most severe cases to the asylums and kept the less severe cases in local workhouses, where the cost was considerably less.

Some officials concluded that insanity was increasing. In 1833 the superintendent of the McLean Asylum noted: "Insanity was once a rare occurrence. . . . Insanity is no longer rare. . . . The increase of this disease since its [the McLean Asylum's] establishment leads to melancholy reflections." Two years later, Amariah Brigham, looking at data on first admissions in Massachusetts, agreed that "insanity is a common disease in that state."[48]

During the early years of the nineteenth century, then, widespread concern emerged that insanity was increasing. This concern became manifest in calls for the creation of public asylums in which insane persons could be housed and treated. The concern was also evident in public discussion of the issue, including an 1817 contribution to the *North American Review* in which an anonymous writer asserted that insanity was much more widespread than officials had said. The solution, the writer facetiously added, was that "instead of an hospital for the *insane,* this establishment be exclusively appropriated to the use of the *sane,*" since the sane would soon be a small minority.[49]

The Contrast between North and South

The apparent increase in Massachusetts in cases of insanity in the 1830s was not necessarily representative of all states of the Union. In South Carolina, for example, the situation was different. At the beginning of the nineteenth century, the state passed an ordinance permitting the confinement in workhouses of "all lunatics or persons disordered in their senses," and seven insane persons were registered in the "lunatic department" of the Charleston workhouse. Like many such facilities, "the lunatic department was apparently an object of particular attraction for locals and tourists alike," and in 1821 visitors were therefore restricted.[50]

After the War of 1812, discussion began regarding the building of an insane asylum. The leaders of South Carolina's society aspired to emulate their northern neighbors, and the group sent a representative to visit the asylums in Philadelphia, New York, and Hartford. The South Carolina state legislature, skeptical of the need for an asylum, conducted a state census in 1818 and found only fifty-five "lunatics and idiots." The population of South Carolina at the time was 503,000, only 20,000 less than the number in Massachusetts. Since the asylum commissioners already had well-developed plans for an asylum for eighty to one hundred patients, this "embarrassingly small" number of insane persons was problematic.[51] The South Carolina Lunatic Asylum was built anyway, and opened to receive patients in May 1828.

Not a single patient was admitted for the first seven months, despite articles praising it and advertisements for patients in newspapers in Charleston and Columbia. In December, the first patient finally arrived. Advertisements were then placed in newspapers in surrounding states, and several patients from North Carolina, Alabama, Georgia, and Florida, states that did not have asylums, were admitted. By 1831 the hospital census reached thirty-five, but "at several points in the early 1830s it was in danger of closing for lack of funds."[52] The full census of one hundred patients was not reached until 1849, more than twenty years after the asylum had opened.

Many reasons were given for the paucity of patients at the South Carolina Lunatic Asylum. Approximately 55 percent of the state population were slaves, who were not eligible for admission. The stigma of having a mentally ill family member was significant, and wealthier families continued to send their insane members to northern asylums. Towns were responsible for the cost of care, similar to Massachusetts and other states, so Charleston and other towns were reluctant to hospitalize insane individuals who could be maintained less expensively in local workhouses. And the South Carolina population growth between 1820 and 1840 was only 18 percent, approximately half the rate of Massachusetts. Despite these factors, there remains a striking contrast between the rapid overcrowding of wards at the Worcester State Lunatic Hospital and the empty wards at the South Carolina Lunatic Asylum in the 1830s.

By the late 1830s, then, there was a concern in some, but not all, states that insanity was becoming more common. This concern was clearly expressed by Amariah Brigham, a physician in Hartford who was specializing in problems of insanity and who would later become the superintendent of the Hartford Retreat and the Utica State Lunatic Asylum. In an 1837 article in the influential *North American Review,* Brigham examined the statistics on insanity and concluded: "These statistics respecting insanity, though few and imperfect, show, that the disease is alarmingly prevalent in this country, especially in the Northern States of the Union. We believe it is not equally so in those of the south and west, though our means of judging are not such as to enable us to speak confidently. From a review of these facts respecting insanity in some of the States, we can hardly avoid the conclusion, that the disease has of late considerably increased."

Brigham attributed the increase both to heredity and to "mental agitation," which he said was caused by such things as "our thousands of newspapers, circulating in all parts of the Union, and their exciting articles read by all classes." The solution to the problem of increasing insanity, he said, was for states to build asylums "where the insane poor can be received and treated properly, and soon restored to society." By effecting cures, such asylums would be, Brigham promised, cost effective. He added that well-run asylums should also have workshops and jobs for patients because "labor is often quite an essential aid and the cure of those who have previously been accustomed to it." However, "patients belonging to the wealthier class, who have never been used to manual labor, require pleasure-grounds, carriages, and horses for experience and amusement."[53]

"The Madman Roams Far and Wide"

In the 1820s and 1830s, as some officials were expressing concern about rising insanity, the public was becoming increasingly interested in the issue. Popular magazines such as *Littell's Living Age* and the *American Magazine of Useful and Entertaining Knowledge* carried detailed and flattering descriptions of the new asylums. In 1837 one magazine enthusiastically claimed: "Perhaps there is no subject in which more has been gained for the cause of humanity, since the commencement of the present century, than in the method of treating persons deprived of the use of reason."[54]

American writers of this period reflected this increasing interest and utilized insanity as a major theme. As Charles Pridgeon noted, "The madman roams far and wide in the literal and symbolic landscapes of early American fiction." One example was John Neal, who in 1822 published *Logan, A Family History.* In it, the fictional Logan "becomes a furious maniac who stalks the forest seeking visitors." The author is said to become "extravagant in his descriptions of hallucinatory states of mind." Thirty years later, Herman Melville would recall Neal's book, comparing Captain Ahab to "that wild Logan of the woods, burying himself in the hollow of a tree. . . . Ahab's soul, shut up in the caved trunk of his body, there fed upon the sullen paws of its gloom."[55]

Richard Henry Dana was another American writer of the 1820s who used insanity as a major theme. Dana was a founder of the *North American Review,* and his son became well known as the author of *Two Years before the Mast.* Dana's novel *Paul Felton* depicts a solitary, brooding, and melancholy protagonist whose blood, in echoes of Benjamin Rush, either moved "sluggishly" or "rushed to the brain, blackening his face." On one occasion, Felton claims to have a fever "that must be cooled quickly or it will sear the brain up."[56] He becomes increasingly delusional that his wife has been unfaithful and receives messages from "a supernatural power" instructing him to kill her, which he does.

James Fenimore Cooper, who became internationally acclaimed for his tales of Native Americans, also utilized a variety of characters with mental aberrations. In *Lionel Lincoln,* for example, the elder Sir Lionel is depicted as a "textbook maniac" who has escaped from an

English insane asylum, gone to Boston, and become "a fanatical Revolutionary." In 1825, the same year that *Lionel Lincoln* was published, a young American poet named Lucretia Maria Davidson wrote of her fear of madness as she lay dying from tuberculosis:

> *There is a something which I dread,*
> *It is a dark, a fearful thing;*
> *It steals along with withering tread,*
> *Or sweeps on wild destruction's wing.*
>
> *That thought comes o'er me in the hour*
> *Of grief, of sickness, or of sadness;*
> *'Tis not the dread of death—'tis more,*
> *It is the dread of madness.*[57]

In the 1830s, insanity was thematically used by several novelists, including James Kirke Paulding, William Simms, and Robert Montgomery Bird. Paulding, who was an associate of Washington Irving's and later U.S. secretary of the navy, "feared what he saw as a general spread of mental derangement throughout the United States,"[58] especially fanaticism and religious mania. He was probably the first American writer to use the term "monomania," which had been introduced by French psychiatrist Jean Esquirol in 1820 to describe a form of insanity characterized by a single overriding delusion.

Paulding's *Westward Ho!* published in 1832, is said to be "one of the most clinically complete descriptions of a madman in nineteenth-century American literature." The protagonist, Dudley Rainsford, is convinced he is destined to become insane since his father and grandfather both did, so he moves west to the American frontier in an attempt to escape his fate. He slowly becomes delusional, however; in Paulding's words, his thinking crosses "the almost imperceptible line, the very hair breadth space which, in the sensitive empire of the brain, separates the fruitful region where the elements act in sweet accord . . . from that of chaos, where nothing but . . . jarring atoms abide." Rainsford becomes convinced that all sexual relationships are evil and that he must kill his fiancée "in order to expiate the curse placed upon him by God." Thus, according to Pridgeon, "Paulding combined two major themes which he recognized as being particularly pertinent in the United States in the 1830s—the promise of the frontier and the growing concern for insanity."[59]

William Simms was best known for his series of melodramatic novels dealing with Native Americans and frontier life. He was especially interested in the criminally insane, and *Martin Faber,* published in 1833, is "a first-person account of how emotional instability evolves into a full-fledged case of insanity." Faber has a delusion that he is possessed by an external force, and "his anti-social acts, including a murder, are part of his inexorable fate which he is acting out." Similarly, in *The Partisan,* published in 1835, Simms depicted the onset of insanity in a man whose pregnant wife had been brutally killed by "a gang of Tories" during the Revolutionary War.[60]

Robert Montgomery Bird's interest in insanity was more clinical, since he had graduated from the University of Pennsylvania Medical School and was close friends with the son of Benjamin Rush. In *Nick of the Woods,* published in 1837, the aptly named Nathan Slaughter has a Jekyll-and-Hyde personality that includes a "homicidal monomania" which leads him to brutally murder Native Americans.[61] Slaughter's insanity was said to be partially caused by a severe blow to the head, a common theory at that time.

By the 1830s, therefore, insanity in the United States had become of increasing concern to public officials and of increasing interest to the public in general, as reflected in popular literature. Insanity was at once both appalling and appealing, evoking fear in people even as they flocked to local asylums to view raving madmen. And throughout this period, both public officials and writers implied that the problem of insanity was increasing.

CHAPTER 10

An Apostle for Asylums

The United States, 1840–1860

Insanity is a terrible calamity at best, but then it was the climax of all human woes, for it contained an ingredient unknown in any other misfortune, —exclusion, not only from hearts and homes to which nature gave a claim, but from the sight of familiar faces, from the ministrations of kindness, and from every circumstance of hope or of joy.

—*North American Review,* 1854

When I say the People abandon'd themselves to Despair, I do not mean to what Men call a religious Despair, or a Despair of their eternal State, but I mean a Despair of their being able to escape the Infection, or to out-live the Plague.

—DANIEL DEFOE, *A Journal of the Plague Year,* 1722

By 1840, the United States was exhibiting many problems of an adolescent nation. Unemployment was high, with lost confidence in the currency following the Panic of 1837. Abolitionists clashed increasingly regularly with pro-slavery supporters as the rhetoric on both sides petrified. The nation continued to move westward, pushing Native Americans aside as it went. Five years earlier, Alexis de Tocqueville had published his *Democracy in America,* highlighting the nation's promise and problems.

Although insignificant in magnitude compared to many other problems facing America in 1840, insanity was a growing concern. Harper and Brothers, whose Family Library series was standard reading in the homes of the educated, decided to publish an entire volume entitled *Imperfect and Disordered Mental Action.*[1] New asylums for the insane had been opened in Maryland in 1834, Vermont in 1836, Ohio in 1838, New York in 1839, and Maine and Tennessee in 1840. Additions had been made to most of the existing asylums, and calls for additional asylums were being heard in virtually every state. Where were all these insane people coming from? some asked.

Since a decennial census was due, it seemed an opportune time to officially ascertain the magnitude of the problem. There had never been a national census of insane persons in the United States. Individual states had made such determinations, and in 1832 the Prison Discipline Society had made rough approximations based upon the number of insane persons in jails and prisons.[2] Therefore, in 1840, U.S. marshals, who were at that time used as census takers, were instructed to count all "insane and idiot" individuals in the course of their household surveys.

The results were less than optimal. The marshals had been given no definition of "insane" or "idiot," and the two categories were combined in census tabulations. A comparison of the census figures with previous enumerations carried out by individual states suggested that the census takers had undercounted in Massachusetts by 36 percent, New York by 43 percent, and New Jersey by 58 percent. This was said to have occurred because the insanity of some individuals "will be concealed by their friends" and because "many monomaniacs and those but little deranged will not be enumerated because [they are] not considered actually insane."[3]

Despite such limitations, the census of 1840 produced some interesting results. When the number of insane persons per total population was examined by state,[4] it was found that Rhode Island (1.3 per 1,000), Massachusetts (1.2), Connecticut (1.1), New Hampshire (0.9), and Vermont (0.9) had the greatest proportion of insane and idiot persons. The rates in Pennsylvania (0.7), Maryland (0.7), New York (0.6), and New Jersey (0.6) were intermediate, and all other states were lower (e.g., Georgia, Alabama, and Mississippi were all 0.2). Insanity was clearly a major problem in New England but a lesser problem in the southern states. This North-South gradient would be found repeatedly in subsequent censuses for the remainder of the nineteenth century.

The count of insane persons in the 1840 census also became an early battleground in the ongoing fight over slavery. As early as 1836, "inquiry was made during the last session of Congress of several members from the slave-holding States respecting the frequency of insanity among the blacks."[5] The 1840 census divided all individuals into whites, free colored, and slaves, thereby making it possible to look at racial differences in insanity rates. The results of the census showed a remarkably low prevalence of insanity among slaves and an extraordinarily high prevalence among free colored persons. Among slaves, there was found to be only one insane/idiot for every 1,558 slaves. In Maine, by contrast, it was said that one in every fourteen free colored persons was insane/idiot; in New Hampshire, one in every twenty-eight; and in Massachusetts, one in every forty-three. For supporters of slavery, the message was clear: freedom begets insanity. *Merchants' Magazine* announced that the census had proven that "slavery appears to be still more favorable" for preventing insanity. The *Southern Literary Messenger* said the census proved that "the negro of the South ... cares not for the morrow. . . . [H]is simple mode of life secures him health." However, when Negroes become free, it said, "they furnish little else but materials for jails, penitentiaries and mad houses."[6]

John C. Calhoun, former vice-president and U.S. senator, was one of the leading defenders of slavery at the time. Shortly after the 1840 census had been carried out, Calhoun was appointed secretary of state. Addressing Congress, Calhoun said of the census: "Here is proof of the necessity of slavery. The African is incapable of self-care and sinks into lunacy under the burden of freedom. It is a mercy to him to give him the guardianship and protection from mental death." And in a subsequent letter to the Speaker of the House, Calhoun added: "The data on insanity revealed in this census is unimpeachable. From it our nation must conclude that the abolition of slavery would be to the African a curse instead of a blessing." Calhoun knew something about insanity because his brother had been committed as insane to the South Carolina Lunatic Asylum six years earlier.[7]

Unfortunately for Calhoun, however, as he was making these remarks, the insanity results of the 1840 census were being completely discredited. Edward Jarvis, a Massachusetts physician with an interest in both insanity and statistics, examined the original census data and found that "the statements in reference to the disorders of the colored race were a mere mass of errors, and totally unworthy of credit." In 110 northern towns, the census listed more insane free colored persons than the total number of free colored who lived in the towns. In Maine, for example, "among the 94 colored lunatics and idiots, 70 are stated to be in towns which have only 8 colored inhabitants."[8] Scarboro, Maine, was recorded as having 6 insane colored, but in fact it had no colored persons living there. In Worcester, Massachusetts, all 133 insane white inmates of the state asylum had been listed as colored.

Jarvis published his findings in medical journals and drafted a petition from the American Statistical Society to Congress asking for an official correction of "the errors, inconsistencies, contradictions and falsehoods" of the census. The fact that virtually all the errors were in a direction that was favorable to the cause of slavery convinced many people that the errors had not been random. The fact that the superintendent of the census in 1840 had been William A. Weaver, "a fellow Southern gentleman" whom Calhoun defended as "a person in every way well qualified to perform the task," convinced the rest.[9]

The myth that slavery was protective against insanity continued to be reported for many years following the 1840 census. In 1855 it was claimed that "as a slave the negro is almost exempt from [insanity]—not only is he far less afflicted than the free negro, but even less than his master." In 1866, after the Civil War had ended, an article sarcastically noted that "the virtuous, upright and intelligent freemen of Massachusetts are shown by this most unimpeachable authority to be 21 times crazier than the negroes of Florida, 38 times crazier than the negroes of Arkansas, and 38 times crazier than the negroes of South Carolina." In 1916, when Henry Hurd published *The Institutional Care of the Insane in the United States and Canada,* he dismissed the 1840 census as "absolutely worthless as regards any correct enumeration of cases of insanity and idiocy."[10]

"Raise Up the Fallen"

The 1840 census helped focus public attention on the insanity problem and prepared the nation for the crusade of Dorothea Dix. When Dix addressed the Massachusetts legislature in 1843, she forcefully brought the problem of increasing insanity to its attention. Not only was the Worcester State Lunatic Asylum severely overcrowded and sending patients back to almshouses and jails, she said, but the almshouses and jails were also teeming with insane persons, many being kept in medieval conditions. Dix had visited the York Retreat in England in 1836 and had a vision of how insane persons should be treated.

Dix's career as a reformer had begun in March 1841, when she had gone to a local jail near Boston to teach a class to women prisoners. She had been horrified by how many of the women were insane and by the conditions in which they were being kept. During the next two years, she had visited every jail and almshouse in Massachusetts. Her 1843 address to the legislature called attention "to the *present* state of Insane Persons confined within this Commonwealth, in *cages, closets, cellars, stalls, pens! Chained, naked, beaten with rods,* and *lashed* into obedience!" She apologized for being "obliged to speak with great plainness, and to reveal many things revolting to the taste.... But truth is the highest consideration." "Men of Massachusetts, I beg, I implore, I demand.... Raise up the fallen; succor the desolate; restore the outcast; defend the helpless."[11]

Dorothea Dix was not the only advocate who in 1843 was urging the Massachusetts state legislature to increase provisions for insane persons. Samuel Woodward, the respected superintendent of the State Lunatic Hospital, acknowledged that in the ten years since the hospital had opened, sixty-four "dangerous insane" patients had been sent from the hospital back to jails and that there were "in the jails and houses of correction . . . as many insane as when the State Lunatic Hospital was established." Robert Waterston, a prominent clergyman, also urged the legislature to act, because "disease should be met with pity, not with punishment; and of all diseases, surely there is none more worthy of compassion than that under which the Lunatic suffers." Samuel Gridley Howe added an eloquent supporting plea: "Come, then, ye whose bosoms heave with just indignation at the oppression of man in distant lands; here are victims of dreadful oppression at your very doors.... Let the State government be urged to make immediate and ample provision for *all* the indigent insane, cost what it may cost. Massachusetts is not too poor to do any thing that can be shown to be her duty."[12]

The increase in insane persons was indeed dramatic. From 1833 to 1836, the earliest years of the State Lunatic Hospital, an average of 88 new admissions per year had been received and the daily census had been 118. From 1843 to 1846, the average annual first admissions had increased to 182, and the daily census was 295. Conditions in the hospital had deteriorated so much that the hospital's board of visitors noted in 1846 that if patients "were not mad when they came to the hospital, they soon would become mad." Only the most severely ill patients and those with good political connections could be admitted; elderly insane persons and other less severe cases were among the more than one hundred cases rejected for admission in the hospital's first decade. Faced with overwhelming evidence of need, the state legislature approved further additions to the Worcester Hospital and later authorized the opening of new hospitals at Taunton in 1854 and Northampton in 1858. Despite these additions, overcrowding persisted. As one official report noted: "Hospitals have been multiplied, but the applicants for admissions have multiplied yet faster."[13]

Dorothea Dix's success in helping to convince the Massachusetts legislature to act launched her on a lifetime career as an apostle for asylums. She went next to New Jersey, which did not yet have an asylum for insane persons, and persuaded the state legislature to build one in Trenton. Dix, a spinster, later called the New Jersey State Lunatic Asylum "my first-born child."[14]

In 1842, Dix spent ten weeks visiting almshouses, jails, and county-houses in New York State. In Albany, she found insane individuals naked in dungeons: "To describe the scenes which were revealed as these loathsome dens were successively thrown open is impossible." She continued:

> In the cell first opened was a madman; the fierce command of his keeper brought him to the door—a hideous object; matted locks, unshorn-beard, a wild wan countenance, yet more disfigured by vilest uncleanness, in a state of entire nudity, save the irritating incrustations derived from that dungeon reeking with loathsome filth: here, without light, without pure air, without warmth, without cleansing, without *anything* to secure decency or comfort, here was a human being, forlorn, abject, and disgusting it is true, but

not the less a human being—nay more, an immortal being, though now the mind had fallen in ruins, and the soul was clothed in darkness.[15]

Dix labeled the county-houses in Oneida, Herkimer, Greene, and Orange Counties as "only *synonyms* for foul crime and base licentiousness." In Rome, Oneida County, Dix was shocked to find two insane women in the county-house who "*have here become mothers*" during their confinement. Those conditions existed in Oneida County despite the fact that the Utica State Lunatic Asylum, which had opened the preceding year and was only twenty miles away, was intended to provide care for such insane women. By the time the Utica Asylum opened, however, "the number of insane persons had risen so sharply that the relative position of the state was not appreciably improved." As Ellen Dwyer noted in her history of the Utica Asylum: "Most New Yorkers thought that they had met the needs of their insane poor for some time into the future [by building the Utica Asylum] . . . and were shocked to learn, almost immediately, that such was not the case."[16]

Other visitors to New York's asylums also noted their shortcomings. For example, in 1842 Charles Dickens, while touring the United States, had visited asylums in New York City and Boston to compare with those he had visited in England. The New York City asylum on Blackwell's Island had opened in 1839. Being somewhat unclear about American geography, Dickens described the asylum as being "on Long Island or Rhode Island." He was, however, completely clear about the conditions in the asylum:

> I saw nothing of that salutary system which had impressed me so favourably elsewhere; and everything had a lounging, listless, madhouse air, which was very painful. The moping idiot, cowering down with long dishevelled hair; the gibbering maniac, with his hideous laugh and pointed finger; the vacant eye, the fierce wild face, the gloomy picking of the hands and lips, and munching of the nails: there they were all, without disguise, in naked ugliness and horror. In the diningroom, a bare, dull, dreary place, with nothing for the eye to rest on but the empty walls, a woman was locked up alone. She was bent, they told me, on

committing suicide. If anything could have strengthened her in her resolution, it would certainly have been the insupportable monotony of such an existence.[17]

When Dorothea Dix addressed the New York state legislature two years later, she again noted the rapidly growing problem of insanity and recommended the building of four to six new hospitals "in convenient sections of the State."[18] Having assumed that they had solved the problem of insanity by building the Utica Asylum in 1843, the legislators were not interested in Dix's proposal. New York City added two new asylums in 1844 (Kings County) and 1852 (Flatbush) to complement the asylum on Blackwell's Island, but no new facility would be added upstate for another twenty-four years.

By the early 1850s, the rising number of insane persons had created a crisis in New York State. In 1855 and 1856, the county superintendents held meetings in Utica "to consider what action they should take to remedy the difficulties they were having in providing for their insane." One superintendent described an insane woman who "had been chained in a garret-room of the poorhouse for eighteen months." Another county had had fifty-three insane persons in the poorhouse, and in a single week twenty-four of them had died from cholera. When the results of the 1850 census were published, it was found that the number of insane persons per population had increased in New York by 40 percent, from 0.58 to 0.81 per 1,000 total population since 1840. With each passing year, it became increasingly difficult to get patients admitted to the Utica Asylum. The pressure on admissions continued to grow despite the fact that either the patient's family or county had to pay most of the cost of their care, a provision that continued in effect until 1890. Counties considered this expense to be a great burden and therefore "transferred pauper lunatics to the state asylum only with great reluctance."[19]

Dr. Cure-Awl

During the 1840s, the United States was growing rapidly in territory and more modestly in population. In 1845, Florida and Texas became states. The following year the United States declared war on Mexico and annexed New Mexico. Two years later Mexico ceded California,

Nevada, Arizona, Utah, and parts of Colorado and Wyoming at the close of the war. During this decade, the population of the country increased 36 percent, from 17.1 to 23.2 million.

The 1840s and 1850s were decades of asylum building, with an average of more than one new state asylum opening each year. The openings of asylums in Maine and Tennessee in 1840 were followed by Georgia and New Hampshire in 1842, New York in 1843, Rhode Island in 1847, and New Jersey, Indiana, and Louisiana in 1848. This surge in new state asylums continued through the 1850s in Pennsylvania, Illinois, Missouri, and California (1851), Ohio and Pennsylvania (1853), Massachusetts and Kentucky (1854), Ohio and Mississippi (1855), North Carolina (1856), Massachusetts and Missouri (1858), and Michigan (1859). A total of twenty-three new asylums had been built in just twenty years. This was almost three times more than had been built in the twenty years prior to 1840 and did not include city asylums, such as those in New York, or the county asylums being built in some Midwestern states.

In reviewing discussions that led up to the building of state insane asylums, one is impressed with the amount of resistance exhibited by many state legislators and officials. Much of this resistance centered on cost. Taxes were very low in most states in the nineteenth century, and it was an important goal of elected officials to keep them that way. In Ohio, for example, it was claimed that 75 percent of all tax revenues were spent on "building and supporting the benevolent institutions, in which are included the insane, blind, deaf and dumb, and idiotic."[20] Economic downturns in the United States from 1837 to 1843 and from 1857 to 1861 put many state budgets in a marginal status, and elective projects such as insane asylums were deferred as long as possible.

Another reason for resistance to asylum building was the public's distrust of some asylum superintendents. In 1844, thirteen superintendents had met in Philadelphia and formed the Association of Medical Superintendents of American Institutions for the Insane (AMSAII), which eventually became the American Psychiatric Association. The leaders of this group, including Amariah Brigham, Luther Bell, Isaac Ray, Samuel Woodward, John Butler, Pliny Earle, and Thomas Kirkbride, were generally respected and considered to be credible when they asked state legislatures for funds.

Other superintendents, however, were not as respected. The first superintendent of the South Carolina Lunatic Asylum "resigned soon after the asylum officially opened after being arrested for an unspecified crime." The superintendent of the Tennessee Hospital for the Insane "was an inebriate." And the superintendent of the Georgia Lunatic Asylum was himself insane and wrote "bizarre and barely comprehensible" reports to the hospital trustees. Dorothea Dix wrote a friend that this superintendent "is really insane, but being harmless, the Trustees consent to his remaining in charge of the Institution."[21]

In addition to problems of the credibility of some superintendents, allegations of favoritism in the letting of asylum contracts and nepotism in the hiring of asylum staff surfaced from time to time. John Bucknill, in his 1876 *Notes on Asylums for the Insane in America,* remarked that "public money [for the asylum] is not expended wisely, nor always even honestly. . . . [T]here is always a tap leaking somewhere." Bucknill said that it was necessary to increase the "confidence on the part of the people and their representatives that the money appropriated to establish and maintain institutions for the insane will be economically and honestly expended."[22]

Despite continuing resistance from state legislators and officials, state asylums continued to be funded and constructed. A major reason for this was the rising number of insane persons who were increasingly visible in the community; the public ultimately demanded that they be accommodated. Many of these high-profile cases involved homicides or other violent behavior. In 1844, for example, the *Southern Literary Messenger* noted that "the plea of insanity in criminal cases has become so common in our courts of law that its bare mention excites a smile." The public was also becoming more sophisticated about the problem of insanity through articles in popular journals. *Harper's Monthly,* for example, in 1851 carried an account of a "mathematical monomaniac" who was completely rational "until it so happened, in the course of conversation, that he mentioned any numerical figure, when his wild imagination was off at a tangent, and he became suddenly as 'mad as a March hare' on one subject." *Chambers' Journal* noted the "startling urgency and importance" of the statistics that "have all but proved that out of every 500 of the population, we have one case of insanity." The *North American Review* commented on "the great prevalence of the disease of insanity, and especially its remarkable apparent increase of late years." And in 1850 the *Home Journal* even published a poem titled "The Ruined Mind":

> *Oh! what a sad and solemn sight,*
> *To see the human mind decay!*
> *To watch its waning, flickering light*
> *Grow fainter, feebler, day by day.*
>
> *To see the bright, the glorious spark*
> *Heaven gave to light, to guide the brain,*
> *Grow glimm'ring, rayless, dim, and dark,*
> *Never to be revived again.*[23]

Four years later, *Harper's Monthly* published an extended account of "A Day in a Lunatic Asylum," describing patients in New York City's Blackwell Asylum. The article noted that the asylum was badly "overcrowded" because "insanity is rapidly on the increase." The patients included a woman who "believed that she was the wife of the President of the United States," a young mother "asserting that the babe in her arms was Jesus Christ," and a man "who imagined that he had charge of the planet Jupiter. . . . Upon him he believed depended the safety of the planet, which, if once destroyed, would plunge the world into irretrievable misery and ruin." Another patient was "a man of almost gigantic proportions, with a strong leather belt fastened around his waist to which his hands were bound by cuffs. . . . There was a mingled expression of wildness and ungovernable passion in his eyes. . . . Among all the inmates of the Asylum there was none to whom the title of madman could be applied with more justice than to him."[24] One hundred years earlier, visitors had been allowed to view the spectacle of insanity by peering through the bars of the inmates' cells. By the 1850s, such visits had become vicarious through the pages of popular journals.

Obtaining public funding for asylum construction was not easy. In Connecticut, for example, a second asylum to complement the Hartford Retreat had been initially proposed in 1837. Additional legislative discussion and proposals took place in 1839, 1851, 1853, and 1855. Finally, in 1866, the Connecticut Hospital for the Insane at Middletown was approved after it was reported that 205 insane persons "were supported and aided by the towns, and that there were 300 others whose status was not known." In New Hampshire, a state asylum had been proposed in 1822, but "it took 11 years of continuous agitation before an institution was established at Concord." In Maine, the construction of an asylum had also been under consideration for many years. It finally opened in 1840 with thirty patients but was immediately overwhelmed by demands for admission. Three additions were added in the first ten years, and by 1850, the census of the hospital had reached 249 patients."[25]

Resistance to asylum building was also significant in many southern states. North Carolina, which had been the third most populous colony when Virginia and Pennsylvania had opened their asylums in 1751 and 1773, did not even begin discussion of an asylum until the 1820s, and it was not approved by the legislature until 1849. Even then the asylum took seven more years to build, because its funding was dependent on special land and poll taxes that could be used only as they accumulated. In Tennessee, "it was not until the 1830s, when the rapidly increasing number of mentally deranged caused general concern for the welfare of society . . . that public apathy gave way to sporadic demands for reform."[26] And in Georgia, proposals to build an asylum had surfaced sporadically since 1834, but nothing happened until the results from the 1840 census of the insane were made public and especially "when the 1841 Legislature received a similar report that approximately 300 white insane persons necessitated immediate care." The Georgia Lunatic Asylum in Milledgeville opened the following year.

An important reason why state insane asylums were ultimately supported by legislators and public officials was the promise by those proposing them that asylums could *cure* insane individuals and therefore would ultimately *save money*. This idea was prominent between approximately 1830 and 1850 in an era that Albert Deutsch a century later labeled "the cult of curability." The idea was based on the increasing prominence of moral therapy, the treatment initiated by Philippe Pinel in France and William Tuke in England, in which patients were treated with kindness but regimented firmness in the isolation of the asylum. In the early years of the nineteenth century, it had generally been accepted that some insane individuals would completely recover from their illness but that the majority of them would be intermittently or continuously sick for many years. At the Pennsylvania Hospital between 1790 and 1830, for example, "the hospital's cure rate remained at around 17 percent and its rate of improvement 12 percent."[27]

The new view on insanity's curability began in 1827 with a report from the Hartford Retreat that twenty-one out of twenty-three admissions that year, 91 percent, had recovered. Insanity, it was claimed, "is equally with other diseases of the human system under the control of proper medical treatment, the proportion of cures being as great." Other asylum superintendents accepted the curability challenge, and in 1843 a clear winner was declared when William Awl, superintendent of the Central Ohio Lunatic Asylum, announced that he had 100 percent recoveries "on all recent cases discharged the present year." Thereafter, he was widely known by his colleagues as "Dr. Cure-Awl"; as Pliny Earle noted, "There was a prophecy even in the sound of his name."[28]

Probably the most influential report on the curability of insanity was issued in 1845 by Samuel Woodward from the Worcester State Lunatic Hospital. Woodward had been elected president of the newly formed Association of Medical Superintendents of American Institutions for the Insane in 1844 and was widely respected. Between 1833 and 1845, Woodward claimed, from 82 to 91 percent of all recent cases (insane for less than one year) had recovered. His report circulated widely and was frequently cited by Dorothea Dix and other proponents of asylum building. As one advocate summarized it:

> Although the immediate expense might be considerable of erecting a new hospital, or of adding new buildings to the hospitals already in operation, yet this step would be, in fact, a matter of real economy. We have seen that under neglect, the disease remains for years, if not for life. In shortening the length of the disease we lessen expense. . . . Dr. Woodward, of Worcester, and Dr. Jarvis, late of Kentucky, and others, have entered into accurate calculations upon this subject, and the result shows, that new hospitals are a great advantage, on the ground of political economy.[29]

It was a promise that would be repeated often but would ultimately come back to haunt the superintendents and significantly impair their credibility.

Poe, Hawthorne, and Melville

From the 1830s to the 1850s, while asylums were being opened and insanity was steadily increasing, Edgar Allan Poe, Nathaniel Hawthorne, and Herman Melville emerged as major American writers and published some of their best-known works. Not surprisingly, insanity was an important theme in the work of all three.

Poe's descriptions of insanity have been widely praised for their realism. According to Charles Pridgeon: "Poe, more than any other nineteenth century American writer, achieved authenticity in identifying and describing the symptoms of mental disorder. . . . Some of his stories read like case histories. . . . Indeed, it would probably not offend medical historians to suggest that in symptomatology Poe rivaled the best known psychiatrists of the day."[30]

Many scholars have speculated whether Poe's interest in insanity arose primarily from his own psychiatric problems. He has been variously alleged to have had epilepsy, brain syphilis, encephalitis, a brain tumor, manic-depressive illness, alcoholism, opium addiction, or some combination of these. It is clear that he had periods of severe depression, and there are suggestions on at least two occasions that he had paranoid delusions. As Poe himself described in a letter: "But I am constitutionally sensitive—nervous in a very unusual degree. I became insane, with long intervals of horrible sanity." The following year, however, he denied insanity in a letter to his mother-in-law, Maria Clemm: "I was never *really* insane."[31]

Although Poe's mental state certainly influenced his writing, his interest in insanity as a subject was also related to its commercial appeal. He was one of the first American writers to support himself entirely by his writing and "hunger was ever at his door." As one critic noted: "Scholars agree that he was acutely attuned to his times, and they commonly note that he was partly motivated to write short stories because they could be written quickly and sold to magazines and that he knew that fiction of this sort was especially salable if it dealt with contemporary issues. . . . From what he read in books and periodicals,

Poe inevitably learned that the abnormal mind was increasingly becoming the subject of formal psychology, the theme of fiction, and the concern of society. He recognized the value of timeliness."[32]

Poe was strongly influenced by other authors who were writing about insanity. He reviewed and reprinted Charles Dickens's "A Madman's Manuscript" in the *Southern Literary Messenger* in 1836 and interviewed Dickens during the latter's 1842 visit to the United States. The use of a first-person narrator in Poe's "Tell-Tale Heart," written shortly after Dickens's visit, echoes "A Madman's Manuscript." Poe also read Brockden Brown, and his "references to Brown's work in [his] criticism . . . [are] respectful and deferential."[33] In addition, Poe corresponded with John Neal, the author of *Logan, A Family History,* which prominently featured insanity.

Some critics have speculated that Poe may also have read psychiatric case histories being published by English and American psychiatrists. For example, there are said to be similarities between the murder committed in "Berenice" and one described by Benjamin Rush in his textbook. Written between 1833 and 1835, "Berenice" was the first story in which Poe used the term "monomania" to describe a fixed delusion. Egaeus, the narrator, refers to himself as a monomaniac and becomes convinced that his cousin's teeth have some magical property. He becomes increasingly psychotic, with symptoms that today would be called schizophrenia: "Then came the full fury of my monomania, and I struggled in vain against its strange and irresistible influence. In the multiplied objects of the external world I had no thoughts but for the teeth. For these I longed with a phrenzied desire. All other matters and all different interests became absorbed in their single contemplation. They—they alone were present to the mental eye, and they, in their sole individuality, became the essence of my mental life."[34]

In 1839, Poe published "The Fall of the House of Usher." The protagonist, Roderick Usher, says that he suffers from an illness that is "a constitutional and family evil, and one for which he despair[s] to find a remedy." Its symptoms include "an excessive nervous agitation," "melancholy," periods of "excited and highly distempered ideality," acuteness of the senses, and auditory hallucinations: "He suffered much from a morbid acuteness of the senses: the most insipid food was alone endurable; he could wear only garments of certain texture;

the odours of all flowers were oppressive; his eyes were tortured by even a faint light; and there were but peculiar sounds, and these from stringed instruments, which did not inspire him with horror." Contemporary critics have suggested that Roderick Usher's illness would meet criteria for the diagnosis of manic-depressive illness.[35]

Poe's "Tell-Tale Heart," published in 1843, is frequently cited as a classic literary description of auditory hallucinations. After brutally murdering an old man and burying him beneath the floorboards of his house, the narrator calmly answers questions being asked by the police until he begins to hear the beating of the dead man's heart: "No doubt I now grew very pale; but I talked more fluently, and with a heightened voice. Yet the sound increased—and what could I do? It was a low, dull, quick sound—much such a sound as a watch makes when enveloped in cotton. I gasped for breath, and yet the officers heard it not. I talked more quickly, more vehemently but the noise steadily increased."[36]

In 1845 Poe published "The System of Doctor Tarr and Professor Fether," a satire on insane asylums and asylum doctors. The narrator visits an asylum in France, where he is treated to dinner by the superintendent, Monsieur Maillard, and his staff. As the story evolves, it becomes clear that the superintendent has himself become insane and that his staff are the patients; the asylum's actual keepers have been confined, "tarred and feathered and kept on a diet of bread and water" by the patients.[37] Like Poe's other stories, this one reflected the contemporary interests of the public, in this case concern about the asylums and skepticism regarding the treatments being used therein.

At the same time that Poe was incorporating the theme of insanity into his writings, Nathaniel Hawthorne was emerging as a writer. A solitary and retiring man, Hawthorne was described by his neighbor and hiking companion Oliver Wendell Holmes as being "like a dim room with a little taper of personality burning on the corner of the mantle." Hawthorne admitted that he sometimes found himself "in the Slough of Despond" and described such feelings: "In moods of heavy despondency, one feels as if it would be delightful to sink down in some quiet spot, and lie there forever, letting the soil gradually accumulate and form a little hillock over us, and the grass and perhaps flowers gather over it."[38]

Hawthorne was very interested in insanity and "was about as

well informed about current trends in psychology and psychiatry as most other American authors of his day, with the exception of Holmes." Isaac Ray, a prominent psychiatrist, had been a fellow student at Bowdoin College, and Horace Mann, who helped found the Worcester State Lunatic Asylum in 1833, was Hawthorne's brother-in-law. Hawthorne recorded several ideas for possible stories about insanity in his notebooks:

> Thanksgiving at the Worcester Lunatic Asylum. A ball and dance of the inmates in the evening,—a furious lunatic dancing with the principal's wife. Thanksgiving in an almshouse might make a better sketch.

> A partially insane man to believe himself the Provincial Governor or other great official of Massachusetts. The scene might be the Province House.

> A dreadful secret to be communicated to several people of various characters, —grave or gay, and they all to become insane, according to their characters, by the influence of the secret.[39]

By 1837 Hawthorne was translating such ideas into stories. "The Minister's Black Veil," for example, was based on the true story of Joseph Moody, a minister who in 1738 became "distracted" and thereafter wore a handkerchief over his face. Hawthorne utilized a black veil instead of a handkerchief and added a happy ending by having the minister cured at the close of the story. In the same year, Hawthorne included a description of an insane asylum in his *Twice-Told Tales:* "Shrieks pierced through the obscurity of sound, and were succeeded by the singing of sweet female voices, which in their turn gave way to a wild roar of laughter, broken suddenly by groanings and sobs, forming altogether a ghastly confusion of terror and mourning and mirth. Chains were rattling, fierce and stern voices uttered threats, and the scrouge resounded at their command."[40]

In 1842 Hawthorne wrote "Egotism; or, The Bosom-Serpent," which described a man who develops a delusion that a snake is living inside him:

"It gnaws me! It gnaws me!" he exclaimed. And then there
was an audible hiss, but whether it came from the apparent
lunatic's own lips. . . .

The man's wife leaves him, and his acquaintances "[think] that their
once brilliant friend [is] in an incipient stage of insanity. . . . He soon
exhibit[s] what most people [consider] indubitable tokens of insanity."[41]

Four years later, Hawthorne included a story in his *Mosses from
an Old Manse* about a man in an asylum who has "long intervals of
partially disordered reason." He experiences auditory and visual hallucinations, including nocturnal visits by Lord Byron, Robert Burns,
Napoleon, and other famous personages: "They visit me in spirit, perhaps desiring to engage my services as the amanuensis of their posthu-
mous productions, and thus secure the endless renown that they have
forfeited by going hence too early." The man concludes the story by
reflecting: "What a strange substance is the human brain! Or rather . . .
what an odd brain is mine!"[42]

Herman Melville was a friend, and for many years a neighbor, of
Hawthorne's. Melville's interest in insanity was a very personal one,
since his father had apparently suffered from mania, his mother from
depression, his older brother had some kind of "nervous condition,"
one son committed suicide, a niece and cousin were both insane, and
Melville himself had periods of instability. In the view of Nathaniel
Hawthorne's son, "There is reason to suspect that there was in him a
vein of insanity."[43]

Kay Jamison wrote that "themes of madness, and its interlacings
with visionary grandness, permeated Melville's writings." Paul
McCarthy, in his book *The Twisted Mind: Madness in Herman
Melville's Fiction*, likewise noted that "the fear of the twisted mind or
of inherited insanity might lie behind the writer's compelling interest
in insanity, his apparent compulsion to learn about the disease, to
observe its effects on the individual and on others, to write about it
repeatedly in his fiction, and to dread its appearance in himself."
Melville read widely on insanity, including Dickens's "A Madman's
Manuscript," Burton's *Anatomy of Melancholy*, and especially the
works of Isaac Ray, "who, more than any other, helped systematize a
previously chaotic assemblage of laws concerning madness."[44] Legal
aspects of insanity were of special interest to Melville, since his father-

in-law was Lemuel Shaw, who was chief justice of the Massachusetts Supreme Court and had written a landmark decision in 1844 clarifying the legal limits for the insanity defense.

In Melville's earliest stories, such as *Typee* (1846) and *Omoo* (1847), "[t]he fictional characters are not necessarily insane, but they appear near the thin red line separating the sane from the insane." By the time Melville was writing *Moby-Dick* in 1851, however, insanity in the form of monomania had become his dominant theme. Although it constituted less than 5 percent of all cases of insanity, monomania was of special interest to writers like Poe, Hawthorne, and Melville since individuals affected with monomania often appear normal except for their fixed delusions. As Melville's father-in-law had written in his 1844 legal decision: "The conduct may be in many respects regular, the mind acute, and the conduct apparently governed by rules of propriety, and at the same time there may be insane delusion, by which the mind is perverted." Noting Shaw's description of the monomaniac's mind as it "broods over *one idea* and cannot be reasoned out of it," one scholar added that "even if the monomaniac can distinguish right from wrong he cannot help doing wrong."[45]

This, then, is Captain Ahab, who destroys his ship, himself, and all his crew except Ishmael in his irrational pursuit of a whale. Charles Pridgeon wrote that "no American writer of the nineteenth century relied more heavily on the term monomania . . . than did Melville in his characterization of Ahab." And Henry Nash Smith, in "The Madness of Ahab," added: "In the course of *Moby-Dick*, Ishmael and other characters declare again and again that Ahab is insane. The Captain is said to be 'crazy' or 'mad' or 'lunatic' or, most often, 'monomaniac.' On at least two occasions, Ahab calls himself 'mad.'" Melville even included a physical basis for Ahab's monomania, saying that it was caused by "the violent circulation of blood which, causing destructive friction, leads to an overheated condition within the physiological system as a whole."[46]

Monomania was also prominent in Melville's next book, *Pierre* (1852), in which the title character, afflicted with a hereditary mental illness, gradually loses his sanity. The book also includes a description of an insane asylum. Pierre's half-sister, Isabel, had been brought up in an asylum, and she describes to him her life in such strange surroundings:

> During my . . . stay, all things changed to me, because I
> learned more, though always dimly. Some of its occupants
> departed; some changed from smiles to tears; some went
> moping all the day; some grew as savages and outrageous,
> and were dragged below by dumb-like men into deep
> places, that I know nothing of. . . . [Inmates] would
> vacantly roam about, and talk vacant talk to each other.
> Some would stand in the middle of the room gazing
> steadily on the floor . . . and never stirred. . . . Some would
> sit crouching in the corner. . . . Some kept their hands tight
> on their hearts, and went slowly promenading up and
> down. . . . But most of them were dumb, and could not, or
> would not speak, or had forgotten how to speak. . . . Some
> were always talking about Hell, Eternity, and God. . . . Some
> harangued the wall; some apostrophized the air; some
> hissed at the air; some lolled their tongues out at the air;
> some struck the air.

Melville probably witnessed such scenes himself, since his niece spent many years hospitalized in New York's Bloomingdale Asylum. *Pierre* was not well received by reviewers. *Graham's Magazine*, for example, noted that "the merit of the book is in clearly presenting the psychology of madness; but the details of such a mental malady as that which afflicts Pierre are almost as disgusting as those of physical disease itself."[47]

In *Bartleby the Scrivener* (1853), Melville drew a portrait of a subtype of insanity that would today be called simple or residual schizophrenia. Bartleby is hired by a law firm, and one of the other employees soon suggests that "I think, sir, he's a little luny." Bartleby slowly slides downhill mentally and finally comes to rest in jail as a vagrant, "strangely huddled at the base of the wall, his knees drawn up, and lying on his side, his head touching the cold stones." Critics have suggested that Bartleby may have been patterned after Melville's boyhood friend Eli James Murdock Fly, who had apparently become insane under similar circumstances and for whom Melville in 1851 had helped arrange for hospitalization.[48]

It should also be noted that both Poe and Melville expressed ambivalence about insanity. It is portrayed as a brain disorder with dire consequences but also as a source of inspiration and creativity. In Poe's "Eleanora," written in 1841, the protagonist says: "Men have called me mad; but the question is not yet settled, whether madness is or is not the loftiest intelligence—whether much that is glorious— whether all that is profound—does not spring from disease of thought—from moods of mind exalted at the expense of the general intellect. They who dream by day are cognizant of many things which escape those who dream only by night."[49] And Melville, in *Pierre*, similarly says: "The intensest light of reason and revelation combined, can not shed such blazonings upon the deeper truths in man, as will sometimes proceed from his own profoundest gloom. Utter darkness is then his light, and cat-like he distinctly sees all objects through a medium which is mere blindness to common vision."[50] A focus upon such positive aspects of insanity, and indeed its romanticization, would recur sporadically but repeatedly throughout the twentieth century.

"The Price Which We Pay for Civilization"

The 1850 decennial census did not bring good news to those who hoped that insanity was not increasing. The census noted that the enumeration of insane and idiot persons in 1840 had "led to very great discussion and excited a good deal of public feeling," so in 1850 "it was deemed important to bestow upon it more than ordinary attention." As one improvement, insane and idiot persons were counted separately. In 1974, Kurt Gorwitz applied the insane-to-idiot ratio from the 1850 census to estimate the proportion for each of them in the 1840 census.[51] Since both enumerations were done by U.S. marshals with neither instructions nor training, the results can only be considered rough approximations. The fact that the results are congruent with much more carefully done counts in the 1880 and 1890 censuses, however, affords them some credibility.

The most striking findings from the 1850 census of insane persons were the increase in the insanity rate since 1840 and the much higher rates in northern states compared to southern states. Using Gorwitz's calculations for 1840, the insanity rate for the United States had increased from 0.51 per 1,000 total population in 1840 to 0.67 per 1,000 in 1850, a 31 percent increase. The New England states had increased 45 percent, while many southern and midwestern states had increased much less. This increase in the insanity rate between the two censuses was consistent with other indicators of increasing insanity. For example, between 1840 and 1850 the average number of annual admissions to state insane asylums increased from 89 to 140, and the average patient census increased from 180 to 333.[52] Previously, there had been widespread agreement among hospital superintendents that no insane asylum should contain more than 250 patients, but by 1850 the majority of asylums had many more.

The higher insanity rates in northern compared to southern states, evident in 1840, were even more clearly demarcated in 1850. For example, the insanity rate in Massachusetts was 1.7 per 1,000, more than four times South Carolina's rate of 0.4 per 1,000. Massachusetts reported 1,680 insane persons in asylums and in the community, while South Carolina reported only 249, despite the fact that the population of Massachusetts was only 5 percent greater. The large number of slaves in South Carolina presumably accounted for some of this difference, but even allowing for that, it must be concluded either that there was a gross discrepancy in ascertainment between the states or the insanity rates were truly different.

Edward Jarvis was concerned by the 1850 census results, and on May 21, 1851, he presented a paper, "On the Supposed Increase of Insanity," before the asylum superintendents. After acknowledging the limitations of the census data for comparing insanity rates over time, he reviewed the dramatic increase in hospitalized insane persons in Massachusetts from 182 in 1832, to 1,015 in 1851. "Beside these," he added, "there is now so great a demand for the admission of patients who cannot be accommodated in these establishments already built. . . . [T]hey increased as fast as rooms in the hospitals increase, and in some places faster."[53]

Given the existing data, Jarvis concluded that "insanity is an increasing disease" and that this conclusion "corroborates the opinion of nearly all writers, whether founded on positive and known facts, on analogy, on computation or on conjecture." The reason for the increase, speculated Jarvis, was "more opportunities and rewards for great and excessive mental action, more uncertain and hazardous employments, and consequently more disappointments, more means and provocations for sensual indulgence, more dangers of accidents and injuries, more groundless hopes, and more painful struggle to obtain that which is beyond reach, or to effect that which is impossible." In summary, he said, "insanity is then a part of the price which we pay for civilization."

The linking of insanity rates to civilization was not a new idea, having been proposed by many British observers and also by Samuel Gridley Howe in Boston eight years previously: "It cannot be denied that civilization, in its progress, is rife with causes which over-excite individuals, and result in the loss of mental equilibrium."[54] But increasing insanity was not a message the asylum superintendents wanted to hear. The superintendents were utilizing the high cure rate reported by Dr. Woodward of the Worcester State Lunatic Hospital to prove to state legislators that insanity could be cured and that asylums would ultimately save money. Jarvis's figures cast substantial doubt on these cure rates and implied that insanity was going to continue increasing whether more asylums were built or not.

The members of the Massachusetts legislature were also concerned about the 1850 census figures and the apparent growing problem of insanity, and in 1854 they appointed a commission "to ascertain the number and condition of the insane in the State . . . [and] to see what further accommodations, if any, are needed for the relief and care of the insane."[55] The three-person Commission on Lunacy consisted of former governor Levi Lincoln, former state senator Increase Sumner, and Edward Jarvis.

Jarvis was determined to carry out the most careful survey of insane persons ever done. He solicited information from all 1,319 physicians in the state, obtaining replies from all except four; all town overseers of the poor; all jails and houses of correction; clergymen; hospital superintendents; officials of neighboring states where Massachusetts citizens might be treated; and "proprietors of all the private houses or establishments devoted to the care of the insane." In addition, one of the commissioners personally visited sixty-five towns to obtain additional information. In a review of the commission's report, Isaac Ray wrote that "never . . . has a statistical inquiry been pursued with such ample provisions against error and imperfections, or with results more worthy of reliance."[56]

Insanity and Idiocy in Massachusetts: Report of the Commission on Lunacy was released in 1855. A total of 2,632 insane persons and

1,087 idiots were identified, making the insanity rate 2.3 per 1,000 total population. Jarvis carefully separated the two diagnoses, counting as an "idiot" only "one who was originally destitute of mind, or in whom the mental faculties have not been developed."[57] Among the insane, 1,141 were in hospitals; 207 in jails, houses of correction, or almshouses; and 1,284 in poorhouses or living at home. Three-quarters of the insane persons were thought to be incurable, which further undermined Woodward's previous claims of high cure rates. The fact that the commission found 952 (57 percent) more insane persons than had been found by the U.S. marshals in the 1850 census suggested that the problem of insanity in Massachusetts was substantially greater than the census had shown.

The report of the Commission on Lunacy received national attention. Isaac Ray, writing in the *North American Review,* concluded that "we have ample ground for our assertion that insanity is more prevalent in Massachusetts than in any other State in the Union," although Ray acknowledged that this was an "unenviable distinction." The Boston Sanitary Association calculated that the annual cost of insanity in Massachusetts, based on the commission's findings, was $6,205,900 (1997 equivalent). This cost was said to be "a matter of terrible interest to the people and the government" and was a "mill-stone hanging on the neck of the body politic."[58]

Immigrants and Poverty

The report of the Commission on Lunacy included analyses of two questions that were increasingly being asked in the 1850s: What was the role of immigrants in the increasing insanity rates, and what was the relationship of poverty to insanity?

Regarding the first, the commission noted "the great number of foreigners among our insane" and speculated that "either our foreign population are more prone to insanity, or their habits and trials, their experiences and privations, and the circumstances which surround them, and the climate of this country, are more unfavorable to their mental health than that of the natives."[59] Specifically, it reported that foreigners constituted 24 percent of insane individuals, but only 20 percent of the Massachusetts population.

Later in the nineteenth century, it would be recognized that when such figures are corrected for age differences in the populations—the immigrants included a higher proportion of young adults in the age range in which insanity is most prevalent—differences in rates were negligible. But correction for age differences was not considered in 1855, and the idea was becoming widespread that immigrants were a major cause of the increasing insanity. As early as 1837, William A. F. Browne had speculated that insanity was common in America because "the refuse of other nations has been poured forth. . . . [T]he tide of population, which has been flowing for so many years uninterruptedly towards America, has been impure and poisoned." In 1849, Isaac Ray had similarly speculated that many of the immigrants had been sent to America "because of their liability to insanity." And in the 1860s, other official reports would describe the immigrants as "ragged and filthy in person as well as diseased in mind" and as "convicts, drunkards, and strumpets, crazed by their crimes."[60]

Insanity among immigrants, according to the Commission on Lunacy report, was especially prominent among Irish immigrants. During 1846, only twelve Irish-born patients had been admitted to the Worcester State Lunatic Asylum; in 1854, ninety-six such patients were admitted, and the hospital's trustees complained that it "is fast becoming a Hospital for foreigners." At the Boston Lunatic Hospital, the percentage of Irish patients increased from 41 percent in 1846 (70 out of 169), to 66 percent in 1848 (124 out of 188), and then to 80 percent in 1851 (164 out of 204), at which time Irish immigrants constituted 31 percent of the city's population.[61]

The Commission on Lunacy offered possible reasons why insanity was more common among Irish immigrants. "Unquestionably much of their insanity is due to their intemperance, to which the Irish seem to be peculiarly prone," it noted. In addition, the Irish were said to "have also a greater irritability; they are more readily disturbed when they find themselves at variance with the circumstances about them. . . . Their lives are filled with doubt, and harrowing anxiety troubles them, and they are involved in frequent mental, and probably physical, suffering." Eight years earlier, George Chandler, a physician in the Worcester State Lunatic Hospital, had speculated that the Irish immigrants' "strong love for their native land, which is characteristic with them [is one of] the fruitful causes of insanity among them."[62]

Massachusetts was not alone in noting an increasing number of foreigners in general, and Irish immigrants in particular, among the insane. At the New York City Lunatic Asylum at Blackwell's Island, 77 percent of all patients were foreign born and 47 percent were from Ireland, although Irish immigrants made up only 28 percent of the city's population. At Butler Hospital in Providence, it was said that "most of the foreigners are Irish." Furthermore, it was noted, "we are not so successful in our treatment of them as with the native population of New England." In Maine, Irish immigrants were also said to occupy a disproportionate number of asylum beds and to be "pre-eminently incurable."[63]

The use of Irish immigrants to explain the increasing number of insane persons was becoming widespread by the 1850s. In 1847, the superintendent of the Worcester Hospital had warned the hospital trustees that "if this bad class continues to press in upon us, I shall be obliged to ask you to send a portion to the jails." The trustees called the Irish immigrants "vicious and depraved. . . . Their misery, their ignorance and their jealousy stand in the way of improvement at the Hospital."[64] Thus, it was not surprising that the Commission on Lunacy also utilized this belief to explain why insanity appeared to be so prevalent in Massachusetts.

This prejudice against Irish immigrants who had become insane was, in fact, part of a broader prejudice against Irish immigrants in general that became prominent in mid-nineteenth-century America. One reason was their increased numbers. In the 1820s, 54,338 Irish immigrants had come to America. This number increased in the 1830s to 207,381, and in the 1840s to 780,719 as the Irish famine took hold. Furthermore, many of the Irish immigrants congregated in specific towns and parts of cities, making them highly visible. New York City had its "little Dublin"; Portland, Maine, had large numbers from County Galway; and Holyoke, Massachusetts, had so many immigrants from County Kerry that they "were Dingle men in everything but geographical location."[65]

Another important reason for the emerging anti-Irish sentiment was religious. Until 1830, three-quarters of all Irish immigrants to the United States had been Protestant, the majority coming from the northern Irish counties of Ulster. During those years, there was said to be a "great disinclination on the part of the Roman Catholics" to emigrate.[66] In the 1830s and 1840s, that changed dramatically, and by the late 1840s, approximately 90 percent of the Irish immigrants to the United States were Catholic.

There was also a class issue associated with the emerging anti-Irish prejudice. The Protestant Irish who had emigrated to America prior to 1830 had been drawn disproportionately from the middle class, including tradesmen and successful farmers. Many of the Catholics who had emigrated in the early years had also come from "the most enterprising, industrious, and virtuous part" of the population. However, "by the mid-1820s a decided shift toward the emigration of poorer classes of Irish seems to have taken place." This became more pronounced during the famine, when a large proportion of the emigrants "were poor smallholders, cottiers, and laborers, often Irish-speakers or their children." Sometimes referred to as "shanty Irish" by other Americans, the newly arrived Irish immigrants, among whom the increasing insanity was observed, were disproportionately poor and unskilled and often lived in cities and towns in overcrowded and unsanitary conditions. In 1850 in New York City, "almost 30,000 people, primarily Irish, lived below ground level in cellars often flooded with rainwater and raw sewage," while among the Irish in Providence "an average of nearly nine persons . . . were packed into one- or two-room dwellings."[67]

In addition to the issue of immigrants, the 1855 Massachusetts Commission on Lunacy discussed the relationship of insanity to poverty. According to the report, insanity is "a part and parcel of poverty," because "both of them grow out of and represent internal mental character." Specifically, "the weak mind" and "the unstable mind" both "fail of securing worldly prosperity, and often bring on poverty and pauperism, and they also often produce insanity."[68] The report noted that "many lunatics by their disease lose their power of self-sustenance" and thereby become paupers, so that on those grounds alone one would expect a correlation between insanity and pauperism.

Since most insane persons sooner or later became paupers, the causal relationship of insanity and poverty was widely debated in the 1850s. Isaac Ray argued that "insanity . . . may be traced, in many instances, more or less directly to poverty." However, he added that "it does not follow that these persons were paupers before becoming insane." In support of this, John Chapin, in a study in New York State, found that 82 percent of insane persons had been self-supporting "previous to the invasion of insanity": "The relation, therefore, that pauperism holds to insanity does not appear to be that of cause and effect, to the degree that many suppose; pauperism being rather a condition involved in the situation of its victims."[69]

In his analysis of the Commission on Lunacy Report, Isaac Ray also touched upon the possible relationship of insanity to industrialization. Since the belief was becoming widespread that increasing insanity was somehow related to advances in civilization, this was a logical relationship to explore. As Ray noted, "It is a popular impression that mental disease is more rife among a mercantile or manufacturing population, peculiarly tried as it is by excessive activity of the mind and frequent reverses of fortune, than in farming communities where life flows on a more even current."[70] Ray examined this question by comparing the 1855 insanity rates in the Massachusetts "counties most extensively engaged in commerce and manufactures" to the "counties most exclusively engaged in agricultural pursuits." He reported no apparent relationship of insanity to industrialization.

Since industrialization and urbanization usually accompany each other, there was also speculation at this time regarding a possible relationship between insanity and urbanization. Such a relationship had been postulated in 1848 by Dorothea Dix: "There are, in proportion to numbers, more insane in cities than in large towns, and more insane in villages than among the same number of inhabitants dwelling in scattered settlements." The reason, Dix said, was because insanity occurs most frequently "wherever the intellect is most excited."[71]

Urbanization in the United States proceeded slowly in the first half of the nineteenth century, but at midcentury it was accelerating. In 1790, only 5 percent of the population lived in towns of 2,500 or more, and there were only six cities with a population of 8,000 or greater. By 1850, 15 percent of the population lived in towns of 2,500 or more, and there were eighty-five cities with populations of 8,000 or greater. New York City had half a million people and was growing at the rate of 50 percent each decade; Chicago was doubling in size each decade.

One concomitant of this urbanization was the crowding of

people together in confined living spaces in apartment buildings, boardinghouses, and tenements. The first apartment building in New York City was erected in 1869; by the end of the century, the buildings had become ubiquitous. Boardinghouses had become common in New York City by midcentury, so much so that in 1856 Walt Whitman, who worked intermittently as a journalist, estimated that seven out of ten family dwellings had been subdivided. Tenement buildings overflowed with immigrants and other poor people. According to Oscar Hamlin: "Some of the earliest buildings [had] no privies at all; the residents [were] expected to accommodate themselves elsewhere as best they could. Tenements from mid-century onward had generally water closets in the yards and alleys, no great comfort to the occupants of the fifth and sixth floors."[72]

The belief that insanity was related to urbanization was not, however, universal. An 1857 article in the *National Magazine* contended that insanity was more common in rural frontier communities because of the "constant exposure to Indian forays and the hardships of pioneer life." Furthermore, because of the individualistic character of Americans, insane persons on the frontier were said to be more violent than their counterparts in Europe.[73]

As the 1850s moved to a close, fears about insanity and other issues were subsumed by the question of slavery. In 1856 John Brown and his followers killed five pro-slavery advocates in Kansas, fusing their irreconcilable opposition to slavery with violence. Three years later, Brown seized the federal arsenal at Harpers Ferry, Maryland. What had been an increasingly uncivil dialogue would soon be a civil war.

CHAPTER 11

"A Very Startling Increase"
The United States, 1860–1890

Of all the afflictions which appeal to human justice and sympathy, none is so anomalous, none so little understood, none so threatening, as insanity. Experts dispute about its definition. Mystery hangs over its cause. Grave doubts obstruct its cure. The common people are perplexed whether to regard it as a mysterious disgrace, a natural disease, or an avenging dispensation of Providence. Judges and juries, in dealing with it, are lost in mazes of metaphysics and in masses of conflicting opinions.

—DORMAN EATON, *North American Review*, 1881

It seem'd enough that all the Remedies of that Kind had been used till they were found fruitless, and that the Plague spread itself with an irresistible fury.

—DANIEL DEFOE, *A Journal of the Plague Year*, 1722

W ars are never kind to individuals with insanity, and the Civil War was no exception. Following closely upon the financial panic of 1857, the war depleted state treasuries, so that asylums lacked basic supplies. With fewer staff, insufficient food, and deteriorating sanitary conditions, infectious diseases spread rapidly among the patients and mortality rates soared. In the South Carolina

Lunatic Asylum, for example, the annual mortality rate had averaged 8 percent between 1853 and 1862 but climbed to 13 percent between 1863 and 1865.[1]

The South Carolina Asylum played a direct role in the war as well. For two months in late 1864 and early 1865, the grounds of the asylum were used by Confederate forces as a prison camp for captured Union officers. One POW later recalled "the numerous doleful sounds emanating" from the asylum. As General Sherman's troops approached Columbia in February 1865, the Union prisoners were moved to Charlotte, North Carolina. As soon as the prisoners left, however, "several hundred Columbians took refuge in the asylum," since its main building was brick "and the nature of its clientele encouraged citizens to believe that it would be spared from enemy attacks." As Sherman's troops burned and looted the city, the citizens of Columbia huddled in the asylum, "their little effects tied up in sheets, and some few had boxes and small trunks."[2] It was difficult to distinguish the patients from the nonpatients.

Another asylum directly affected by the politics of the Civil War was Virginia's Lunatic Asylum west of the Allegheny Mountains. When the war had begun in 1861, the asylum's construction had been almost complete, but it had not yet been opened for patients. The majority of residents living in the western part of Virginia opposed the state's secession from the Union, and in 1862, forty counties voted to become West Virginia. When the new state was officially admitted to the Union in 1863, it inherited the new asylum as its only government building, which was then opened as the West Virginia Hospital for the Insane the following year.

The West Virginia Hospital was the only asylum that began operations during the war. In the ten-year period following the war, however, twenty-two additional asylums opened: four in New York, two each in Illinois, Virginia, and Missouri, and one each in Rhode Island, Massachusetts, Connecticut, New Jersey, Pennsylvania, Kentucky, Wisconsin, Minnesota, Iowa, Kansas, Nebraska, and Oregon. The twenty-two asylums were half as many as the total number that had opened in the preceding one hundred years.

In each state, "patients endlessly appeared at the doors of the newly opened asylums such that overfilling arose in two years or less. . . . Each new hospital was rapidly filled as if from an endless hidden reservoir." The average census for the hospitals for the insane increased from 369 patients in 1860 to 473 in 1870, the average thus being almost twice what had been set as a hospital maximum just twenty years before. By 1870, two hospitals—the New York City Lunatic Asylum at Blackwell's Island and the Insane Asylum of California at Stockton—each had more than one thousand patients. The number of annual admissions per hospital grew from 142 in 1860 to 182 in 1870, an increase of 28 percent.[3]

The consequences of these increasing numbers were not pleasant for the patients. An English visitor to the New York City Lunatic Asylum in 1868 found 304 patients sleeping on the floor and observed: "Never, in fact, have I visited any institution for the insane where the noise and confusion were so bewildering, nor where I experienced the same feeling of relief on leaving." Patient suicides by drowning in the East River, which ran next to the asylum, were said to be "rather frequent."[4]

In Connecticut in 1867, "the pressure for admission . . . has been so great as often to compel us to discharge those who are more quiet and less troublesome and dangerous; receiving in their stead, with no greater profit to the institution, those who were dangerous to themselves or others." Predictably, patient attacks on other patients, including homicides, were not rare. At the Asylum for Chronic Insane at Tewksbury, Massachusetts, patient mortality for 1873 was 13 percent—60 out of 435—due to "lack of proper medical supervision and of sanitary provision." At the South Carolina Lunatic Asylum, which had had to advertise for patients when it had originally opened, by 1875 the patients were crowded "like sheep on the floors, in the corridors, and in rooms that are only large enough for one, or two at most."[5]

These asylum conditions in the 1860s and 1870s suggested to many that insanity was increasing. This suspicion was strengthened by the realization that the number of insane individuals in poorhouses, almshouses, and jails was as great, or even greater, than it had been forty years earlier. The original impetus to build asylums had been to provide humane care for insane persons who were being held in such facilities, but forty years of asylum building had produced no change. In 1864 the *Atlantic Monthly* noted that "as statistics reveal the late gradual and general increase of insanity, it becomes a provident people to consider what may be the ultimate results, if this increase should happen never to be checked." If everyone becomes mad, nobody would know it. "Should a whole community become insane, it would nevertheless vote itself wise."[6]

The number of insane persons in jails continued to be problematic. For example, an 1873 survey of Wisconsin jails reported:

> Men and women unable to take care of themselves in pens with loose straw for beds and only a blanket to cover their naked bodies. . . . In one county an insane man and an insane woman were found nude, covered with their own excrement, huddled in a pile of straw above a pig pen. . . . A sick woman was found in a dark cell in the cellar of a county jail. She received her food through a hole in the floor, much like a wild animal receiving food from its keeper. . . . Inmates frequently killed each other and black eyes and bruises were evidence of fights and abuse of the keepers.[7]

Walter Kempster, the superintendent of the Northern Hospital for the Insane, responded to the report as follows: "Who can think of the number of unfortunate beings now confined in the receptacles of the different counties of this state, and realize in the most remote degree, the sorrowing hearts their misfortunes have created; of hopes once bright now dashed; of the ambitions that lured beyond strength; of life's work begun but left unfinished. . . . Who can think of these things, *of the measureless calamity of insanity,* and turn idly away, closing eye and hand, withholding that which is known to be required to make life comfortable?"[8]

The number of insane persons in county poorhouses also continued to be problematic. In 1864 the New York state legislature ordered Sylvester Willard, secretary of the State Medical Society, to ascertain the number of insane persons in these institutions. Willard's report the following year included facts "too appalling to be forgotten and too important to be thrown aside." There were, he said, 1,345 insane persons in county poorhouses, not including those in New York City and Kings County. Jefferson County, for example, had sixty-one insane inmates in the poorhouse. In Greene County, "Six lunatics are confined in cells, five of them are in chains, including two women." In Delaware County, "the sufferings of these unfortunates, from whom air and the light of heaven are shut out, would form a dark chapter of human misery, could it be written."[9] Each time insane inmates were transferred from the county poorhouse to the Utica State Lunatic Asylum, others appeared to take their places. Then, as the Utica Asylum became overcrowded, these inmates were often sent back to the county poorhouses, exacerbating the crowding there still further.

The outcome of the Willard report was authorization by the New York state legislature to build a new asylum for 1,500 chronic patients. It would be the largest asylum in the nation, and it was "confidently expected that the questions of providing for the dependent insane with a maximum of humanity, efficiency and economy had been at last satisfactorily solved." The asylum was built, named after Willard, who had died shortly after submitting his report, and opened in 1869. It filled to capacity almost immediately with "chronic cases transferred from Utica and from local poorhouses and jails." The pool of insane persons appeared to be endless. In desperation, the New York State Legislature authorized the building of four more asylums, which were opened in Poughkeepsie (1871), Middletown (1874), Binghamton (1879), and Buffalo (1880). Despite these increased beds, an 1880 survey of county poorhouses still reported that 24.3 percent of the inmates were insane.[10]

The decennial censuses of 1860 and 1870 provided some clues regarding the origins of the apparently endless pool of insane persons. The population of the United States had increased from 17.1 million to 39.9 million between 1840 and 1870, thus slightly more than doubling. On the basis of population alone, therefore, a twofold increase in the number of insane persons needing treatment would have been expected. Yet the number of insane persons in hospitals and asylums had increased from 2,561 in 1840 to 17,735 in 1870, an increase of almost sevenfold.[11]

In New York State, the total population had been 2.5 million when the Utica State Lunatic Asylum opened in 1843. The Utica Asylum and the New York City Lunatic Asylum together had 600 patients at that time.[12] By 1870 the state population had increased to 4.4 million, not quite double. However, by 1870 in upstate New York, there were over 600 patients in the Utica State Lunatic Asylum, 1,500 in the

Willard Asylum for the Insane, 1,345 in county poorhouses, and uncounted others trying to gain admission. In New York City, there were an additional 1,250 insane individuals in the New York City Lunatic Asylum and 600 in the Kings County Lunatic Asylum. Clearly, the increase in the general population could account for only a small proportion of the increasing number of insane persons.

The 1860 and 1870 censuses confirmed that insane persons were increasing in number much faster than the general population. Overall in the United States, the number had increased from 0.67 per 1,000 total population in 1850 to 0.97 in 1870; for every two insane persons per population in 1850, there were three in 1870. The New England states continued to have the greatest number of insane persons—1.67 per 1,000 in 1870, compared to 0.54 for states in the South. Although methodologically the counting of insane persons in these early censuses was less than optimal, the results were remarkably consistent in showing a continuing increase.

"The Craziest People in the World"

The most unexpected finding in the 1860 and 1870 decennial censuses was the high rate of insanity in California. In 1860, California's rate of insane persons was 1.20 per 1,000 total population, ranking behind just four New England states. By 1870, California's rate had almost doubled, to 2.05 per 1,000, and only Vermont's rate was higher. In the 1880 census, California ranked third, but by 1890 it had achieved the dubious distinction of leading all states, with a rate of 2.98 insane persons per 1,000 total population. By that time, Californians were widely referred to as "the craziest people in the world."[13]

The increase in California's overall population during these years was startling. In 1848, before John Sutter discovered gold, the state's total population had been approximately 20,000, with only 900 living in the village of San Francisco. As word of the gold strike spread, a wave of humanity poured over the mountains and arrived by ship, 40,000 people disembarking in San Francisco in 1849 alone. By 1850, the state's population was 93,000, and over the next ten years it increased fourfold again to 380,000. By 1880, California's population reached 865,000, representing a more than fortyfold increase in thirty-two years.

As fast as the general population increased, the number of insane persons increased even faster. Initially, there were only a few, arrested under an 1849 San Francisco city ordinance that permitted the police to detain "any suspicious, insane or forlorn persons found strolling the city at night." In 1849 and 1850, such individuals were detained in a British ship that had been captured in the War of 1812 and moored in downtown San Francisco for use as a jail. By 1851 the insane detainees were transferred to the new jail, where it was said "they were confined with criminals and in a noise and din that would almost make a sane man crazy." The following year California established three general hospitals in San Francisco, Sacramento, and Stockton; in a forerunner of a financing system that would become popular more than a century later, the San Francisco Hospital allowed for "any healthy person by paying the sum of $5, [to be] thereby entitled to a year's hospital care, should it be necessary."[14]

Initially, all three general hospitals admitted insane patients, but even in 1852 newspapers commented on the "surprisingly . . . great number of insane persons." By 1853 a decision was made to convert the hospital at Stockton for exclusive use by insane persons. Like its eastern counterparts, this hospital rapidly filled to overflowing, and as California's population increased, additional state hospitals were built at Napa (1876), Agnew (1889), Mendocino (1893), Patton (1894), and Norwalk (1916). Each filled rapidly, and overcrowding continued to be such that "many were temporarily bedded on mattresses spread on the floor," so that "at night one [could not] walk across certain wards without stepping over these recumbent bodies."[15]

Why did the number of insane persons in California increase so much faster than the general population, so that by 1890 it led the nation? One reason in the early years was demographics—the men and women who initially came to seek gold were mostly in their twenties and thirties, the age of peak onset of insanity. By 1880, however, the age distribution in California had become similar to that of the eastern states.[16]

Many people believed that individuals inclined to become insane were more likely to go to California. John Robertson, superintendent of Napa State Hospital, called California "the dumping ground for the off-scourgings of creation." William A. White referred to Californians as "the wandering, unsettled, riffraff of the country."

Many new Californians had also come from New England, an area with a high rate of insanity; the influence of New Englanders can still be seen in the architecture of towns such as Mendocino. Overtly insane individuals would not have been able to get themselves to California, however. And many others who became insane were sent home, such as the "promising young physician from New Orleans" who was sent home under guard, and the first insane person admitted to Stockton State Hospital, who was repatriated to his native France.[17]

Other people, including the superintendent of the Stockton State Hospital, believed that "disastrous enterprises, sudden reverses of fortune, intemperance, fast living, and an unsettled condition of life [were] the chief causes of mental disorder on the Pacific Coast." However, it was noted even by 1870 that miners were not disproportionately represented among insane persons; in fact, the Chinese, who in some areas made up more than half of the miners, had the lowest rate of insanity of any group of Californians by far.[18]

Still others argued that California appeared to have more insane persons per population because it had fewer almshouses and therefore the state hospitals admitted "imbeciles, dotards, drunkards, simpletons, fools; a class, in fact, of harmless defectives usually found in poorhouses elsewhere." This point was strongly emphasized by Richard Fox in his analysis of San Francisco's insanity records in *So Far Disordered in Mind*. Against this argument is the fact that a diagnostic breakdown of records from Stockton State Hospital does not appear to differ significantly from hospital records from eastern asylums.[19] And in the national censuses of 1880 and 1890, when California was a leader in the number of insane persons per population, insane persons in the community were being counted as well as those in the hospitals.

Many people in California also blamed the high insanity rate on foreigners, just as others were increasingly doing in the eastern states. An 1870 survey provided support for such a theory; the insanity rate among individuals who were foreign born was 1.8 per 1,000, whereas among the native born it was 0.5 per 1,000. If such figures had been age corrected, however, the differences would have been much less. In the 1870 survey, the highest insanity rates occurred among those who had come from Norway and Sweden (4.5 per 1,000), Scotland (3.6), France (3.2), and Ireland (3.2). The rate among Chinese immigrants was 0.3 per 1,000, even lower than for those born in the United States.[20]

It should also be noted that, contrary to what is generally assumed, the population of California was highly urban. "During the second half of the nineteenth century . . . the American West included the fastest-growing cities in the nation, and by 1890 had become more heavily urban than any other region except the Northeast."[21] Since it is now known that urban living is a risk factor for insanity, this fact must also be included in any assessment of possible causes of California's high rate of insanity.

In the end, however, there is no definitive answer why Californians became "the craziest people in the world." One can select any one of the many theories proposed at that time, including even "Mormonism" and the "excessive use of tobacco and mint candy."[22]

"Could It Be Madness?"

The years of the Civil War saw the publication of Oliver Wendell Holmes's novel *Elsie Venner* in 1861, which also marked the termination of insanity as a major theme in American literature. Since Brockden Brown's *Wieland* in 1798, insanity had been prominently featured in the works of many authors, including Neal, Dana, Cooper, Paulding, Simms, Bird, Poe, Hawthorne, and Melville. But by the 1860s, insanity was no longer unusual and therefore would have been of interest primarily to authors who themselves feared its symptoms or who had family members afflicted by it.

Holmes was interested in insanity from a medical viewpoint. During his training to become a physician, he had studied the pathology of brain diseases and had read the works of Burton, Maudsley, Pinel, Rush, and Tuke. In 1840 Holmes had served with Edward Jarvis on a committee of the Massachusetts Medical Society to investigate the 1840 census results, which had grossly overcounted the number of insane free colored persons. Three years later, he and Jarvis had also worked together on a classification of mental diseases.[23]

By the time Holmes wrote *Elsie Venner,* his first novel, he was established as an essayist and poet as well as being a professor of anatomy at Harvard Medical School. He was convinced that insanity was caused by "something wrong in their nervous centers," caused either by heredity or organic disease. The title character in *Elsie Venner* is afflicted by "a form of congenital moral insanity" because her mother had been bitten by a snake during pregnancy. In much of the book, various characters discuss whether or not Elsie can be held responsible for her behavior. As summarized by Charles Pridgeon, "*Elsie Venner*, more clearly than any other American novel written in the 1800s, provides a microcosmic view on the moral implications of insanity."[24]

At the same time as Oliver Wendell Holmes was publicly expressing his views on insanity in Boston, Emily Dickinson was privately recording her views at her home in Amherst. Dickinson was apparently normal until her twenties, at which time she became increasingly reclusive, eventually not even leaving the house for fifteen years. Biographers have debated whether she had periods of true insanity, suffered from agoraphobia, or both. Dickinson's abundant correspondence reflects rational thinking, but her poems, which she did not intend to publish and which became known only after her death, reflect an intense interest in insanity.

For example, in "The First Day's Night Had Come," written in 1862, Dickinson describes her fears of insanity:

> *My Brain—began to laugh—*
> *I mumbled—like a fool—*
> *And tho' 'tis years ago—that Day—*
> *My Brain keeps giggling—still.*
>
> *And Something's odd—within—*
> *That person that I was—*
> *And this One—do not feel the same—*
> *Could it be Madness—this?*

And in "I felt a Funeral in My Brain," also written in 1862, she describes thought processes that are similar to those described by some insane persons:

> *I felt a funeral in my brain,*
> *And mourners, to and fro,*
> *Kept treading, treading, till it seemed*
> *That sense was breaking through.*

And when they all were seated,
A service like a drum
Kept beating, beating, till I thought
My mind was going numb

And then I heard them lift a box,
And creak across my soul
With those same boots of lead, again.
Then space began to toll

As all the heavens were a bell,
And being, but an ear,
And I and Silence some strange Race
Wrecked, solitary, here.

Psychotic thought processes were also the subject of Dickinson's "I felt a Cleaving in My Mind," written in 1864:

I felt a cleaving in my mind
As if my brain had split;
I tried to match it, seam by seam,
But could not make them fit.

The thought behind I strove to join
Unto the thought before,
But sequence ravelled out of reach
Like balls upon a floor.

In contrast to Emily Dickinson, who never expected her ruminations on insanity to be made public, Charlotte Perkins Gilman specifically wrote *The Yellow Wallpaper* to be published and to embarrass the eminent neurologist S. Weir Mitchell, who was her doctor. Perkins was suffering from severe postpartum depression in 1887 when Mitchell was enlisted to treat her. Mitchell recommended a rest cure, which Gilman found made her symptoms much worse. She therefore wrote her story of a woman's slow descent into insanity as the narrator sees a woman's figure trapped behind the wallpaper in her room:

> There is one marked peculiarity about this paper, a thing nobody seems to notice but myself, and that is that it changes as the light changes. . . . That is why I watch it always. . . . At night in any kind of light, in twilight, candle light, lamplight, and worst of all by moonlight, it becomes bars! The outside pattern I mean, and the woman behind it is as plain as can be. . . . But there is something else about that paper—the smell! . . . It is not bad—at first, and very gentle, but quite the subtlest, most enduring odor I ever met. . . . The front pattern does move—and no wonder! The woman behind shakes it! . . . I think that woman gets out in the daytime! And I'll tell you why—privately—I've seen her! I can see her out of every one of my windows! It is the same woman, I know, for she is always creeping, and most women do not creep by daylight.[25]

Gilman sent a copy of her story to Mitchell, but he did not reply. She subsequently recovered and became a prominent feminist social critic.

Emily Dickinson and Charlotte Perkins Gilman, then, represented a new group of American writers whose preoccupation with their own feelings of insanity led them to incorporate the theme into their writings. This would remain true in the twentieth century as well. Other than for writers directly or indirectly affected by it, insanity has not been a major theme in American literature since the middle of the nineteenth century.

An Angry Woman and a Psychiatric Judas

In addition to bringing hardship to America's insane, the Civil War also brought hardship to the superintendents of the asylums. Up to that time, the superintendents had enjoyed some degree of trust and respect from the public and from state legislators, even if insanity itself was poorly understood. The Civil War and the years following it would prove to be a watershed for asylum doctors' esteem, which would continuously diminish until the end of the century.

The first problem was attacks on asylum doctors by former patients. There had been occasional attacks in the past; for example, in 1833 Robert Fuller had published *An Account of the Imprisonments and Sufferings of Robert Fuller of Cambridge*, in which he had compared his involuntary hospitalization at McLean Asylum to the Spanish Inquisition. In 1849 in Philadelphia, a man had charged his family with unjust involuntary hospitalization, leading a local newspaper to headline: "A Sane Man Confined as a Lunatic." Similarly, in 1852 Isaac Hunt had published *Three Years in a Madhouse!* in which he accused Isaac Ray, superintendent of the Maine Insane Hospital, of having forcibly given him "poisonous medicines."[26]

These were mere flea bites, however, compared to the attack unleashed by Elizabeth Packard in 1866. Involuntarily hospitalized by her clergyman husband in 1860 in the Illinois State Hospital, she claimed that she had been hospitalized only because she disagreed with him on religious matters. She further alleged that the hospital medical director, Andrew McFarland, had made sexual advances to her and that she had been abused by hospital attendants. Her allegations were printed in Chicago newspapers, which led to a legislative investigation and a five-day trial that received national publicity. The jury declared her sane, and she was released, despite the fact that she had once claimed to be "the third person in the Holy Trinity and the mother of Jesus Christ" and had previously been psychiatrically hospitalized.[27]

Mrs. Packard thereupon divorced her husband and embarked on a national crusade to tighten commitment laws. In Iowa and Illinois, she succeeded in implementing so-called Packard Laws under which no person could be committed to an insane asylum without first having a jury trial. Several other states modified their laws at her urging, and Congress in 1875 even considered, but ultimately rejected, a national version of her proposed commitment statute.

Mrs. Packard also sought revenge on Dr. McFarland by persuading the state to investigate him. For six months a panel heard highly publicized allegations of illegal commitment practices by the doctor, who complained to a friend that "the whole legislative body is at the feet of a crazy woman." "I have drunk at the very deepest wells of humiliation," he added, "and am humiliated."[28] McFarland later committed suicide.

Elizabeth Packard's campaign against commitment laws and asylum superintendents was reinforced by other events. In 1864 *Hard Cash*, Charles Reade's novel about a sane man's false commitment to an English asylum, achieved as much success in America as it had in England. Four years later, the *Atlantic Monthly* published "A Modern Lettre de Cachet," which included numerous accounts of false commitment for the personal gain of relatives. Additional highly publicized cases continued to surface, such as a case against the superintendent of the Michigan State Insane Asylum in which the jury awarded the plaintiff $75,000 (1997 equivalent), and the case of Susan Dickie, in which a New York psychiatrist admitted to having spent less than fifteen minutes examining Dickie before committing her and acknowledged that he had been hired to commit her by her sister. As one hospital trustee noted, "It seems as if the public believe that every man connected in any way with a hospital had entered into a conspiracy to deprive the patients of all their rights."[29]

In addition to the commitment laws, the asylums themselves were increasingly attacked following the Civil War. Such attacks were inevitable, given markedly overcrowded conditions, lack of effective treatment, and high staff turnover. Asylum attendants worked fourteen or more hours each day, and their leave was restricted to two evenings a week, one Sunday, and one other half-day each month. In 1875 at the New York City Lunatic Asylum, "only two attendants had served for more than twelve months." An official in New York noted that on many asylum wards "the sight was most repulsive, and the odors intolerably sickening. . . . Some of the patients were literally wallowing in their own excrements." The *New York Tribune* claimed that such wards were "holes not fit for a dog." In 1887 *New York World* writer Nellie Bly had herself committed to the New York City Lunatic Asylum and then published a damning series called "Ten Days in a Mad-House." Indeed, from the Civil War onward, "asylum exposés became a nationwide, indeed international, phenomenon."[30]

Attacks on the asylum doctors and asylums were also reinforced by revelations about the asylum doctors themselves. Prior to 1860, the asylum superintendents had been a small, tightly knit group who had often referred to themselves as "the brethren." In 1861 William Prince, superintendent of the Northampton State Lunatic Asylum, married one of his patients, "causing great surprise in the village and intense horror among its marriageable ladies." In 1866 Thomas Kirkbride, superintendent of the Pennsylvania Hospital for the Insane and a leader among his peers, also married a former patient, who was twenty-seven years younger than he was, and subsequently had four children by her.[31] Three years later, Kirkbride's reputation suffered further when Ebenezer Haskell, a former patient, published a bitter attack on both him and his asylum.

Revelations about and attacks on asylum superintendents became increasingly commonplace. In 1865 Merrick Bemis, superintendent of the Worcester State Lunatic Hospital, was himself hospitalized for severe depression and alcohol abuse. Andrew McFarland in Illinois and D. T. Brown in New York both took their own lives after resigning from their posts as asylum superintendents. And in Washington, D.C., Charles Nichols, superintendent of the Government Hospital for the Insane, was investigated by the government in 1869 and again in 1876 for allegations of theft of public funds and other crimes.[32]

Probably no single event, however, shattered the reputation of "the brethren" as effectively as a paper, "The Curability of Insanity," read by Pliny Earle before his colleagues in December 1876.[33] The idea that insanity was curable had been a cornerstone for the asylum movement since its earliest days, used by Dorothea Dix and others to justify building and staffing ever more buildings. The asylums would ultimately *save* money, state legislators were promised, because active treatment would cure those affected and prevent chronicity.

Armed with statistics, Pliny Earle completely shattered the myth of curability. He showed convincingly that previous claims of high cure rates had been achieved "by repeated recoveries from the periodical or recurrent form of the disease in the same person." In one hospital, five patients had accounted for thirty-three recorded cures; in another, five patients were responsible for fifty-two cures. A woman at the Worcester State Lunatic Hospital "within a period of twenty years and two months recovered twenty-two times," even as she was spending more than eleven of those years in the hospital. Earle attributed the previous inflated claims to "zeal and . . . rivalry," the shadow of Dr. Cure-Awl. Earle also cited data showing that recoveries had "been constantly diminishing during a period of from twenty to fifty years," suggesting that insanity had become less curable even apart from the earlier inflated claims. As a member of the original thirteen founders of the Association of Medical Superintendents of American Institutions for the Insane and an asylum superintendent himself, Earle's public contradiction of his colleagues' sacred shibboleth made him nothing less than a psychiatric Judas.

Barbarians at the Psychiatric Gates

Pliny Earle's 1876 claim that most cases of insanity were not curable could not have come at a worse time. The fortress of the asylum super-intendents was under siege by the newly emerging neurologists, who were claiming that insanity really belonged to them. It was a bitter fight that lasted from the early 1870s until the mid-1880s and almost succeeded in merging the professions of psychiatry and neurology.

The leader of the neurologists was forty-eight-year-old William Hammond, who in 1874 had been appointed to the first professorship in nervous and mental disease in the country and who had been one of the seven founders of the American Neurological Association. Like other fledgling neurologists, Hammond was a veteran of the Civil War, during which he had acquired his neurological skills treating war injuries. His 1883 book, *Treatise on Insanity and Its Medical Relations,* was the first American textbook on insanity since Benjamin Rush's 1812 publication.

Hammond was said to be "an uncommonly tall and large man with a voice so powerful that it could be heard up-wind in a hurricane." He was also said by some to be "pompous and arrogant." During the Civil War he had risen to be surgeon general of the Union Army until 1864, when he had been court-martialed on charges of "irregularities in granting contracts for hospital supplies." He had then established his practice of neurology in New York and was known to be exceedingly wealthy, charging very high fees and making "well over $50,000 per year [$835,000, 1997 equivalent] at the peak of his career."[34]

Hammond and his colleagues in the emerging neurological profession did not restrict their practice to organic conditions of the brain. They believed that all disorders of the brain belonged legitimately to them, including insomnia and various forms of neuroses. Indeed, neurologist George Beard coined the term "neurasthenia" in 1869 and advocated "mental therapies" that today would be categorized as psychotherapy. Similarly, the neurologists argued that "the study of insanity should be considered a subdivision of neurology. . . . Neurology deals with the whole nervous system, mental pathology merely with a part."[35] The problem with this was that asylum doctors had already laid claim to insanity and were not pleased to see their neurological colleagues invading their professional territory.

The leader of the asylum superintendents was fifty-one-year-old John Gray, superintendent of the Utica State Lunatic Asylum, editor of the *American Journal of Insanity*, ubiquitous expert witness in trials involving insanity, and adviser to government officials, including President Lincoln. He was also known for his 300-pound girth and was said to be "autocratic," "socially conservative," "a staunch upholder of religion, social, and traditional morality," and "an enduring hater." It was additionally alleged that "the powerful and manipulative Gray" had taken "an active role in the unseating of his superior," Nathan Benedict, the previous superintendent of the Utica Asylum.[36]

This, then, was the lineup in 1876: William Hammond versus John Gray, two titans whose physical presence was overshadowed only by the magnitude of their egos. The prize would be professional jurisdiction over the insane, including the control of state asylums and the teaching of mental disorders in schools of medicine. Both men had their followers, some of whom were known to be as tactically devious as their leaders. Other members of the medical profession anticipated the inevitable clash.

An initial encounter had occurred in 1871 in the trial of David Montgomery, who had been accused of having killed his wife. Gray had testified that Montgomery suffered from childhood epilepsy, had a "strong hereditary tendency to insanity," and had been insane at the time of the murder. Hammond had testified that Montgomery had been "perfectly sane" at the time of the crime and had added that Gray's testimony was due to his "want of practical experience with epilepsy or insanity."[37] The jury had sided with Hammond and had found the defendant guilty of first-degree murder.

Three years later, in 1874, Hammond was appointed to a professorship in nervous and mental disorders at the University of the City of New York, and in 1876 was named to a second professorship at Bellevue Hospital Medical College. Also in 1876, English psychiatrist John Bucknill published his *Notes on Asylums for the Insane in Amer-*

ica, which was sharply critical of the use of restraints and other practices of American asylum superintendents. Finally, in December 1876, Pliny Earle publicly proclaimed that insane asylums had failed egregiously in their efforts to cure insanity. As one physician wrote to Earle: "It becomes an important social problem whether the large and costly modern asylum is not a mistake if four-fifths of the insane are incurable."[38]

In March 1878, Hammond and his colleagues attacked the asylum superintendents directly. The designated gunman was Edward Charles Spitzka, a twenty-three-year-old German-trained neurologist who read a paper, "The Study of Insanity Considered as a Branch of Neurology," before the New York Neurological Society. Spitzka attacked Gray personally as "an indifferent, superficial man, owing his position merely to political buffoonery." He further accused Gray of having "harmoniously confused if not falsified the [asylum's] financial statements" and "manipulated statistics . . . to strew sand in the eyes of the public and to serve as an excuse for preposterous demands."[39]

Spitzka also included Gray by implication when he claimed that most asylum superintendents had been selected "on grounds of nepotism and political favor." The "average articles" in their asylum journals, he added, seldom rise above "occasional melancholy lucubrations over deceased and lamented brother superintendents." There was, Spitzka claimed, virtually no research or scientific activity in the asylums, and he censured "the apathy and ignorance manifested by those concerned in this dereliction of scientific duty." In the annual asylum reports, the superintendents were said to "wax enthusiastic over the prizes gained by their hogs and strawberries at agricultural fairs":

> Judging by the average asylum reports, we are inclined to believe that certain superintendents are experts in gardening and farming (although the farm account frequently comes out on the wrong side of the ledger), tin roofing (although the roof and cupola is usually leaky), drain-pipe laying (although the grounds are often moist and unhealthy), engineering (though the wards are either too hot or too cold), history (though their facts are incorrect, and their inferences beyond all measure so); in short,

experts at everything except the diagnosis, pathology and treatment of insanity.

The obvious solution, concluded Spitzka, was to terminate the "self-implied omnipotence" of asylum superintendents and subsume insanity "as a subdivision of neurology."[40]

The absence of ambiguity in the neurologists' intentions was confirmed the following month at the next meeting of the Neurological Society. A committee recommended launching a crusade for "asylum reform" in order "to rectify if possible the evils" that Spitzka had cited. In elections held that evening, anti-asylum activists were chosen "as president, first and second vice-presidents, treasurer, and to fill three seats on its council."[41] A petition was forwarded to the New York State legislature requesting an official investigation of the asylums and their management. Later in 1878, Spitzka was awarded a Neurological Society prize offered by William Hammond for outstanding scientific work.

A rapid response to the neurologists' challenge came from John Gray and the asylum superintendents in May 1878. The surrogate assassin was Eugene Grissom, a friend and classmate of Gray's at the University of Pennsylvania School of Medicine and superintendent of the Raleigh Insane Asylum. In a paper read before the Association of Medical Superintendents of American Institutions for the Insane, Grissom attacked Hammond as a "criminal" and "poisoner of the fountain of justice." Hammond was said to be an "atheist . . . to whom Christianity . . . is but a myth," in contrast to Gray, who was devoutly pious. Hammond was also labeled "a great magician" with an ability to "hoax a great metropolitan educative power like the [New York] Herald."[42]

But the major recurring theme of Grissom's attack on Hammond was his reputation for charging high fees. Hammond was said to "prostitute science in the market, and smother her pure light under his greed for pelf." As such, Hammond was "the Benedict Arnold of his profession" and "a Judas Iscariot to humanity, selling the blood of her children for thirty pieces of silver." Grissom concluded his description of Hammond as follows:

> It is not that as we remember the victims already buried,
> that we see Draco reappear, with swift condemnation upon

his lips, it is not that the scales of justice drip with blood from hands already dyed in gore, but that behind the black robe of the semi-judicial expert, may be heard a sound, more fearful than the groans of suffering humanity, more ominous than the click of loaded arms, a sound that chills the marrow as with the breathing of a fabled vampire, it is the clink of money under the girdle. Now at last we shudder as we recognize that the false expert is no man at all, but a moral monster, whose baleful eyes glare with delusive light; whose bowels are but bags of gold, to feed which, spider-like, he casts his loathsome arms about a helpless prey.

Grissom's paper was said to have been "greeted with thunderous applause by the Association."[43]

The paper was published in the July issue of the *American Journal of Insanity*. Hammond promptly sued Gray for libel as the journal's editor and also because Gray was widely assumed to have written the paper. Details of Grissom's attack appeared in medical and lay publications, and the charges were widely discussed. Spitzka prepared the neurologists' response to Grissom for the October meeting of the Neurological Society, and "the Society's rules were suspended to permit newspaper reporters to attend the meeting."[44]

Spitzka opened his response by deploring Grissom's "purely personal attack" on Hammond, which was, he said, "in its language exceeding anything which has yet appeared in a professedly medical publication." He also criticized Grissom for failing to address any of the substantive issues regarding the shortcomings of the asylums, "although the absence of argument is liberally made up for by personal insults."[45]

After claiming the high ground, Spitzka then attacked the asylum superintendents as "shallow pretenders and ignorant indifferentists," including "one prominent superintendent" who was being investigated for "extravagances and looseness in [financial] accounts" and two other superintendents who had been dismissed "for being repeatedly intoxicated." He then detailed "an asylum whose record of accidents during the current year . . . sounds like the list of casualties of a Bulgarian campaign" and specifically accused the superintendent of falsifying death certificates to hide patient abuses by his staff: "Three patients beaten to death, one of whom had twelve broken ribs! One patient boiled to death, by having the hot water turned on him in a bath, while the attendant went out of the asylum building, leaving the helpless paralytic to his horrible fate." Spitzka concluded: "We already perceive the dawn of the day when incompetence and unreliability in high places will cease to exist. . . . Hard, earnest labor alone will be able to draw the field of psychiatry from the slough of despond into which it has sunken in every scientific and administrative respect." The following day, the *New York Times* reported Spitzka's remarks favorably under the headline "A Plea for Asylum Reform."[46]

In addition to Spitzka's rejoinder, William Hammond also published "An Open Letter to Eugene Grissom" as a pamphlet. In it, he "defended his practice of accepting large monetary rewards for the valuable services that his scientific knowledge enabled him to render" and further detailed the shortcomings of the asylum superintendents. As for Grissom, Hammond suggested that he himself might possibly be insane.[47]

The immediate effect of the neurologists' attack on the asylum superintendents appeared to be favorable for the neurologists. Hammond claimed to have received "hundreds of letters" of support and was invited to address the Connecticut Medical Society, where he again urged that "the absolute and irresponsible power of the superintendents . . . be taken away, and hospitals for the insane . . . be organized exactly as are all other hospitals." In Michigan also "a special committee of the state legislature conducted an inquiry into the Asylum for the Insane at Kalamazoo." Many newspapers wrote in support of asylum reform, including the *New York Times,* which detailed abuses under the headline "Bad Management of Blackwell's Island Asylum."[48] For a brief period, it appeared that the neurologists might indeed oust the asylum superintendents and add the province of psychiatry to their own territory.

But the superintendents were not to be underestimated. They had been organized for forty years more than the neurologists and had accumulated a backlog of IOUs from politically important people, often for having provided care for a family member. When the neurologists submitted their 1878 petition to the New York State Legislature requesting an investigation into the asylums, it was referred to a two-man committee, one member of whom was from Utica. And, when in

1879 the New York Commissioners of Charity and Corrections appointed a board to investigate the asylums, the only member with any psychiatric expertise was Allan Hamilton, whom Hammond was at that time suing for plagiarism. The board, complained Hammond, "could not have been more favorable to the superintendents if the latter had themselves, as was very likely, selected the names of the appointees."[49]

Hammond and his neurologist supporters continued attacking the asylum superintendents at every opportunity. In 1879, in the highly publicized Susan Dickie case, Hammond testified against the psychiatrist who had committed her to an asylum. In 1880, Hammond testified against several asylum superintendents who had claimed that a patient named Abraham Gosling, accused of destruction of property, was sane. Hammond claimed that Gosling had paralytic insanity (syphilis) and stated: "[If he] does not die . .. within three years, I will burn my diploma and retire from the medical profession." Gosling was judged to be insane and died shortly after the trial.[50]

In late 1879, the neurologists devised a new strategy to attack the asylum superintendents. With the cooperation of social workers and laypersons interested in asylum reform, they organized the National Association for the Protection of the Insane and the Prevention of Insanity (NAPIPI). The constitution of the organization included an assertion that insanity had increased and had become more difficult to cure; an editorial in the first issue of its journal, the *American Psychological Journal,* noted "the alarming increase of insanity." Several neurologists played leading roles in NAPIPI as it advocated investigations into asylum management and state commissions to oversee asylums and even introduced a bill in Congress to investigate the causes and treatment of insanity in the United States.

In 1884, the NAPIPI journal attacked John Gray directly, accusing him of "deception and concealment," "cooking . . . its [the asylum's] accounts," and being "a political boss" and noted that he was under investigation for the fourth time by the state legislature. In another NAPIPI article, a neurologist said that "the growth of cabbage and currants interests this official [the superintendent] more than morbid growths within the encephalon" and "the location of turnip or potato patch interests him more than the localization of cerebral lesions." The asylum superintendents strongly opposed NAPIPI, which was said to be "really for the purpose of concentrating and organizing hostility to present institutions and present methods" for treating insanity.[51]

In December 1880, Hammond, Spitzka, and six other neurologists finally got the opportunity they had requested to testify before a New York State senate investigation committee on asylum management. The hearings, held in New York City's Metropolitan Hotel, "were crowded to overflowing with witnesses and interested spectators," including many representatives of the media. Hammond cited his usual litany of asylum abuses and drew laughter, according to the *New York Times,* when he suggested that asylum medical superintendents should be abolished and "a lay superintendent appointed to raise turnips, lobby the Legislature, and entertain the friends of visitors." Spitzka accused the asylum superintendents of perjury in their testimony against him and said that "he had done nothing to provoke these unseemly personal squabbles which had been thrust upon him." Overall, however, the hearings were not a success from the neurologists' point of view. They offered remarkably few suggestions for improving the asylums, "failed to establish themselves as the sole authorities on the treatment of the insane, and even appeared to be somewhat irresponsible and sensationalist."[52]

The battle for control of insanity was not going as the neurologists had hoped, but they pressed on. In March 1881, lawyer and social activist Dorman Eaton published an article, "Despotism in Lunatic Asylums," in the widely read *North American Review.* He quoted the New York governor's claim that "the rapid increase of insanity is truly alarming" and then castigated asylum superintendents as examples of "unparalleled despotism" and for being "autocratic—absolutely unique in this republic." The asylum superintendent, Dorman asserted, "is the monarch of all the surveys, from the great [asylum] palace to the hencoops": "The superintendents represent, not the inmates, not the people, not helplessness that needs protection, but only those in authority who maintain all secrecy, who are responsible for all that is wrong, who are interested in all that is corrupt, who are themselves the very persons who need to feel the force of public opinion and to have their doings inspected and laid open to view."[53]

Eaton's attack was immediately answered by Orpheus Everts, superintendent of the Cincinnati Sanitarium, who excoriated the "professed neurologists and flippant neurospasts" who, "arrogating to themselves all knowledge of psychology and psychiatry, have by sneers, innuendo, and direct assault . . . done what they could do toward the disparagement of hospital [asylum] reputation."[54]

On July 2, 1881, one month after Everts's impassioned defense, President James Garfield was shot by Charles Guiteau. Following Garfield's death two months later, Guiteau was brought to trial on charges of murder. The two-month trial became yet another occasion for the neurologists and asylum superintendents to fight, and the entire country watched this round.

John Gray was the chief psychiatric witness, and throughout the trial he sat at the prosecution table, "even preparing specific questions for use in cross-examination."[55] The prosecution claimed that Guiteau was perfectly sane, a position held by Gray, most other asylum superintendents, and most of the public. The defense contended that Guiteau was mentally ill and called upon Spitzka and four other neurologists to support their position.

Spitzka proved to be a most effective witness for the defense, despite constant disparaging questions from the prosecution. Since he had served as a professor of comparative anatomy at the Columbia Veterinary College, the prosecution referred to him as a "horse doctor." In discussing Spitzka's credentials, a member of the prosecution team asked Spitzka whether he had treated horses:

A. I never have treated any other animal but the ass, and that animal had two legs, and therefore, I could not consider myself a veterinary physician, but a human professional.

Q. You are a veterinary surgeon, are you not?

A. In the sense that I treat asses who ask me stupid questions, I am.

Spitzka testified confidently that Guiteau probably had "a congenital malformation of the brain" and was therefore not responsible for his actions. Hammond did not testify but commented publicly that Guiteau was affected with "reasoning mania." Gray, seizing the opportunity to discredit the neurologists, derided Hammond for inventing "a new discovery in the fauna of insanity," which Gray called "Guiteau-mania." "Reasoning mania," said Gray, "is synonymous with what he might as correctly call arrant roguery."[56]

Guiteau was found guilty, and on June 30, 1882, he was hanged. An autopsy of Guiteau's brain reported "chronic degeneration of gray cells and small blood vessels" and "asymmetry of the convolutions." A more recent review of the neuropathological findings concluded that there was "fairly good evidence for syphilitic involvement of the brain."[57] Many medical publications concluded that, in retrospect, Spitzka and the neurologists had been correct.

The neurologists, then, technically won the battle, but they lost the war. Their defense of Guiteau had been highly unpopular with the public because Guiteau appeared to be sane. Infighting among the neurologists further weakened their efforts. By 1883, the neurologists, social workers, and laypersons who had founded NAPIPI were at odds, and within a year the organization was defunct. Also in 1883, New York State created a State Lunacy Commission, as the neurologists had requested, further defusing the asylum issue. Reformers generally had tired of the problems of the insane, for nothing seemed to help, and they had moved on to issues such as women's rights, temperance, and the problems of immigrants. Even Dorothea Dix had been swallowed up by the Civil War as the superintendent of Union army nurses, and there was no strong advocate to take her place.

Perhaps the neurologists' greatest weakness, however, was that they had no comprehensive plan to improve the treatment of insanity and were perceived as acting primarily in their own self-interest. This was clear as early as 1879, when the *New York Times* referred to them as "a clique of physicians who are radically opposed to everything in existing asylum management because they are not themselves the managers at liberal salaries."[58]

In one of the many ironies of the neurologists–asylum superintendents fray, two months after the Guiteau trial ended, John Gray was shot by Henry Renshaw, who had been one of Gray's patients. The newspaper noted that the case had "a resemblance to that of Guiteau." Gray eventually died in 1886 from complications of his wounds. In another irony, Eugene Grissom, who Hammond had publicly speculated might be insane, did indeed later become insane with brain syphilis, and in 1902, "he committed suicide by firing a pistol into his brain."[59] Hammond and Spitzka both went on to have eminent careers as neurologists, dying, respectively, in 1900 and 1914. But their attempt to seize insanity and the insane asylums for themselves was never forgotten by the asylum superintendents and the emerging profession of psychiatry.

The 1880 and 1890 Censuses

The 1880 census provided strong evidence that insanity in the United States was truly increasing. Coming as it did in the middle of the war between the neurologists and asylum superintendents, it received less professional attention than it might have under other circumstances. But its methodology was so thorough and its results so striking that it continued to influence thinking about insanity for many years. Never before and never since in the United States has the counting of insane persons been as complete as it was in 1880.

The director of the 1880 census was Francis Walker, an economist with a special interest in the role of immigrants. His experience with the 1870 census had "brought the realization that the ethnic composition of the American people was undergoing a radical change."[60] Because of this concern and the increasingly widespread belief that insanity was increasing, Walker recruited Frederick Wines, a statistician and social reformer, to conduct a special census of all "defective, dependent, and delinquent classes," including the insane, the blind, and idiots and deaf-mutes.

Wines insisted that an accurate count must include the whole American population, not merely institutionalized individuals. Census enumerators were therefore given extra pay and special forms to ask each household and were told "to counsel with [local] physicians upon this point, to make inquiries of neighbors, and to report all [insane persons] whether the information respecting them should be derived from the family to which they belong or to other sources." To supplement the direct census information, all 100,000 physicians in the United States were sent a letter asking them to report "all idiots and lunatics within the sphere of their personal knowledge"; over 80 percent of the physicians responded. All duplication between enumerator and physician lists was eliminated "by employing a sufficient number of clerks to scrutinize the returns, . . . and great pains were taken with this branch of the work."[61]

Information on insane persons was collected by age, sex, marital status, race, native or foreign born, and age of onset; whether or not they had insane relatives on the mother's, father's, or both sides; where they were residing (in a hospital or asylum, almshouse, jail, or other institution, or at home); and by state and county of origin ("redistributing to their places of permanent residence all who were temporarily absent from their homes, either in institutions or elsewhere"). Insanity was also classified into seven subtypes "on consultation with the members of the New England Psychological Association and with other expert alienists (who concurred in this opinion)," using the information obtained from physicians to assign most cases.[62]

A total of 91,997 separate insane individuals were identified by the 1880 special census, yielding a rate of 1.83 per 1,000 total population, or almost double the 0.97 per 1,000 rate that had been reported in 1870 (fig. 11.1). Since case finding was much more complete in 1880, it was expected that the 1880 rate would be higher. However, the number of insane persons in hospitals and asylums alone had grown from 17,735 in 1870 to 40,942 in 1880, an increase of 131 percent. The Willard Asylum for the Insane was the largest, with 1,513 patients, although two other New York State asylums and the Insane Asylum of California each had more than 1,000 residents as well.

Diagnostically, 38 percent of the insane were said to suffer from mania and 29 percent from dementia, although it was added that "not more than one-fifth of the insane have reached the final stage of dementia." In addition, 19 percent were diagnosed with melancholia, 9 percent with epilepsy, 2 percent with paresis (syphilis), 2 percent with monomania, and 1 percent with dipsomania (alcoholism). Idiots were clearly differentiated from insane persons by having been affected since childhood, and all mentally ill children under age twelve were also automatically assigned to the idiot classification.

In addition to the high number of insane persons, the two most striking findings from the 1880 special census were the unequal geographical distribution of the insane and their overrepresentation among immigrants. Geographically, New England, the Middle Atlantic states, and California had the highest rates. Vermont (3.1 per

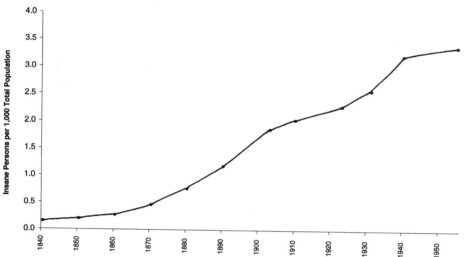

FIG. 11.1. United States: Insane Persons in Psychiatric Hospitals per 1,000 Population, 1840–1955. Data on which the graph is based are taken from Atlee L. Stroup and Ronald W. Manderscheid, "The Development of the State Mental Hospital System in the United States: 1840–1980," *Journal of the Washington Academy of Sciences* 78(1988): 59–68.

1,000 total population), New Hampshire (3.0), Massachusetts (2.9), California (2.9), Connecticut (2.8), and New York (2.8) had rates that were approximately six times higher than those for Colorado, Arizona, Nevada, Idaho, and North Dakota (all 0.5 per 1,000). As noted in figure 11.2, insanity appeared to be disproportionately concentrated in the Northeast, confirming the trend reported in 1840 and observed in every subsequent census. As described by one of the asylum superintendents in 1887, "Dividing the country into two great belts of north and south, there is an almost regular proportionate decrease of lunacy as we leave the older settled parts of the country along the Atlantic coast, till we reach the extreme western slope."[63]

The 1880 census also noted "the extraordinary ratio of foreign insane," a finding that was undoubtedly of great interest to census director Francis Walker. Foreign-born individuals had a rate of insanity of 3.9 per 1,000, more than double the rate for native-born individuals of 1.5 per 1,000. At that time, foreign-born individuals constituted just 13 percent of the total population, yet they accounted for 19 percent of the total insane. No attempt was made at that time to correct these figures for differences in the age distribution in the foreign-born and native-born populations.

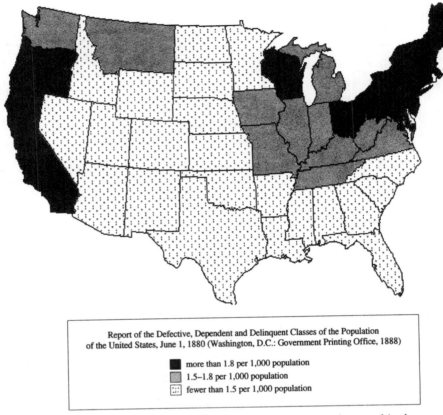

Report of the Defective, Dependent and Delinquent Classes of the Population
of the United States, June 1, 1880 (Washington, D.C.: Government Printing Office, 1888)

■ more than 1.8 per 1,000 population

▨ 1.5–1.8 per 1,000 population

⠿ fewer than 1.5 per 1,000 population

FIG. 11.2. United States: Insane Persons per 1,000 Population in Asylums and in the Community, 1880.

Newspapers reported the 1880 census as showing "a very startling increase in the number of insane. . . . While the population during the last decade increased by 30 percent, the apparent increase of the insane was a little over 155 percent." They also observed that "the tendency to insanity in the foreign population . . . is very remarkable."[64]

A few asylum superintendents publicly addressed the census findings. Foster Pratt, superintendent of the Michigan Asylum for the Insane, said that the increasing insanity was an "important and alarming fact . . . a great question of public health that demands careful study." He noted the North-South geographical disparity and speculated that much of the increasing insanity was due to "race taint" by immigrants: "Immigration, to us, is more like the 'flood' of a great river, occasionally overflowing its banks and leaving behind it a sediment that generates a pestilential malaria, dangerous to the physical, mental, and moral health." Pliny Earle, who had broken from his colleagues by publishing data proving the low cure rate of insanity, also acknowledged that "all the known data ... very clearly lead to the inference that insanity in the United States is increasing, not merely absolutely in correspondence with the increase of population, but relatively as compared with the number of inhabitants."[65]

The official reaction to the 1880 census from the Association of Medical Superintendents of American Institutions for the Insane was silence. Under siege by the neurologists and fighting for their professional lives, the superintendents had understandably little interest in focusing on any issue that implied they were failing. In 1883, the *American Journal of Insanity* even reprinted an article from *The Lancet*, questioning whether insanity was really increasing: "It does appear passing strange that people persist in distressing themselves about the 'increase of insanity' without making sure that there is an increase. ... It is better to ascertain definitely whether it be a fact that the fish does weigh heavier in water before brains are worried and hearts made to ache by the endeavor to solve a problem which, possibly, is not seriously proposed." The following year, William Godding, superintendent of the Government Hospital for the Insane, defended his fellow superintendents at the association's fortieth anniversary celebration. After acknowledging the apparent increase in insanity over the previous four decades, he said that "the medical superintendents ... have put themselves on record again and again as demanding that the State should make the best possible provision for every insane person within its jurisdiction. ... The brethren have stood shoulder to shoulder on this high ground of principle." Don't blame us, Godding said, if provisions are inadequate. Blame instead the "Boards of State Charities ... legislatures ... [and] a sovereign people, indifferent also to true economy in the future on this growing problem of insanity. ... Let every ass bear his own burden."[66]

Alarmed by the reports of increasing insanity, many states began compiling their own data to ascertain the magnitude of the problem. In Massachusetts, for example, first admissions to the state asylums were found to have almost doubled in the seventeen years between 1868–1869 (616 and 695, respectively) and 1885–1886 (1,100 and 1,120), although the increase in the general population had been only 54 percent. In 1885, the *Boston Medical and Surgical Journal* acknowledged that "the increase in the number of the insane has been exceptionally rapid in the last decade." Overcrowding of the asylums was so pronounced that at Danvers State Lunatic Hospital "from one hundred to nearly two hundred [patients] have been obliged to occupy beds placed upon the floors of wards at night." The 1887 report of the State Board of Lunacy and Charity noted that "the statistics collected by this board since 1880 tend to indicate a considerable, though not uniform, increase, even in recent insanity, out of proportion to the gain of population. . . . This would indicate that recent insanity is increasing more than twice as fast as the whole population."[67] Similar increases were published in annual reports from other state boards during this period.

Between 1880 and 1887, an additional fifteen public asylums opened, including some in the emerging territories of the West, such as the Dakotas and Idaho. Most of the older asylums continued enlarging, and as soon as they did, their beds were filled. Few persons were surprised, therefore, when the 1890 census reported a total of 74,028 insane persons in hospitals and asylums, an increase of 81 percent from the 40,942 reported in 1880; during the decade, the population of the United States had increased 25 percent. Seventeen asylums now had more than 1,000 patients each, whereas ten years earlier, only four had had that many patients. The total number of asylum admissions had increased from 16,617 in 1881 to 25,645 in 1889.

The 1890 census did not solicit information from physicians in the community, so the enumeration of the noninstitutionalized population was less complete than it had been for the 1880 census. The 1890 census did, however, collect more detailed information on the foreign-born population, which continued to have a greater representation of insane persons (3.8 per 1,000) compared to the native-born population (1.3 per 1,000). The 1890 census ascertained the birthplace of the mothers of all insane persons and found that "among the children of Irish mothers, the number of insane was much above the average."[68]

The 1890 census also provided a comparison of insane persons by cities of 50,000 or more total population. The figures included not only the insane persons presently living in a particular city "but also those insane persons in asylums and institutions who were reported as belonging to that city." The overall rate of insanity in the cities was 2.3 per 1,000, compared to 1.8 for the country as a whole. "The largest proportions of the insane to population are found in the eastern cities, San Francisco [in the West] being the marked exception."[69] Troy, New York (4.6 per 1,000) had the highest rate, followed by New York City (3.9), Allegheny, Pennsylvania (3.5), Worcester, Massachusetts, (3.5), San Francisco (3.2), and Boston (3.1).

The idea that insanity was more common in urban areas was being publicly discussed at this time. Living in a city somehow increased one's risk for becoming insane. Urban living did not increase one's liability to mental retardation, however, since the 1890 census showed idiots to be underrepresented in cities compared to rural areas. In 1885 an article in *The Nation* stated clearly that "the liability of city people to insanity is much greater than that of the rural population." One reason, it speculated, was the urban "noises which do not allow an overworked brain to enjoy a really sound and dreamless sleep." Others suggested that residents of cities were more prone to insanity because of their exposure to "sewer gas" or lack of exposure to fresh air.[70]

What is clear is that the urbanization of America was taking place at the same time as insanity was rapidly increasing. Horse-drawn streetcars had became prominent in the 1850s, allowing cities to expand into suburbs from which individuals could commute. In 1840 there had been just 1,845 towns in the United States with a population of 2,500 or greater. By 1890, there were 22,106 such towns, and by 1910, there were 41,999. In 1840 only 10 percent of the population had lived in such towns, but by 1900, 40 percent did. The growth of large cities was even more dramatic: in 1840, just 3 percent of the population lived in cities of 100,000 or more, but by 1900, 19 percent of the population lived in such cities. Between 1880 and 1890, Chicago more than doubled in population, while Minneapolis and St. Paul grew threefold. A few people wondered whether urbanization and insanity might indeed have some relationship to each other.

CHAPTER 12

"The Apocalyptic Beast"
The United States, 1890–1990

Of all the ills which flesh is heir to, there is perhaps none so dreadful as insanity. Utter poverty, hideous deformity, mutilation of limbs, deafness, blindness, all these, sad as they are, leave alive the human affections, and admit the consolations of sympathy and love; while insanity not only makes man utterly dependent upon others for the supply of his physical wants, but it strips him of the noblest attributes of humanity.

—SAMUEL GRIDLEY HOWE, 1843

But the Physicians being sent to inspect the Bodies, they assur'd the People that it was neither more or less than *the Plague*, with all its terrifying Particulars, and that it threatened an universal Infection.

—DANIEL DEFOE, *A Journal of the Plague Year*, 1722

By 1890 the asylum superintendents were exhausted by the continuing increase of insanity. The hope and therapeutic optimism of their earlier years had been suffused by relentless waves of patients and by criticism from the public. Their mood was reflected by William Godding in an 1890 address to his colleagues:

All my term as a superintendent I have known no hospital but a crowded one. Erecting buildings all the time, the incoming flood has still kept in advance of construction. I have had dreams of classification of which the thronged wards would never permit the realization. Day by day, year after year, I have seen the individualized treatment of special cases swamped by the rising tide of indiscriminate lunacy pouring through the wards, filling every crevice, rising higher and higher until gradually most distinctions and landmarks have been blotted out. Twenty years I have battled with this flood.[1]

Four years later, the asylum superintendents invited the distinguished neurologist S. Weir Mitchell to address the celebratory fiftieth annual meeting of their association. After reminding the superintendents that in 1889 they had had responsibility for 91,152 insane patients in 160 hospitals "at a cost of $10,692,000, over and above $2,209,000 spent that year in building," Mitchell told them in no uncertain terms that they had failed:

With you, it has been different. You were the first of the specialists and you have never come back into line. It is easy to see how this came about. You soon began to live apart, and you still do so. Your hospitals are not our hospitals; your ways are not our ways. . . . The cloistral lives you lead give rise, we think, to certain mental peculiarities. . . . I think asylum life is deadly to the insane. . . . Frankly speaking, we do not believe that you are so working these hospitals as to keep treatment or scientific product on the front line of medical advance. Where, we ask, are your annual reports of scientific study, of the psychology and pathology of your patients? It is a grave injustice to insist that you shall conduct a huge boarding house—what has been called a monastery of the mad—and keep yourselves honestly able to move with the growth of medicine.[2]

In the published version of his talk, Mitchell appended letters he had solicited from twenty-four leading American physicians, offering their opinion of American psychiatry. Typical was the response of Abraham Jacobi: "The actual fact is that our asylums have always been more or less gentle and genteel prisons for the mentally sick rather than hospitals."[3]

One had to feel some sympathy for the asylum superintendents. They had started working fifty years earlier with the best of intentions and with abundant promises of cures. From the day they opened their asylum doors, they had been overwhelmed with an endless flood of patients. They had had no effective treatments and were being criticized on all sides for asylum conditions over which they had had little control. As Walter Channing stated in a published reply to Mitchell: "From that day [1844] to this the pressure has never relaxed for more accommodations." The superintendents had done the very best they could, Channing added. "They have not sat blind-folded, or played puss-in-the-corner, or milked the cows."[4]

It must have seemed to the asylum superintendents in the 1890s that, professionally, things could not get any worse. But they could, and they did. Patients kept appearing at their doors, increasing in numbers, every month, every year. Two patients would be discharged, but then three new patients would appear. Shortly thereafter, one of the discharged patients would return. In 1894 Franklin Sanborn, an inspector on the Massachusetts Board of Health, Lunacy and Charity, published a detailed analysis of state data showing that "the insane have increased twice as fast as the whole people. . . . We find this insane accumulation going on as fast as fifty years ago."[5]

The magnitude of the continuing increase became even more apparent in the special censuses of 1904 and 1910. Attempts to count insane persons living in the community, as had been done in 1880 and 1890, were discontinued because, according to the census of 1904, "it is not the function of a statistical bureau to inquire into the subtler aspects of insanity as a disease." The special census was instead restricted to an enumeration of individuals in "public and private hospitals treating only the insane or having a separate department for the treatment of this class of patients." The officials did not even include insane persons in almshouses or jails, despite the acknowledgment in the 1904 census that "the statistics of paupers in almshouses for 1904 give 11,807 inmates as insane."[6]

The figures on the number of hospitalized insane alone were

startling. In 1890, there had been 74,028 insane persons in 162 hospitals (119 public, 43 private). In 1903 this had increased to 150,151 insane persons, and in 1910 the count was 187,791. Between 1890 and 1910, then, the number of hospitalized insane individuals in the United States had increased by 154 percent, whereas the general population had increased from 63.1 to 92.4 million, or 46 percent. Hospitalized insanity was increasing more than three times faster than the general population, a trend that the census itself called an "extraordinary increase" and a "phenomenal accumulation."[7]

Equally arresting was the increasing size of the hospitals and asylums. In 1870, there had been just two hospitals with more than 1,000 patients. By 1880, the number had doubled to four, and by 1890, there had been seventeen. But by 1910, the number of hospitals with more than 1,000 patients was seventy-five. Of these, nine held over 2,000, four others held over 3,000, and one—Manhattan State Hospital—had a patient census of 4,400.[8] It appeared that the "monasteries of the mad" were being replaced by institutions that were more like Gothic cathedrals.

Some asylum superintendents and other writers attempted to minimize the importance of the increases. For example, in 1899 the *Catholic World* claimed that whether or not insanity was increasing was "open to dispute" and recommended "more fresh air, more bicycle riding, more field sports, and above all more holidays," so that in the new century Americans would be "the sanest people on earth." In 1905 *The Nation* assured the public that "there is no real increase in the number of the insane." And in 1916 the *North American Review* advised readers not to believe the dire warnings about rising insanity, which it called "the Apocalyptic Beast." "It is true that some statistics are somewhat startling; or are made to appear so, which is a very different thing," it said. But: "Let us be tranquil. The human race is not all going mad."[9]

An alternative but equally optimistic approach was to claim that increasing insanity was simply a concomitant of civilization. This idea had circulated throughout the nineteenth century in both Europe and America but gained greater sophistication and currency as the realization of increasing insanity loomed larger. It postulated that civilization produced an overload of the brain, causing it to fail. An 1859 article in the *North American Review* had compared the brain to muscles that "may be weakened or disordered" if "exercised beyond their strength." An 1885 article in *The Nation* compared the brain to a razor that "is, in its place, a stronger implement than an axe, but it is more easily spoiled if improperly used." Given the development of electric lights, telegraphs, radios, and even cars, increasing insanity appeared inevitable, as noted by J. S. Jewell: "I will state my belief, derived from considerable observation and study, that, taken as a whole, nervous and mental diseases are increasing, and must, as things now stand, increase with the advance of civilization."[10] Others accepted the inevitability of increasing insanity, but more reluctantly: "Yet it appears to be a humiliating admission to make, that, with all the increase of mental power and range of thought, with acquired power over the forces of nature, with ability to convert the hidden treasures and forces of nature, into the means of supplying wants and ministering to comfort, and, with the vast storehouse of mental wealth which comes into the possession of mankind through the influences of civilization, there should, somehow, necessarily come with them, greater liability to such a calamity as insanity."[11] And for a few, the increasing insanity was even an honor: "A high insane ratio does not necessarily mean either a nervously bankrupt nation or merely one whose statistics have been carefully tabulated. It means much more: not only a nation civilized, but, to the highest degree, humanized. It is a badge of honor to a nation, as the gold medal is given to the life-saver, and the more highly this spirit is developed, the better for the public at large as well as for the individual."[12]

The Appeal of Eugenics

Trying to persuade the public that increasing insanity was an honor was, however, a hard sell, so the asylum superintendents looked elsewhere for possible explanations. An obvious answer presented itself in the censuses of 1880 and 1890: increasing insanity was caused by immigrants.

The idea was not entirely new. The 1858 Massachusetts Commission on Lunacy had reported that foreigners constituted a disproportionate share of insane individuals in that state, with Irish immigrants being especially prominent, and similar reports had followed from other states. By 1883, asylum superintendent Foster Pratt had been certain that individuals hereditarily predisposed to insanity were being "shrewdly selected" by European officials to emigrate and become "a plague spot on our vital and social conditions, and a blot on our vital statistics." Then "insanity is increased among our native whites by intermarriage with this tainted foreign element."[13]

In the 1890s, the immigrant explanation for increasing insanity moved to the forefront. As the economic depression of 1893 to 1897 took hold and job actions such as the Homestead and Pullman strikes spread, immigrants were blamed for almost everything wrong in the nation. In 1894, the Immigration Restriction League was founded in Boston; within a year its literature was being reprinted by more than five hundred daily newspapers, and Senator Henry Cabot Lodge was serving as its Washington spokesperson. Populism tinged with bigotry spread quickly, and in Iowa, "the governor outlawed the use of all foreign languages even over the telephone." As Thomas Watson summarized a popular feeling: "The scum of creation has been dumped on us."[14]

The man who claimed to know the most about the relationship of immigrants to insanity was Francis Walker, superintendent of the censuses of 1870 and 1880 and president of the Massachusetts Institute of Technology from 1881 to 1897. In a June 1896 issue of the *Atlantic Monthly*, Walker derided immigrants as "ignorant and brutalized peasantry . . . degraded below our utmost conceptions," with "habits repellant to our native people." Unless restrictions were placed on immigration, Walker warned, "there is no reason why every foul and stagnant pool of population in Europe . . . should not be decanted upon our soil."[15]

The prevention of insanity and idiocy was an effective argument used by supporters of the Immigration Restriction League. After the turn of the century, "League leaders stressed the 'vast inheritance of insanity, imbecility and feeble-mindedness' which the United States was garnering. . . . They propagandized through the committee of the National Association of Mental Hygiene, the Boards of Charities, the Commission of the Alien Insane in the various states . . . [and] the Immigration Committee of the American Medico-Psychological Association," the new name for the organization of the asylum superintendents. Scandinavians were said to be predisposed "toward melancholy and insanity." Jews were said to be "very prone to mental diseases." The Irish were said to be "notably numerous amongst the asylum population." William Godding even suggested that Irish patients could not recover in American asylums because they felt uncomfortable in nice surroundings: "Darby and his Joan, Bridget and Patrick, who all their lives have been happy in houses of the most primitive architecture with but one room, or at the best with a ground floor and an attic, with the goats and the pigs, and the children together, now find themselves in the midst of oppressive splendor, vast hall spaces lined with settees, in stately gothic, mediaeval in their discomfort."[16]

By 1908, when Congress set up an Immigration Commission to ascertain whether immigrants were physically and mentally debasing the native American population, it was widely assumed that immigrants were in fact the most important cause of increasing insanity. A 1912 article in *Harper's Weekly,* "Importing Our Insane," claimed that "one alien out of every 50 becomes a lunatic; the ratio among native Americans is one in 450." It continued:

> All over the United States today a protest is rising against the practice of this country in admitting and acting as the benevolent and gratuitous guardian and supporter of these tens of thousands of mental incompetents who are the subjects of other nations. Each of these defectives costs the State about $3,500 to maintain until his existence ends. If no more aliens were admitted to the institutions, the total bill for the maintenance of those already there would be in the neighborhood of $175,000,000. It will continue to increase each year until some adequate remedy is found.[17]

Such thinking was consonant with the rising tide of anti-immigrant bias and increasing calls for restrictions on immigration. When Madison Grant's *The Passing of the Great Race* was published in 1916, it quickly sold more than 16,000 copies and was reviewed in *Science* as "a work of solid merit." Grant excoriated the immigrants, especially "the Polish Jew whose dwarf stature, peculiar mentality and ruthless concentration of self-interest are being engrafted upon the stock of the nation." Grant's solution was sterilization of "an ever widening circle of social discards, beginning always with the criminal, the diseased and the insane."[18] Grant's book circulated widely in Germany and was later quoted by Nazis seeking a final solution to the problem of insane persons.

The 1910 special census included a discussion of the role of immigrants in causing insanity. Among foreign-born whites, the rate of hospitalized insanity was 4.1 per 1,000, whereas among native-born whites the rate was 1.7 per 1,000. Thus, while immigrants constituted only 15 percent of the general population, they accounted for 29 percent of asylum inmates. However, the census also noted that these numbers were "misleading," since much of the difference could be accounted for by age differences in the populations. "The native population includes large numbers of children, while the foreign-born population comprises comparatively few, most immigrants being past the period of childhood when they arrive in the United States." The census then compared insanity rates for specific age groups and found that the rate among foreign-born individuals was only approximately 15 percent higher among comparable age cohorts of adults.[19]

The necessity of age-correcting insanity prevalence rates was widely recognized following the 1910 census. H. L. Reed, in a 1913 article in the *Journal of Political Economy,* noted this necessity. Aaron Rosanoff, in his 1915 article "Some Neglected Phases of Immigration in Relation to Insanity," discussed age differences and other factors as explanations for the higher insanity rates of immigrants and concluded: "Upon eliminating the errors resulting from these disturbing factors there remains but a slight difference between the native- and foreign-born parts of the population in the incidence of certified insanity."[20]

But by 1910, it was too late for such rational discussion. The eugenics train had left the station and was moving rapidly across America. Restriction on immigration was only one car on this train. Restriction on marriage of insane persons was another eugenics approach; in 1896 Connecticut had been the first state to pass such legislation, and other states quickly followed. The superintendent of the Stockton State Hospital in California even suggested that marriage licenses in the general population should not be given to anyone with "a taint of insanity in his or her family" unless the person had first undergone sterilization.[21]

Sterilization was another approach to eugenics, and it became increasingly popular after the turn of the century. Legislation to permit the sterilization of individuals with mental retardation was introduced in Michigan in 1897 and in Pennsylvania in 1901 but failed to be enacted. Indiana in 1907 became the first state to implement mandatory sterilization for "idiots and imbeciles," and insane persons were added shortly thereafter. By 1928 twenty other states had passed similar legislation. In some states, the mandatory sterilization net was cast much more broadly; Iowa, for example, included "orphans, ne'er-do-wells, the homeless, tramps and paupers," and Missouri tried unsuccessfully to include individuals convicted of "chicken stealing [or] theft of automobile."[22]

Between 1907 and 1940, a total of 18,552 insane individuals were sterilized in the United States. Half of the procedures were done in California, and a quarter more in Virginia and Kansas together. Many asylum superintendents supported such measures because once insane persons had been sterilized, "it could legitimize the discharge of large numbers of patients from overflowing asylums." It was also believed that sterilization would reduce the number of insane persons requiring admission in the future, since it was widely claimed that the high incidence of insanity was due to "our past custom of permitting defectives to reproduce without restriction."[23]

Eugenics, then, held a strong appeal in the opening years of the twentieth century to people looking for solutions to the problem of increasing insanity. As Nathan Hale noted in *Freud and the Americans,* "Logically, only eugenics programs could halt the apparently mounting incidence of insanity." Barbara Sicherman, in *The Quest for Mental Health in America: 1880–1917,* similarly observed that "most psychiatrists were greatly interested in the scientific study of eugenics." And historian Ian Dowbiggin added: "In recent years the history of eugenics around the globe has received increasing attention from scholars, nearly all of whom cite the disproportionately high number of physicians in general, and psychiatrists in particular, within the ranks of the eugenics movement. . . . Asylum psychiatrists in particular found these eugenic solutions tempting." The official organization of America's psychiatrists, then called the American Medico-Psychological Association, created a Committee on Applied Eugenics, and a few leading psychiatrists joined other eugenics organizations. Adolf Meyer, for example, was a member of the Committee on Eugenics of the American Breeders' Association,[24] an organization that included Madison Grant and other avowed racists.

Given the problems they were facing, it is not surprising that many asylum superintendents found eugenic arguments increasingly attractive. Ian Dowbiggin cogently illustrated "how psychiatric acceptance of eugenics was shaped to a great degree by the conditions that characterized occupational practice." To illustrate this, Dowbiggin documented the shifting opinions of Alder Blumer, superintendent of the Utica State Lunatic Asylum from 1886 to 1899 and the editor of the *American Journal of Insanity*. In 1890, when the asylum had fewer than six hundred patients, Blumer claimed that insanity was due to "an environmental stress [on the brain] which is disproportionate to our present stage of evolution." He specifically rejected the hereditarian arguments of his colleagues, saying that such hereditary effects were merely "a drop in the bucket."

In 1890 New York State passed legislation mandating the transfer of all insane patients from county almshouses and other facilities to state hospitals. The census at the Utica Asylum almost doubled to 1,119 patients by 1899, overwhelming the hospital. By 1897 Blumer was more enthusiastic about hereditarian arguments, claiming, "I am the last man in the world . . . to belittle the effects of heredity." And by 1900 he was claiming that "all diseases are hereditary," praising the ancient Scots for "burying alive babies and their epileptic or mentally ill mothers" and praising Michigan's proposed legislation "for the emasculation and spaying of all chronically insane dependent men and women." As president of the American Medico-Psychological Association in 1903, Blumer proposed legislation that would make it illegal for individuals with a family history of insanity to marry.[25]

Although such eugenic solutions to the insanity problem continued to appeal to some psychiatrists, others slowly lost faith in them. Restricting marriages was viewed as largely ineffective, since marriage was not necessary for procreation. Restricting immigration also became less appealing after the census of 1910 demonstrated that once age correction was considered, immigrants were not, in fact, a major factor in the increasing insanity. Sterilization continued to have its adherents, but many psychiatrists found it to be draconian, and some leaders, such as William A. White, opposed it vehemently: "I do not believe that there is the slightest particle of justification for the mutilating operations that are being advocated."[26]

Preventing Insanity

Another solution to the insanity problem was needed. The United States had emerged from the depression of 1893–1897, defeated Spain in the Spanish-American War of 1898, and extended its borders to the Pacific Ocean. The country had truly become a nation, and "publicists were savoring the word 'nation' in this sense of a continent conquered and tamed. It was a term that above all connoted growth and development and enterprise. The talk had such a breathless quality: so much so fast, with so much still coming."[27] Surely people who had conquered a continent as well as the Spanish could also solve the insanity problem.

In the opening decades of the twentieth century, American psychiatrists slowly reached consensus on a final solution to the problem of increasing insanity—they would prevent it. Many infectious diseases were being prevented by vaccinations, the Association for the Study and Prevention of Tuberculosis was formed in 1904, and the American Association for the Study and Prevention of Infant Mortality began operation in 1909. Why should insanity not also be prevented?

In February 1909, a National Committee for Mental Hygiene was organized by psychologist William James, psychiatrist Adolf Meyer, and former psychiatric patient Clifford Beers. Beers's primary interest was in reforming mental hospitals such as the one in which he had been a patient, but "his doctor friends of those days were more interested in the possibility of *preventing* mental illness, inspired by the examples set in the control of epidemic diseases through sanitation and immunization."[28] The precise means by which insanity was to be prevented were initially unclear but came into better focus in September 1909, when Sigmund Freud, a Viennese physician, addressed a gathering at Clark University. Both James and Meyer were among those attending Freud's lectures and heard him expound on the importance of individual experiences, especially those occurring in childhood, in causing insanity and other mental disorders. If that were true, then by altering childhood experiences, one could prevent insanity.

The mental hygiene movement was enormously attractive to psychiatrists looking for a definitive solution to the insanity problem. Many who were promoting eugenic solutions, such as Alder Blumer, were among its earliest supporters. Others viewed mental hygiene as an alternative to eugenic solutions. For example, William A. White, who strongly opposed sterilization, became an early supporter of mental hygiene, began using Freud's psychoanalytic techniques to treat insane patients at the Government Hospital for the Insane, and in 1913 published the first American psychoanalytic journal.

The mental hygiene movement also attracted those who were promoting restrictions on immigration. Thomas Salmon, who had been an examiner of immigrants on Ellis Island and who was sharply critical of the nation's liberal immigration policies, which he said were causing increasing insanity, became the director of the National Committee for Mental Hygiene. Salmon was an enthusiastic Freudian who claimed that "errors of education, unsuitable environment, and the acquisition of injurious habits of thought and the suppression of painful experiences, usually in the sexual field, . . . later in life form the bases for psychoses." Salmon called these early experiences "psychic infections" and recommended psychotherapy and child guidance clinics to treat and prevent insanity.[29]

By 1913 the mental hygiene movement was advertising itself as "a well-organized endeavor to reduce the alarming amount of mental impairment in the United States." It referred to the 1910 census figures showing "187,454 insane persons in institutions in the United States," a number that was said to be "increasing rather than decreasing." The cost of these patients was said to be "over $32,000,000 a year . . . [which] is greater than the Government's expenditure this year on the Panama Canal, the greatest engineering work in the world's history." The mental hygiene movement, under the direction of the National Committee of Mental Hygiene, promised to reverse insanity's relentless increase: "Thus the present campaign against insanity is undertaken in line with every recent successful war upon disease. We have learned that tuberculosis can be cured if taken in time, but better far, we have learned that it can be absolutely prevented by stamping out the sources of infection."[30]

World War I brought additional reminders why the prevention of insanity was needed. In Massachusetts and New York, four out of every 1,000 men were rejected for military service because of "mental alienation," leading observers to conclude that there were "at least as many men with mental diseases . . . outside the hospitals for insane in New York as there were patients in the hospitals." Psychiatric hospitals in the United States, unlike those in England, did not have to be used for military purposes, so the hospital census did not decline. The influenza pandemic of 1919 killed some patients—in New York State, the excess death rate was 21 percent in 1919, compared to the years immediately preceding and following—but insanity was increasing so rapidly that the difference was barely noticeable. Between 1897 and 1917 both the number of hospital admissions and the total number of inpatients in New York State almost doubled.[31]

The national 1923 census of hospitalized insane persons caused further alarm. The number of psychiatric patients in the United States had grown from 187,791 in 1910 to 255,245 in 1923, an increase of 36 percent; during the same time period, the population had increased only 21 percent. Earlier in 1923 a French psychologist, Emil Coué, had arrived in the United States and started a health fad whereby each person was to repeat daily: "Every day in every way I am getting better and better." From the vantage point of the 1923 census, that did not appear to be the case.

The increase in the number of hospitalized insane persons in the 1923 census provided additional impetus to eugenicists, who were promoting sterilization, and to anti-immigrant adherents, who were promoting the abolition of immigration. The Immigration Act of 1921 had partially closed the immigration door. A 1921 series of articles in the *Saturday Evening Post* attacking immigrants as "streams of undersized, peculiar, alien people" and a 1922 article in the *Atlantic Monthly* alleging that more than 60 percent of Eastern European immigrants had been classified as "morons" on IQ tests provided additional fuel. Calvin Coolidge had said that "our country must cease to be regarded as a dumping ground,"[32] and when he ascended to the presidency in 1923, following Warren Harding's death, additional immigration restrictions were assured. The Johnson-Reed Act passed the following year and effectively reduced Eastern European immigration by 89 percent.

The hope that the new restrictions on immigration would reverse increasing insanity proved vain. Existing data from the Immigration Services made clear that this was most unlikely, since among all immigrants debarred from entering the United States at the time the immigration restrictions went into effect, less than one percent were being rejected for reasons of insanity. In 1923, for example, when a peak of 30,284 immigrants were debarred, only seventy-two of them were debarred for being insane.[33] If immigrants were causing the increasing insanity, then it must be because they had become insane after they had entered the country.

In fact, the restrictions on immigration appeared to have no effect whatever on the rate of insanity. The numbers of insane persons continued to steadily increase, apparently unaffected by World War I, Prohibition, or the Great Depression. Subsequent censuses of the public mental hospitals reported that the number of hospitalized patients increased from 255,245 in 1923 to 318,821 in 1931 and then to 423,445 in 1940. The seventeen-year increase from 1923 to 1940 was 66 percent, during a time when the general population increased only 18 percent. Between 1931 and 1940, thirty-two additional patients were added to America's mental hospitals *each day*. And in the sixty-year period between 1880 and 1940, the rate of hospitalized psychiatric patients had almost tripled, from 1.18 to 3.21 per 1,000 total population.

The consequences for the hospitals were predictable. In 1938 a federal study found that the average daily population of mental hospitals exceeded their capacity by 11 percent, and in three states the excess was more than 40 percent. Some persons blamed the overcrowding on the Depression, but in fact it was the continuation of a trend that had existed for a hundred years. The Metropolitan Life Insurance Company in 1938 calculated that "more than 5 percent of the children born alive in New York State and Massachusetts will spend some part of their lives in a mental hospital." The federal government estimated that the annual cost of hospitalization of mental patients was between $150 million and $200 million. And almost everyone agreed with the 1938 assessment that "from the standpoint of prevalence, as well as economic loss, the problem of mental disease is without question one of the major issues facing medical science and political organization as well as modern society."[34]

During the 1920s and 1930s, a few physicians turned to surgery as a means to alleviate the rising insanity problem. Foremost among these was Henry Cotton, who removed teeth, tonsils, and parts of the intestine from hundreds of patients at the Trenton State Hospital in New Jersey. Cotton claimed that there were foci of infections in these organs that were causing the insanity and that removal of the infections would produce clinical improvement. Using his surgical techniques, he asserted, "the alarming increase in insanity will be checked."[35] It was a truly desperate treatment for what appeared to be a desperate problem.

Another response to the rising rates of insanity in the 1920s and 1930s was to simply deny their validity. For example, in 1927 Henry Elkind, the medical director of the Massachusetts Society for Mental Hygiene, published a paper asking whether mental disease was on the increase. He reviewed rates of first admissions to mental hospitals in New York, Massachusetts, and Rhode Island and noted that the rates had been steady between 1912 and 1923. The rising rates prior to 1912 Elkind labeled "a statistical illusion." Elkind's paper was commended by some of his colleagues as a proper response to "the alarmists who are constantly proclaiming the great increase of insanity as shown by their shallow study of poorly prepared statistics."[36]

Elkind published another paper, "The Alleged Increase in the Incidence of the Major Psychoses," in 1936. After acknowledging that "a cursory examination of these data might lead one to infer increases both in the general and specific rates of mental disease," he showed that there had been no increase in first admissions for schizophrenia or manic-depressive illness in Massachusetts and New York between 1920 and 1933. Also at this time, Ellen Winston published a paper, "The Assumed Increase of Mental Disease," in the *American Journal of Sociology*. Winston's paper, which was widely cited in subsequent years, concluded that "the present evidence . . . leads one definitely to question the assumption of an increasing rate of mental disease throughout the United States." The data in her paper, however, showed a 13 percent increase in first admissions to state mental hospitals, from 6.7 per 10,000 in 1922 to 7.6 per 10,000 in 1931.[37]

In the late 1930s, then, the question of increasing insanity was continuing to be widely debated both by mental health professionals and by the public. *Scribner's Magazine* published an article asking, "Is Civilization Driving Us Crazy?" and answered: "The truth is that we are living in a world that is hard to adjust to. Some of us have more trouble in adjusting than others. Those that have the hardest time are popularly described as crazy." *Harper's Monthly* magazine published an article, "The Age of Schizophrenia," in which it described schizophrenia as being caused by repressed "infantile unconscious" mental processes and concluded: "If we could give free vent to every emotional urge, we should not have schizophrenia." An article entitled "But *Is* the World Going Mad?" argued that insanity was not increasing but was merely being brought out of people's back rooms; the apparent increase in insanity in fifty years merely meant that "fewer families have afflicted relatives hidden away in the attic or the back bedroom."[38]

In examining the data on increasing insanity in the United States between 1920 and 1940, three aspects are prominent. First, some of the increased hospitalization rates were due to increased numbers of elderly patients being admitted for conditions that were then called "senile psychosis" and "cerebral arteriosclerosis." In 1923 these two diagnoses contributed 14 percent of public mental hospital admissions, but by 1943 that had increased to 27 percent. This increase was consistent with the number of individuals age sixty-five and over in the general population, which increased from 5.4 million in 1923 to 9.9 million in 1943. Many of these patients would today be diagnosed with Alzheimer's disease and vascular dementia. Medicare and Medicaid for the support of such individuals in nursing homes would not begin until the 1960s, and so the majority of them were admitted to public mental hospitals. As will be discussed in chapter 14, such admissions of elderly individuals were therefore responsible for a portion of the increasing psychiatric hospital admission rates after 1920.

Another aspect of insanity that stands out in the period between the wars is the higher rates for individuals living in cities compared to those living in rural areas. This had been documented in the 1890 census and again in the 1910 census, at which time it was noted that first admissions to psychiatric hospitals from large cities (500,000 and over) were two and a half times higher than from rural areas. That census had concluded that "there is relatively more insanity in cities than in country districts and in large cities than in small cities."[39] After 1910, the urbanization of America continued. By 1920, 26 percent of the population lived in cities of 100,000 or more; in 1840, only 3 percent of people had lived in such cities.

In 1921 a New York State study compared first admissions to mental hospitals for residents of New York City to first admissions for the rest of the state. The admission rate for city residents was almost twice as high for schizophrenia and manic-depressive illness, but no such difference existed for other diagnoses. Similarly, in Chicago in 1939, Robert Faris and Warren Dunham published their widely cited study of mental hospital admissions from different areas of that city. They reported that insanity was more common in the more crowded and poorer areas and attributed the high rates to "extreme social disorganization." *Time* magazine reported this work as having established "insanity zones" in cities and included a map of Chicago's "geolunatics." Half a century later, Dunham recanted his sociological explanation, acknowledging that "there is hardly a shred of hard evidence" to support it.[40] The idea that cities somehow spawn insanity had been clearly established, although what was cause and what was effect was open to debate.

A third aspect of insanity that stands out in the 1920–1940 period is the continued reporting of its uneven geographical distribution. Consistent with studies dating to 1880, the highest reported first admission rates for schizophrenia from 1923 to 1940 were in the northeastern and West Coast states, although rates in midwestern states such as Illinois, Wisconsin, Michigan, and Minnesota were also increasing. This distribution was consistent with the increasing urbanization of these states compared to states with lower first admission rates for schizophrenia.

"The Versatility of Madness"

The representation of insanity in American literature in the first half of the twentieth century contrasted sharply with its representation a century earlier. In the early nineteenth century, insanity was omnipresent in literature, consistent with the intense public interest in it as a new phenomenon. By the late nineteenth century and throughout the twentieth century, the thematic use of insanity was restricted mostly to writers who themselves had major psychiatric problems or who had an intimate association with insanity through a family member.

Eugene O'Neill, for example, is said to have "introduced insanity to modern American drama."[41] In *Strange Interlude*, which won a

Pulitzer Prize in 1928, the aunt of Sam Evans lives in the attic and is hopelessly insane, while his grandmother and great-grandfather both died in insane asylums. O'Neill himself suffered from severe recurrent depressions, tried suicide on at least one occasion, and had a son who committed suicide.

At the time that *Strange Interlude* was being acclaimed, Zelda Fitzgerald was showing increasing signs of psychiatric illness and in 1930 was admitted to the first of what would be many psychiatric hospitals. She was variously diagnosed with schizophrenia and manic-depressive illness during her several hospital admissions, and she incorporated descriptions of her psychotic symptoms into her 1932 book, *Save Me the Waltz:* "Meaningfully the nurses laughed together and left her room. The walls began again. She decided to lie there and frustrate the walls if they thought they could press her between their pages like a bud from a wedding bouquet."[42]

F. Scott Fitzgerald exploited his wife's illness extensively in *Tender Is the Night,* published in 1934. The two main characters, Nicole and Dick, are thinly disguised surrogates for Zelda and Scott, with many details of Nicole's illness closely paralleling Zelda's. On one occasion, for example, Nicole grabs the steering wheel of their moving car, causing it to crash into a tree: "She was laughing hilariously, unashamed, unafraid, unconcerned. No one coming on the scene would have imagined that she had caused it."[43] Zelda had, in fact, done the same thing. Similarly, parts of letters written by Zelda to Scott while she was hospitalized were incorporated into the novel as letters from Nicole to Dick.

F. Scott Fitzgerald was intrigued by insanity, both by its power and by its destructive effects. In *Tender Is the Night,* he noted: "But the brilliance, the versatility of madness is akin to the resourcefulness of water seeping through, over and around a dike. It requires the united front of many people to work against it." Like many educated people of his generation, Fitzgerald generally accepted the currently fashionable psychological explanations of insanity, and in *Tender Is the Night,* Nicole's schizophrenia is said to have been caused by incest. At other times, however, Fitzgerald wondered if Zelda's illness had biological origins, as he expressed in a letter to her psychiatrist: "I can't help clinging to the idea that some essential physical thing like salt or iron or semen or some unguessed-at holy water is either missing or is present in too great quantity."[44] Fitzgerald himself suffered from severe alcoholism and periods of depression, and on several occasions he made suicide attempts and was psychiatrically hospitalized. In 1936, he published an autobiographical story, "The Crack-Up," in which he described his periods of depression.

Tennessee Williams was another American writer who suffered from both alcoholism and depression and who was psychiatrically hospitalized. His mother was diagnosed with psychosis, and his sister, Rose, was afflicted with severe schizophrenia and underwent a lobotomy. According to Jacqueline O'Connor: "It was because of Rose that he wrote so often about insanity: not merely because he was obsessed with her madness, but because her madness strongly suggested that his lurked around the corner, and that somehow he must evade it, outrun it, keep it from conquering him."[45]

Insanity is a recurring theme in Williams's plays, including the madness of Lucretia in *Portrait of a Madonna* (1947), Blanche's slow descent into madness in *A Streetcar Named Desire* (1947), the chronic psychosis and proposed lobotomy of Catherine in *Suddenly Last Summer* (1958), the repeated mental breakdowns of the Reverend Shannon in *The Night of the Iguana* (1961), and the arguments between a brother and sister regarding which one is truly insane in *The Two Character Play* (1967).

Like Tennessee Williams, Conrad Aiken had both a parent and a sister who became insane. His father, a successful surgeon, killed his wife and then himself because of a delusional belief that his wife was going to have him committed to an insane asylum. Aiken, then age eleven, found their bodies. His younger sister became insane in her early twenties and spent much of her life hospitalized. Aiken himself had periods of depression and made at least one serious suicide attempt. He lived his life fearing that he, too, would become insane and in 1932 wrote "Silent Snow, Secret Snow," which he acknowledged was "a projection of my own inclination to insanity." It is an account of the onset of schizophrenia in a twelve-year-old boy:

> Not a moment too soon. The darkness was coming in long white waves. . . . The snow was laughing; it spoke from all sides at once: it pressed closer to him as he ran and jumped exulting into his bed.

"Listen to us!" it said. "Listen! We have come to tell you the story we told you about. . . . Lie down. Shut your eyes. . . ."

A beautiful varying dance of snow began at the front of the room, came forward and then retreated, flattened out toward the floor, then rose fountain-like to the ceiling.[46]

The Era of Deinstitutionalization

Two events during World War II profoundly changed the face of mental illness in America. The first was the fact that 18 percent of all men rejected for induction into the armed forces were rejected because of mental illnesses—the largest single cause. Gen. Lewis Hershey, the director of the Selective Service System, testified at congressional hearings in September 1945 that "mental illness was the greatest cause of noneffectiveness and loss of manpower that we met." Two months later, President Truman publicly sounded the alarm: "Accurate statistics are lacking, but there is no doubt that there are at least two million persons in the United States who are mentally ill, and that as many as ten million will probably need hospitalization for mental illness for some period in the course of their lifetime."[47]

The other event that influenced the debate about mental illness was the assignment of approximately 3,000 conscientious objectors—mostly Mennonites, Quakers, and Methodists—to alternate duty in state mental hospitals. The "conchies," as they were often called, were appalled by the conditions in the hospitals. Their reports to the media formed the basis for a series of exposés after the war in *Life* magazine and *Reader's Digest* and eventually led to the publication of Albert Deutsch's *The Shame of the States* and Mary Jane Ward's novel *The Snake Pit*. The last was an apt description of conditions in most state mental hospitals at that time and provided a rationale for the subsequent deinstitutionalization of patients that would continue for the remainder of the century.

The question of increasing insanity was addressed one last time following World War II. In 1949, concerned about the high number of inductees and military personnel who had been affected with severe mental illnesses, the U.S. Department of Defense gave a contract to the

Rand Corporation to ascertain whether or not insanity was increasing. The study was carried out by Herbert Goldhamer, a social psychologist, and Andrew Marshall, a statistician who had just completed his training. Their published study, *Psychosis and Civilization,* concluded that insanity had not increased. The study was subsequently cited by multiple psychiatric textbooks and psychiatric historians as having laid to rest the myth of increasing insanity.[48]

Psychosis and Civilization is a curious book. It shows clearly increasing first admission insanity rates between 1840 and 1885 for all age groups, from 3.9 to 6.2 per 10,000, but then dismisses these rates as "essentially misleading." It then proceeds to compare selected nineteenth-century rates with selected twentieth-century rates, making some remarkably liberal assumptions in the process. For example, it deletes 85 percent of all insane persons reported as having been in nineteenth-century almshouses, because it assumes they had also been hospitalized, and thus double-counted, despite abundant evidence that many such insane persons had remained in the almshouses exclusively. In another example, the authors "assume that the opportunity for hospitalization and incentives for hospitalization" in the first year of a hospital's opening were the same as "those that exist today."[49] Given the tremendous backlog of unmet needs when most hospitals opened in the nineteenth century, this is analogous to comparing the number of shoppers, many of whom have been waiting outside, that rush through the doors as a department store opens for a large sale to the number of shoppers entering several hours later.

The most troubling aspect of *Psychosis and Civilization,* however, is the authors' selective use of comparison data. As summarized by sociologist William Eaton in a 1980 critique: "At several points in the text, it becomes obvious that the comparisons are selected carefully, and one has no way of knowing which comparisons they attempted but did not include in the text." Eaton also noted that Goldhamer and Marshall "consistently ignore factors that might inflate the nineteenth-century rates ... and they ignore factors that might deflate the present-day rates. ... It is also clear that they wish to support the hypothesis that the rates have not changed."[50]

Psychosis and Civilization concludes on an optimistic note that "there has been no long-term increase during the last century in the incidence of the psychoses of early and middle life," a conclusion the authors themselves label as "astonishing." Their Freudian theory bias is suggested by their observation that "theories that view the functional psychoses as resulting from repression of basic human drives . . . may possibly be thought of as being more especially consistent with our findings," since such "early psychic traumas" were assumed to have changed little during the period of their study.[51]

Since the publication of *Psychosis and Civilization* in 1949, there has been virtually no discussion of increasing insanity in the United States. The number of mentally ill hospitalized individuals continued increasing until 1955, when it totaled 558,922, or 3.38 per 1,000 total population. The hospitalized rate had thus increased from 0.20 per 1,000 in 1850 to 1.86 in 1903 and then to 3.38 in 1955, a seventeenfold increase in just over one hundred years.

State hospitals such as Pilgrim on Long Island had as many as 14,000 patients and were cities unto themselves; twenty other hospitals had over 4,000 patients each. Overcrowding ranged from 20 to 74 percent, and the cost of the state mental hospitals consumed on average 8 percent of total state budgets.[52] Diagnostically, 62 percent of all patients were diagnosed with "functional psychosis," 13 percent with "diseases of the senium" (mostly Alzheimer's disease), 7 percent with "mental deficiency," and 5 percent with "syphilitic psychosis."

There are suggestions that insanity continued to increase in the United States until at least 1960. The first admission rate for schizophrenia, for example, increased from 1.3 per 10,000 in 1939–1941 to 1.7 in 1949–1951 and 2.0 in 1959–1961. Studies of specific geographical areas also suggest a continuing increase. For example, a 1938 study of all individuals with psychoses in Williamson County, Tennessee, reported 6.3 per 1,000 total population, compared with 1.6 per 1,000 for the same county in the 1880 census. And the 1950 Hollingshead and Redlich study of New Haven reported a rate of 4.2 individuals per 1,000 with schizophrenia and affective psychoses who were in treatment.[53] This rate is almost double the 2.5 per 1,000 rate for New Haven in the 1880 census, which included *all* individuals with psychoses, those who were in treatment and those who were not.

Beginning in the late 1950s, the census of American mental hospitals began decreasing as deinstitutionalization got underway. The falling census eradicated any remaining interest in the question of whether insanity had been, or still was, increasing. By 1961, when the congressionally appointed Joint Commission on Mental Illness and Health issued its final report, the falling census was noted and the question of increasing insanity was not even mentioned in its 298-page report. By this time, American psychiatrists were also abandoning the state mental hospitals that had been their main work venue for over one hundred years; in 1940, 68 percent of psychiatrists still worked in the hospitals, but by 1957, the figure had fallen to 17 percent.[54] With both patients and psychiatrists leaving the hospitals, who could worry about increasing insanity?

As we enter the twentieth-first century, however, we have no clear assessment of the number of insane person in the United States today. If, in the year 2000, we had the same number of persons in public mental hospitals as we had hospitalized in 1955, allowing for the increase in population that has taken place, the census of state mental hospitals would be approximately 932,000. As in 1955, however, there would also be a significant number of insane persons not hospitalized, some being treated and some not being treated, so the total number of insane persons would be much higher.

The best estimates of the prevalence of insanity in late-twentieth-century America came from the Epidemiologic Catchment Area (ECA) study, carried out from 1980 to 1985 in New Haven, Baltimore, Durham, St. Louis, and Los Angeles. Based on interviews with a sample of 20,291 individuals, the ECA study reported that 2.2 percent of adults (ages 18 and over) were diagnosed with schizophrenia or manic-depressive illness (bipolar disorder).[55]

Since the ECA study was carried out a century after the 1880 census of insane persons, it is instructive to compare the two results. Based on 1980 census figures, the 1980s ECA study identified 3.6 million adults as having schizophrenia or manic-depressive illness, or 15.9 per 1,000 total population. In 1880 the census had found 91,997 individuals with insanity, or 1.8 per 1,000 total population. The 1980s study included some individuals who would not have been counted as insane in 1880 (bipolar disorder II, depression with hypomania), and the 1880 study counted some individuals as insane who would not have been included in the ECA study (e.g., epilepsy with insanity). Even allowing for methodological problems and diagnostic differences, however, the almost ninefold greater prevalence in 1980 is both impressive and a source of concern.

Another means of approximating contemporary insanity rates is by ascertaining the number of individuals who are receiving federal disability assistance for "mental disorders other than mental retardation" from the Supplemental Security Income (SSI) or the Social Security Disability Insurance (SSDI) programs. In 1997 the total number of such individuals was 2.5 million,[56] and this number did not include individuals in state mental hospitals, those receiving Veterans Administration benefits, and those who were homeless or in jail and who had not applied for such benefits. Most individuals receiving SSI or SSDI for "mental disorders other than mental retardation" would have been counted as insane in 1880. The "insanity" rate for these 2.5 million individuals receiving SSI or SSDI *alone* in 1997 was 9.4 per 1,000 total population, more than five times the 1.8 per 1,000 rate reported in 1880.

The most remarkable thing about insanity in contemporary America, however, is that its existence as an epidemic is unknown. Despite the evidence of its startling increase over two centuries, despite its enormous fiscal and human costs, and despite the fact that *it still may be increasing*, there is virtually no interest in this issue. Insanity has become accepted, like an unwelcome guest who slowly settles into the household and eventually is thought of as a member of the family. AIDS, tuberculosis, and cancer continue to evoke adversarial feelings—they do not *belong*. Insanity, by contrast, is widely thought of as part of the human condition and assumed to have always been with us in its present form. Such acceptance of insanity betrays a fundamental misunderstanding of its essence.

CHAPTER 13

Why Is the Epidemic Forgotten?

The Politicalization of Insanity

How many wretched beings do the wards of a public lunatic asylum enclose, who, having been once as we are, are now reduced to a state of worse than brutal ferocity. . . . In the great round of human misery and woe, there cannot surely be found any case that comes at all near to this in dreadful and heart-appalling interest.

—Anonymous, *Eclectic Review,* 1816

It seems that the Government had a true Account of it, and several Counsels were held about Ways to prevent its coming over; but all was kept very private. Hence it was, that this Rumour died off again, and People began to forget it, as a thing we were very little concern'd in, and that we hoped was not true.

—Daniel Defoe, *A Journal of the Plague Year,* 1722

Living amid an ongoing epidemic that nobody notices is surreal. It is like viewing a mighty river that has risen slowly over two centuries, imperceptibly claiming the surrounding land, millimeter by millimeter. The people who once lived on the land have either died or moved away, and few of their relatives are aware that the river was once much smaller. Humans adapt remarkably well to a disaster as long as the disaster occurs over a long period of time.

Since the middle of the twentieth century there has been virtually no discussion of epidemic insanity. Like the mighty river, the high prevalence of insanity is accepted as a given and assumed to be similar to the prevalence of insanity of one hundred, five hundred, even one thousand years ago. The possibility of its having been otherwise is not considered and, when raised for discussion, is met with incredulity. Haven't you seen the river? How could you think that it was ever otherwise?

The question of increasing insanity is even ignored by mental illness professionals. When discussed at all, it is usually dismissed with a standard litany, as in this 1967 psychiatric textbook: "Hospital records provide evidence that the incidence of schizophrenia in the United States has probably remained unchanged, at least for the past 100 years and possibly throughout our entire history, despite tremendous socioeconomic and population changes." The usual reference for such declarations is Goldhamer and Marshall's *Psychosis and Civilization*, the seriously flawed 1949 study in which the authors' conclusions are contradicted by their own data. American historians such as Gerald Grob in *The State and the Mentally Ill* and David Rothman in *The Discovery of the Asylum* have cited the Goldhamer and Marshall study as demonstrating "convincingly that the rate of insanity in this country has remained constant from before the Civil War to the present." English historians such as Ida Macalpine and Richard Hunter similarly declared the idea of epidemic insanity "laid to rest and not heard from again."[1] With so many respected individuals having asserted increasing insanity to be a non-issue, it has become so.

Another factor that has discouraged discussion of epidemic insanity is that the idea of increasing insanity is inconsistent with theories about insanity's causation that dominated professional thinking during the twentieth century. For example, one theory was that adverse early childhood experiences caused insanity. Although there was no scientific evidence to support it, this theory strongly influenced thinking about insanity in the United States and, to a lesser extent, Europe for over fifty years. Therefore, if insanity was increasing because of adverse childhood experiences, then childhood experiences must have been getting progressively worse. There were no data to support this, and it also conflicted with beliefs about human progress.

Another major theory was that insanity is caused by genes. Although it is now well established that genes play some role in causing both schizophrenia and manic-depressive illness, viewing these disorders as primarily genetic diseases is incompatible with the increasing prevalence described in the preceding chapters, for reasons to be discussed in chapter 14. Why, for example, should insanity have increased most rapidly during the years when most individuals with insanity were institutionalized and thereby prevented from reproducing?

The Myth of Mental Illness

The major reason, however, why increasing insanity became a non-issue in the latter half of the twentieth century was the emergence of historical theories that appeared to negate it. If there had been any hope of seriously examining the question of epidemic insanity, that hope died in 1961 with the publication of three books: Michel Foucault's *Histoire de la Folie* (translated in 1965 as *Madness and Civilization*), Thomas Szasz's *The Myth of Mental Illness,* and Erving Goffman's *Asylums.* These books and their successors dominated thinking about insanity for most of the remaining twentieth century in both Europe and North America. Epidemic insanity was subsumed by discussions of whether insanity even existed, and if it did exist, whether it was the product of social or economic forces. In viewing insanity's history, this period will likely be regarded in retrospect as both partisan and puzzling.

Foucault, who earned degrees in philosophy and psychology in Paris, was strongly influenced by Marxist thought. He became a French cultural official, with postings in Sweden, Poland, and Germany, and died of AIDS in 1984. According to his biographers, Foucault was emotionally unstable, made multiple suicide attempts, and, in the view of one friend, "all his life . . . verged on madness."[2]

In his influential *Madness and Civilization,* Foucault argued that insanity had always existed but had been accepted as an alternative lifestyle until the seventeenth century. Because of social and economic changes at that time, insane persons started to be institutionalized, along with paupers, vagrants, beggars, criminals, and prostitutes, and the era of "the great confinement" began. As Foucault noted, this was "the moment when madness was perceived on the social horizon of poverty, of incapacity for work, of inability to integrate with the group."[3] The insane replaced lepers as the outcasts of society, symbols of economic parasitism and nonproductivity.

Foucault's account of history has been widely criticized. Andrew Scull, for example, asserts that Foucault's "reconstruction of the encounter of (Western) civilization and madness remains deeply and fundamentally flawed" and accuses Foucault of attempting "a peculiar marriage of history and French structuralism in a style evocative of James Joyce at his most obscure." German Berrios and Hugh Freeman, more politely, observed that Foucault "as a historian, was economical with the facts." In replying to such criticisms, Foucault claimed that it was unfair to oppose "little true facts against big vague ideas."[4]

But there is no gainsaying the fact that Foucault's work had a profound influence on historians in general and on American intellectuals in particular. Marlene Ariano claimed that "since Foucault burst upon the scene, all writers on the subject have traveled in the wake of his work." And the *New York Review of Books* noted in 1982 that Foucault "has set the agenda for the last fifteen years of research." The appeal of Foucault's book was not only its benign view of madness but also, in Scull's words, "its metaphysical subtleties, its flamboyant romanticism, and its dazzling prose." Foucault dressed insanity in its best philosophical finery: "The symbol of madness will henceforth be that mirror which, without reflecting anything real, will secretly offer the man who observes himself in it the dream of his own presumption. Madness deals not so much with truth and the world, as with man and whatever the truth about himself he is able to perceive."[5] Foucault thus had great appeal to a generation that often mistook obscurantism for wisdom.

For Thomas Szasz, the question of increasing insanity has been remarkably easy to answer—insanity cannot possibly be increasing because it does not exist. In his *Myth of Mental Illness* and voluminous writings that have continued to the present, Szasz has persistently argued that "the phenomenon psychiatrists call 'schizophrenia' is not a demonstrable medical disease but the name of certain kinds of social deviance." He acknowledges that some "persons often behave and speak in ways that differ from the behavior and speech of many (though by no means all) other people in their environment," but he argues that such behavior is a consequence of "desocialization" that begins during adolescence.[6]

Szasz, trained in psychiatry and psychoanalysis, began his career as a psychiatrist in the United States Navy. As such, he encountered many individuals who were faking psychiatric symptoms to obtain discharges or disability pensions. After leaving the military, Szasz went into the private practice of psychotherapy, seeing few, if any, individuals who suffered from insanity.

In recent years, Szasz has claimed that homeless individuals who appear to be mentally ill are really, "by the inexorable standards of social reality, losers. . . . Others [among the homeless] are simply people who develop in such a way that their desires or demands hopelessly exceed their achievements or expectations." "Mental illness," he has endlessly argued, "is undefined, undefinable, and, in my opinion, nonexistent," and the psychiatrist is simply a "nanny for troublesome adults."[7]

In the present era, in which magnetic resonance imaging and neuropathology have unequivocally established that schizophrenia and manic-depressive illness are diseases of the brain, it would be easy to dismiss Szasz's writings as simply historical anomalies. But that would be to underestimate the profound influence he has had on contemporary thinking about insanity. By questioning its very existence, Szasz has cast a pall over inquiries regarding insanity's origins and historicity. And that is quite apart from his influence on the civil libertarian movement to abolish all involuntary treatment of insane persons, on the antipsychiatry Church of Scientology's Citizens Commission on Human Rights, which has sometimes claimed him as a founder, and on romantic narratives that have depicted hospitalized psychiatric patients as normal individuals being persecuted by evil psychiatrists, such as Ken Kesey's *One Flew over the Cuckoo's Nest*.

Simultaneous with the publication of Szasz's *The Myth of Mental Illness* in 1961 was the publication of Erving Goffman's *Asylums*. Goffman was a sociologist who spent several months observing patients in a mental hospital. Like both Foucault and Szasz, Goffman viewed the hospital "as one among a network of institutions designed to provide a residence for various categories of socially troublesome people."[8] Insane behavior, reasoned Goffman, was a response of patients to being confined in a "total institution." If the gates of the hospital were to be opened, therefore, the patients would return to the community and live happily ever after, as they did in the movie *King of Hearts*.

Foucault, Szasz, and Goffman are the forerunners of a continuing corps of European and American intellectuals who have depicted insanity not as a brain disease but rather as the consequence of labeling for social or economic reasons. Ronald Laing, an English psychoanalyst, came to prominence in 1964 with an article in the *New Left Review* in which he claimed that what people called schizophrenia was really a useful voyage to "inner space": "I do not myself believe that there is any such 'condition' as 'schizophrenia.' Yet the label is a social fact. Indeed, this label as social fact is a *political event*."[9] Three years later, Laing's *The Politics of Experience* was published, and he emerged as a guru of the New Left movement. His claim that insanity was a rational adjustment to an insane world resonated with the political exhortations of the sixties radicals, and Laing participated in the 1969 Dialectics of Liberation Congress with radical leaders such as Herbert Marcuse, Stokeley Carmichael, and Paul Goodman.

Laing, in fact, was convinced that insane behavior was really caused by parental pressure on children. As Laing's protégé Joseph Berke explained it, "The one family member who happened to have been diagnosed schizophrenic or neurotic or whatever was not necessarily the most disturbed person in the family." This belief made for an especially painful experience for Laing in 1977, when his eldest daughter became insane and had to be hospitalized. By then Laing's mother, who "was deeply ashamed and perfectly aware, through local reviews and gossip, of what her son was saying about families," had told him never to contact her again. Laing had problems with alcoholism and drug use that worsened as he grew older, and his license to practice medicine was eventually revoked. By 1982 Laing appeared confused and dejected and in an interview stated: "I don't think I could pass an exam question on what is R. D. Laing's theory. I was looked to as one who had answers, but I never had them."[10]

Social Control and Marxist Economics

As the 1960s brought Foucault, Szasz, Goffman, and Laing to address the history of insanity, so the 1970s added David Rothman, Andrew

Scull, and Gerald Grob. Rothman, an American historian, came to prominence in 1971 with the publication of *The Discovery of the Asylum*. He was impressed by the number of states that had begun opening asylums in the 1830s, during the presidency of Andrew Jackson, and assumed that their opening was linked to contemporary social unrest, "the frantic spirit at loose in the community." Insane asylums were thus "an effort to ensure the cohesion of the community in new and changing circumstances":

> The response of the Jacksonian period to the deviant and the dependent was first and foremost a vigorous attempt to promote the stability of the society at a moment when traditional ideas and practices appeared outmoded, constricted, and ineffective. . . . The asylum was to fulfill a dual purpose for its innovators. It would rehabilitate inmates and then, by virtue of its success, set an example of right action for the larger society. . . . The well-ordered asylum would exemplify the proper principles of social organization and thus ensure the safety of the republic and promote its glory.[11]

Rothman's explanation of insanity's history was thus a Jacksonian version of Foucault's "great confinement," the incarceration of society's deviant and unproductive members so as to promote social stability. It views asylums essentially as units of social control, to impose order on the disordered masses. Rothman did not believe that insanity was really increasing, and he cited Goldhamer and Marshall's *Psychosis and Civilization* as evidence; rather, insanity was merely being viewed differently.

Rothman has been criticized for his interpretation of history. Jacques Quen, in a review, claimed that Rothman's book "demonstrates a deplorable selective inattention to historical data" and "must be embarrassing to the professional historian." Norman Dain characterized Rothman as a "scholarly romantic" who, like Michel Foucault, assumed the existence of a golden age in the pre-asylum years when insane persons lived happily in the community. Andrew Scull accused Rothman of using "quasi-magical incantations and invocations of demographic and economic developments" to try to make his thesis fit historical facts. And all three critics accused Rothman of having a strong anti-institutional bias; Rothman did nothing to mitigate this charge when he praised Thomas Szasz, joined the boards of the New York Civil Liberties Union and the Mental Health Law Project, and urged his colleagues to "work toward decarceration—toward getting and keeping as many people as possible out of institutions."[12]

Andrew Scull was also profoundly influenced by his political beliefs in his analysis of the rise of insanity. An English sociologist, Scull acknowledged his early debt to Foucault, Szasz, and other writers of the 1960s: "I began work on madness and its place in the social order in the early 1970s, the heyday of a romantic antipsychiatry. . . . It would be disingenuous to pretend that this intellectual climate was somehow irrelevant to my own concerns and emphases."[13] He entered the debate about insanity with a series of papers and then, in 1979, with the publication of *Museums of Madness*, later revised and republished as *The Most Solitary of Afflictions*.

Scull has asserted that the main impetus to the building of insane asylums, and thereby to the incarceration of insane persons, could be explained by Marxist economics: "I suggest that the main driving force behind the rise of a segregative response to madness (and to other forms of deviance) can much more plausibly be asserted to lie in the effects of a mature capitalist market economy and the associated ever more thoroughgoing commercialization of existence." Prior to the rise of the market economy, "mad people for the most part were not treated even as a separate category or type of deviants": "Beginning in the late eighteenth century, however, capitalism broke the social bonds that had formerly held it in check. There occurred a massive reorganization of society as a whole along market principles. . . . The old social order was undermined and then destroyed, and profound shifts took place in the relationships between superordinate and subordinate classes: changes we may sum up as the movement from a paternalistic social order dominated by rank, order, and degree to a society based on class."[14]

According to Scull, "The emergence of a market economy, and more particularly, the emergence of a market in labour, provided the initial incentive to distinguish far more carefully than heretofore between different categories of deviance . . . the able-bodied from the non-able-bodied poor."[15] Jails, workhouses, and insane asylums therefore emerged as government solutions to the different types of deviance, with the last being the institution for those individuals who were least able to contribute economically.

Scull's explanation for the apparently rising number of insane persons and rapidly expanding asylums was that such people had always existed but had not been collected together. In one of his first papers, he said that prior to the eighteenth century, "lunatics were generally treated no differently from other deviants: only a few of the most violent or troublesome cases might find themselves confined." With the changing economy, however, it became necessary to collect them together. Scull cited approvingly the 1870 lumber room analogy offered by Andrew Wynter, the founder of the *British Medical Journal*: "The very imposing appearance of these [asylum] establishments acts as an advertisement to draw patients towards them. If we make a convenient lumber room, we all know how speedily it becomes filled up with lumber. The county asylum is the mental lumber room of the surrounding district; friends are only too willing, in their poverty, to place away the human encumbrance of the family in a palatial building at county expense."[16]

The corollary to the lumber room thesis is that, as the availability of asylums became increasingly known by the community, families sent less disabled family members to fill them. Within a market economy, Scull noted, "family members unable to contribute effectively towards their own maintenance must have constituted a serious drain on family resources." This led to "an ever-wider practical application of the term mental illness. The asylum provided a convenient and culturally legitimate alternative to coping with 'intolerable' individuals within the family."[17] The lumber room, initially reserved for large pieces of wood, increasingly became a storage center for ever smaller pieces.

There is one additional aspect of Andrew Scull's economic thesis that he has used to explain the apparent rise of insanity. This is the economic advantage to psychiatrists themselves as experts in treating insanity. The earliest private insane asylums in the eighteenth and early nineteenth centuries were, according to Scull, "generally a very lucrative investment" and "it was precisely at this stage that the medical profession began to assert an interest in lunacy." Scull has repeatedly returned to what he has called "one centrally important feature of this whole process: just how that segment of the medical profession we now call psychiatry captured control over insanity." The subsequent building of public asylums "provided the incentive, in the form of a guaranteed market for the experts' [psychiatrists'] services," and psychiatrists, in turn, confined society's unproductive members. Scull thus viewed psychiatrists as classic capitalists who have made handsome profits by ridding society of some of its deviant members "who had been placed in an institution because of their failure to conform to the ordinary rules and conventions of society." Rather than seeing psychiatrists as motivated by a desire to improve the lives of insane persons, Scull was impressed by their economic self-interest "to manage and clothe with a veil of legitimacy their expanding empire": "My work, like that of the antipsychiatrists, is thus marked by a pronounced skepticism concerning psychiatry's self-proclaimed rationality and disinterested benevolence, a skepticism rooted in what is, on the whole, a dismal and depressing historical record."[18] In Scull's view, as psychiatrists expanded their empire, insanity thus appeared to become increasingly more common.

The validity of Scull's lumber room thesis, and its corollary of an expanding diagnostic spectrum, will be discussed further in chapter 14. However, Scull has been criticized on other grounds as well. Michael MacDonald noted that asylums could not have been a consequence of the new capitalist economy because "there were already many asylums in England before the social effects of industrialization were widely felt in the first half of the nineteenth century." Harold Merskey claimed that "Scull has grossly misinterpreted the nature of major advances. . . . No scholar who took the minimum of care to appreciate the nature of his topic should have reached such conclusions. . . . Scull's writing offers a sort of sophisticated mayhem." Edward Shorter in his *History of Psychiatry* includes Scull among the "lost generation" of psychiatric historians who "have chosen to pursue puffs of smoke, displaying no interest in the question of just what happens historically to make the mind and brain go away." And Kathleen Jones, in an article entitled "Scull's Dilemma," chastened him for being critical of both hospital care and community services for insane persons and for having no alternative solutions to offer. Scull's reply affirmed for many that he had, in fact, no answers: "How we are to reach such a Utopia, when the alternatives history presents us with are inadequate, often inhumane, and always underfunded mental hospitals or a grossly underdeveloped and frequently nonexistent system of community care, is dare I say it, not Scull's dilemma but yours—and that of the all-too-indifferent larger society in which we both reside."[19]

Gerald Grob, an American historian, was the third major writer on the history of insanity to emerge in the 1970s. His 1973 book, *Mental Institutions in America: Social Policy to 1875,* has been followed by a plethora of articles and books on related subjects.

In marked contrast to Andrew Scull, Gerald Grob viewed the building of asylums in the nineteenth century as an attempt by well-meaning psychiatrists to provide treatment for mentally ill individuals. Most of the psychiatrists, he claimed, "were primarily concerned with uplifting the mass of suffering humanity and were not particularly aware of political or economic considerations." "The most impressive fact," Grob added, "is the relative absence of malevolence."[20]

Grob's writings have clearly detailed the rise of asylums and their subsequent failure as therapeutic institutions despite the good intentions of asylum superintendents. Grob did not believe that insanity was truly increasing and cited Goldhamer and Marshall's study to support his view. Like Scull, he accepted the "lumber room" thesis to explain the rising number of hospitalized patients: "The presence of a mental institution had the inadvertent effect of altering both the expectations and behavior of the surrounding population. When offered an alternative to home or community care, many families and local officials opted to use institutional facilities with far greater frequency than was originally anticipated. New asylums, therefore, found that admissions tended to exceed capacity." With the availability of asylums, "families that had once been reluctant to send loved ones to substandard institutions [e.g., workhouses] were now more willing to consider the possibility of institutionalization." Furthermore, the building of asylums led to "increased societal awareness of mental disease, and undoubtedly some who had been considered quaint or odd were now looked upon as insane."[21]

Grob has also suggested multiple explanations for the increasing failure of asylums in the latter part of the nineteenth century. These included insufficient funding, an increasing heterogeneity of patients, and the failure of the leaders of American psychiatry during those years. Grob concluded that the outcome is a "tragedy, in which most participants, to a greater or lesser degree, were well intentioned but their actual behavior gave rise to less than desirable results."[22]

Grob has been criticized, one might say ridiculed, for his meliorist views by Andrew Scull: "Apparently, the history of lunacy reform records the efforts of a largely well-intentioned group of men (and the occasional woman) whose endeavors mysteriously always produced accidental and unintended unpleasant consequences." Scull said Grob "seems extraordinarily concerned to rescue the reformers' reputations for humanitarianism and benevolence" and criticized "the shrillness with which Grob insists upon the primary, the virtually unqualified, hegemony of benevolent motives."[23]

Captains of Confinement

Writers on the history of insanity in the 1980s and 1990s almost all followed the lead of Foucault, Szasz, Rothman, and Scull. Foremost among these was Roy Porter, an English historian whose *Mind-Forg'd Manacles* and *A Social History of Madness* displayed an impressive erudition that established him as a dominant voice in the insanity debate.

Porter shared many of Andrew Scull's assumptions about the rise of insanity, including the importance of economic antecedents. Psychiatry, said Porter, was generated by the laissez-faire economy of the late eighteenth and nineteenth centuries:

> In a buoyant market, entrepreneurs sprouted in many fields, from mills and music to madness, combining business acumen with technical skills, to provide services for which there were at least potential buyers. Madhouses and mad-doctors arose from the same soil which generated demand for general practitioners, dancing masters, man midwives, face painters, drawing tutors, estate managers, landscape gardeners, architects, journalists and that host of other white-collar, service, and quasi-professional occupations which a society with increased economic surplus and pretensions to civilization first found it could afford, and soon found it could not do without.[24]

Porter also shared Scull's assumptions regarding the self-interest of psychiatrists: "All the same, the emergence in England of institutions for the mad is best regarded not as an act of state, not as a work of social control or medical police, nor even as bowing to necessity—the sheer pressure of madness!—but rather as triumph of these captains of confinement."[25]

Porter also appears to have shared Thomas Szasz's fundamental doubts regarding the very existence of insanity. "A sizable section of those who experienced themselves as going mad," he claimed, "were undergoing what in previous ages would have been seen as a fairly routine—if in some cases heretical—drama of the soul's wrestling with sin and the Devil, its search for faith, justification, grace and salvation." Porter's skepticism about insanity was illustrated by an analysis he did of the symptoms of John Clare, the English poet who in the early nineteenth century had been institutionalized for twenty-seven years. Clare had had delusions of being Lord Byron, Lord Nelson, and other famous personages and also exhibited classic symptoms of a thought disorder characteristic of some forms of insanity. For example, Clare claimed, "They have cut off my head and picked out all the letters of the alphabet—all the vowels and consonants—and brought them out through my ears." Porter speculated that Clare may not have been insane at all but was merely playing with words, and that Clare's psychiatrists, "so resistant to the play of the literal and figurative, . . . failed to see the joke." Rather than harboring delusions, Porter suggested that Clare may have been adopting Byron and Nelson as "a disguise": "Identity confusion? Tease? A coded message about Clare's place in the canon? Who is to say?" And in an echo of Ronald Laing, Porter added that "if Clare really went mad, it seems fairly safe to suggest this was a *consequence* of being buried, in the prime of his life, in an institution he detested."[26]

Other recent commentators on the issue of increasing insanity have included Richard Warner and Elaine Showalter. Warner, in his 1985 book *Recovery from Schizophrenia: Psychiatry and Political Economy*, followed Andrew Scull closely in linking schizophrenia to social and economic stress. Showalter, in her 1985 book *The Female Malady: Women, Madness and English Culture, 1830–1980*, praised Foucault who, she says, "brilliantly exposed the repressive ideologies that lay behind the reform of the asylum." She then proceeded to put a feminist patina on the Foucault-Scull thesis: "In the most obvious sense, madness is a female malady because it is experienced by more women than men. The statistical overrepresentation of women among the mentally ill has been well documented by historians and psychologists. By the middle of the nineteenth century, records showed that women had become the majority of patients in public lunatic asylums."[27] Joan Busfield and Andrew Scull have pointed out the fallacy in Showalter's thesis.[28] The "statistical overrepresentation" was caused entirely by the fact that women lived longer than men and therefore outnumbered them in many asylums. Schizophrenia, the single largest contributor to insanity, is well documented to occur both earlier and more severely in men.

There have been very few dissenting views in recent years to such social and economic interpretations of insanity's history. One such dissent was put forth by the senior author in 1980 in *Schizophrenia and Civilization,* which included a preliminary analysis of the nineteenth-century insanity data and concluded: "Throughout the nineteenth century, there was evidence in Europe that insanity (presumably including schizophrenia) was rapidly increasing. Evidence suggests that there was also a dramatic increase in insanity in the United States. Several possible explanations for the late appearance of schizophrenia and its apparent nineteenth-century increase have been offered. The explanation that the late appearance and increase are real phenomena is at least as persuasive as other explanations."[29]

Another dissent from the dominant socioeconomic view was registered by the late Edward Hare, a prominent English psychiatrist who, in 1983, published a paper entitled "Was Insanity on the Increase?" in which he made a strong case for the validity of increasing insanity. He concluded, "there appears to me to be a strong case for thinking that a considerable, perhaps a major, part of the increase in the asylum admission rate was due to a real increase in the incidence of insanity, of a kind not less severe than formerly." The following year, Andrew Scull responded with "Was Insanity Increasing? A Response to Edward Hare." Scull reiterated his previous contention that the broadening of diagnostic criteria for mental illness and the hospitalization of increasingly milder cases were primarily responsible for the rising insanity rates in the nineteenth and early twentieth centuries.[30]

And here the debate has rested.

CHAPTER 14

Possible Causes of Epidemic Insanity

The way society handles its mentally ill has been the subject of scandalized public attack many times. Humane, healing care for the mentally ill . . . remains the great unfinished business of the mental health movement. . . . A large proportion of mental patients at present, as in the past, are not treated in accordance with democratic, humanitarian, scientific, and therapeutic principles. We have substantially failed them on all counts.

—*Final Report of the Joint Commission on Mental Illness and Health*, 1961

We continued in these Hopes for a few Days, But it was but for a few; for the People were no more to be deceived thus; they searcht the Houses, and found that the Plague was really spread every way, and that many died of it every Day.

—Daniel Defoe, *A Journal of the Plague Year*, 1722

The foregoing analysis of insanity rates in England, Ireland, Canada, and the United States suggests that the prevalence of insanity, as a rate per population, increased at least sevenfold between the mid–eighteenth and the mid–twentieth centuries; in Ireland and the United States, the increase appears to have been even greater. If this increase was real, we have argued, then we are now in the midst of an epidemic of insanity, an epidemic so insidious that most people are even unaware of its existence. It is doubtful whether there has ever been any disease in Western history that has affected so many lives, yet been so profoundly misunderstood.

Occasional cases of insanity have always existed, caused by infectious agents, brain trauma, tumors, metabolic and toxic disorders, and other conditions, as detailed in appendix B. These conditions disrupt brain chemistry and may cause delusions, hallucinations, disordered thinking, and mood swings—the symptoms of insanity. At any given time, these known causes of insanity, many of which are transient, cause approximately one case of insanity among every 1,000 adults, or 0.5 cases per 1,000 total population. This is the baseline rate of insanity.

At the end of the sixteenth century, additional cases of insanity began to appear. These were initially few in number but provoked some discussion among the public. The overall prevalence of insanity, however, remained low. Then, in the later years of the eighteenth century, the prevalence of insanity began noticeably to increase. Among the four countries studied, the increase occurred first in England and Ireland, and by the early years of the nineteenth century the term "epidemic insanity" was being heard in both London and Dublin. In the United States and Canada, the increase occurred three or four decades later, and throughout the nineteenth century the slope of increasing insanity in the United States and Canada appears to lag behind that for England and Ireland.

By the second half of the nineteenth century, insanity was increasing rapidly in all four countries, with prevalence rates often doubling over twenty or thirty years. The increase was a cause of major concern for many, and alarm for a few. Others attempted to rationalize the increase as being a statistical artifact, or said that it was caused by immigrants, alcohol, inbreeding, degenerating morals, or other things. A few patriots insisted that insanity simply *could* not be increasing in their country, because it *should* not be increasing.

The existing evidence suggests that insanity continued to increase rapidly in all four countries throughout the nineteenth century and the first half of the twentieth century, uninfluenced by social or economic crises. The Irish Famine, the American Civil War, World

War I, independence for the Irish Republic, the Great Depression, and World War II all appeared to have had no impact on insanity's steady and relentless rise. The only event that slowed this inexorable ascent was the influenza pandemic of 1918, which temporarily decreased the prevalence of insanity by killing large numbers of patients in the asylums.

As the twentieth century progressed, insanity appeared to increase at a decreasing rate. Precisely what happened to insanity's prevalence in the second half of the twentieth century is unclear, however, because patients were deinstitutionalized from asylums to the community, making accurate counts more difficult. Also, remarkably, governments failed to collect the relevant data needed to ascertain the prevalence of insanity. In England and Ireland, existing data suggest that the prevalence of insanity leveled off. In Canada and the United States, there are no such suggestions, and the vague indicators that do exist point in the opposite direction. The presence of multitudes of insane persons living on the streets and filling jails and prisons in the closing years of the twentieth century again raised the question heard throughout the nineteenth century: Where did all these people come from?

As we move into the twenty-first century, two questions demand our attention: Is the epidemic real? If so, what might be causing it?

The Lumber Room Thesis

Almost everyone who has written about insanity in the past half-century has assumed that insanity's increase was not real. Rather, they have subscribed to some variant of the lumber room thesis, initially proposed by Andrew Wynter in 1870: "If we make a convenient lumber room, we all know how speedily it becomes filled up with lumber. The county asylum is the mental lumber room of the surrounding district."[1] Foucault, Szasz, Goffman, Laing, Rothman, Scull, and Porter all have accepted the lumber room thesis, although they have differed somewhat regarding *why* the lumber room became filled.

The lumber room thesis assumes, quite simply, that insane asylums were originally built for social or economic reasons and then, once built, were filled with individuals with varying types of mental illness or troublesome behavior. Andrew Scull stated it as follows: "On the whole it was the existence and expansion of the asylum system which created the increased demand for its own services, rather than the other way around." Trevor Turner similarly claimed that "a Parkinson-like law, namely 'lunatics increase to fill the number of spaces available for them'" was the driving force behind increasing insanity.[2] Michael Foucault's theory of the "great confinement" created asylums; then they were filled with the human dregs of society in order to promote social stability and economic progress. Since the lumber room thesis has dominated discussions about insanity's increase, it bears close examination.

The first problem that becomes apparent with the lumber room thesis is the problem of cause and effect. The thesis states that approximately the same number of insane persons existed two hundred years ago as exist today, and that they lived in the community. Then, in the early nineteenth century, social and/or economic changes occurred (e.g., Rothman's Jacksonian social unrest, Scull's movement to a market economy), which, it is claimed, stimulated authorities to build asylums in which to confine insane persons.

When the historical record is examined, however, it becomes apparent that the original stimulus to building the asylums was the *perceived needs* of insane persons, who appeared to be increasing in number. In Manchester and York, Dublin and Cork, Halifax and St. John's, and Philadelphia and Boston, the principal concern of authorities was the increasing number of insane persons in the almshouses and jails. In many places, in fact, the leadership for building asylums came from those who were most familiar with conditions in the almshouses and jails. It was not merely that the preexisting insane individuals were being perceived differently, as the lumber room thesis posits. Rather, it was that insane individuals *were* different, and there were many more of them.

The lumber room thesis is also inconsistent with the reaction of the general public to the asylums, once built. In London, Philadelphia, and other cities, the newly opened asylums became major attractions for visitors. The public flocked to the asylums, especially on holidays, in order to glimpse insane men and women. If these same insane persons had been living in the community for hundreds of years, as the lumber room thesis contends, the public would have been more familiar with their behavior. The fact that insane persons were regarded by the public as a novelty in the early nineteenth century suggests that they *were* in fact a novelty.

The building of asylums in response to social or economic imperatives, as the lumber room thesis contends, is also not consistent with the intense local resistance to their construction. Kathleen Jones is not correct in implying that in England it was relatively easy to build asylums in the nineteenth century because "building costs were low and land was cheap." Similarly, Gerald Grob is not correct in claiming that in the United States "Dorothea Dix encountered little opposition in persuading state legislatures to appropriate funds for mental hospitals."[3] During the nineteenth century, the cost of building asylums fell primarily upon the shoulders of city, county, and state governments, and local taxpayers did not hesitate to express their opposition to any proposals that would increase their taxes.

In England, in Suffolk there were "concerted local campaigns of petitions and protests" against building an asylum. In Sussex, "there was clearly a highly organized campaign against building a county asylum." In Buckinghamshire "six hundred ratepayers, led by Benjamin Disraeli, renewed their opposition [to an asylum], complaining that they had already been taxed for a new jail and judges' lodging, and were now being asked to underwrite another expensive capital project." In Ireland, in Ulster there were "protests by Derry ratepayers against the new county asylum," and "the County Councils of Leitrim and Sligo refused to supply the funds for carrying out the work [of building an asylum]." In Canada on Prince Edward Island, in Newfoundland, and especially in Nova Scotia there was substantial and prolonged resistance to allocating public funds for building asylums. In the United States, in Connecticut twenty-nine years elapsed between the initial proposal to build an asylum and its opening, while in Massachusetts the delay continued for fifty-five years, from 1763 until 1818. Dorothea Dix encountered major opposition to her asylum-building plans in most of the states and Canadian provinces to which she took her campaign. Economic opposition to the building of more asylums continued into the twentieth century in states like Massachusetts, where in the 1930s "the Department of Mental Diseases absorbed about 25 percent of the state's income."[4] Viewed against this backdrop of widespread and persistent opposition to the building of asylums, the lumber room thesis appears simplistic.

Another assumption of the lumber room thesis is that insane asylums were expressly built to isolate the human flotsam and jetsam of society. For Foucault, this included people unable to work or "integrate with the group." For Goffman, asylums were intended to isolate "various categories of socially troublesome people." For Rothman, asylums came into being to isolate "the deviant and the dependent." And for Scull, asylums were built to provide social control for "the non-able-bodied poor," who were unable to contribute to the emerging market economy.[5]

Analyses of patients entering insane asylums in the nineteenth century, however, provide no support for this thesis. In England, John Walton, in his analysis of admissions to the Lancaster Asylum in the 1840s, reported that the majority of patients had been employed prior to the onset of their illness. He concluded that "most of those who were admitted and remained within its walls were not so much 'inconvenient people,' in Scull's terminology, as impossible people in the eyes of families, neighbors, and authorities. . . . The county asylum provided relief for desperate families rather than an easy option for the uncaring or irresponsible." Leonard Smith also contended that "the early nineteenth-century [English] asylum was not a receptacle for those who were merely deviant, odd, eccentric, or socially unacceptable."[6]

In Ireland, Lindsay Prior, in examining early admissions to the Omagh Asylum, concluded that "there is little evidence . . . that they [admissions] were either physically decrepit or economically useless. . . . The detail gives lie to the notion that asylum inmates were in any way drawn disproportionately from the feeble, infirm, and severely deprived strata of Irish society." Similarly, in Canada it was noted that "no evidence has been found to suggest that . . . the Newfoundland government or public-at-large was a part of any conspiracy merely to hide away misfits and non-conformists." And in the United States, John Chapin reported that 82 percent of asylum admissions in New York State in the 1850s had been self-supporting "previous to the invasion of insanity." In summary, there is no evidence to support the belief that asylums were built to house "various categories of socially troublesome people," and there is much evidence to the contrary. As

Edward Shorter noted in his book *A History of Psychiatry:* "It is astonishing that this interpretation could have achieved such currency as there is virtually no evidence on its behalf."[7]

If the main purpose for building insane asylums in the nineteenth century was to isolate deviant and troublesome individuals, as the lumber room thesis contends, then one might expect the prison population to have similarly increased. In an analysis of such data in the United States, John Sutton showed that between 1880 and 1923 "the number of asylum inmates increased more than sixfold, from around 40,000 . . . to over 263,000," but during this period the number of people in state and federal prisons was unchanged as a rate per population. In Ireland in the late nineteenth century, the prison population declined as the general population declined, but the population of the insane asylums increased rapidly.[8]

Another assumption of the lumber room thesis is that, once the asylums had been built, families readily availed themselves of the opportunity to get rid of troublesome family members. In England, it has been asserted that families "were compelled to send the insane or imbecile members of their families to asylums" because the family members were increasingly working in factories or other venues away from home. In Ireland, it has been claimed that "many took advantage of the comparative ease with which persons could be accepted as insane and admitted to the asylum to rid themselves of relatives and friends who were a burden or a nuisance." And in the United States, it has been said that "asylums reduce people's level of tolerance of deviants. . . . People are no longer willing to put up with lunatic relatives."[9]

In a variation on this theme, Nancy Tomes, in her book *A Generous Confidence: Thomas Story Kirkbride and the Art of Asylum-Building, 1840–1883,* claimed that "the greater emphasis upon the family as an affective and educational unit may have changed popular attitudes toward home care of the insane," reducing "the family's willingness to tolerate lewd, noisy, profane behavior" in an effort to meet "increased expectations of the intimacy and moral uplift of domestic life."[10] Simply translated, this says that foul-mouthed and eccentric Uncle John could no longer stay in the guest room because the family was changing, so he was shipped off to the Pennsylvania Asylum.

Although the contention of decreased stigma and increased acceptability of insane asylums is repeated by virtually every supporter of the lumber room thesis to partially explain why the lumber rooms filled so quickly, there is virtually no evidence to support it. It is true that there was optimism regarding the curability of insanity for a brief period in the middle of the nineteenth century, but this optimism died quickly when it became apparent that the asylum cure rates were being vastly inflated. And it seems doubtful whether the stigma against insane asylums decreased much, if at all, between the early 1800s and the middle 1900s.

An analysis of existing studies of asylums suggests that most families were, in fact, reluctant to send their family members to the asylums. "There is ample evidence from Victorian letters, diaries, and autobiographies that upper and middle-class families regarded the asylum as a place of last resort," said Charlotte MacKenzie in a study of a private English asylum. "The asylum was not resorted to lightly by families and Poor Law authorities. It was the final resource when all else had failed," claimed John Walton in his study of the Lancaster Asylum. "Family members were reluctant to send their relatives to the asylum," added Samuel Thielman in his study of asylums in Virginia and South Carolina. And Gerald Grob, who has probably examined more original data on American asylums than anyone, noted that "relatives began the process of institutionalization as a last resort."[11]

It is also not true that families sent troublesome family members to insane asylums so that the married women in the family could go to work in factories or offices, rather than look after their insane relatives. The women who took those jobs in the nineteenth and early twentieth centuries were almost all single, and most of them stopped working once they married. A national study in the United States in 1900 reported that only 4 percent of all married women worked outside the home. In 1920 the rate was 8 percent, and "as late as 1940 the proportion of white married women who worked outside the home was not greater than 12 percent of the total."[12]

Proponents of the lumber room thesis also write as if it were relatively easy to get troublesome or eccentric individuals admitted to the insane asylums, and that as time went on an increasingly broad diagnostic spectrum of individuals was deemed eligible for asylum placement. As Andrew Scull phrased it, "The asylum provided a convenient and culturally legitimate alternative to coping with 'intolerable' individuals within the family," and over time this led to "an ever-wider practical application of the term mental illness."[13]

Advocates for this view cite individual cases, such as the "two women who were confined in McLean Asylum in the 1820s because they confessed to despising their husbands." They also cite Richard Fox's *So Far Disordered in Mind: Insanity in California, 1870–1930.* Fox, an admirer of Foucault's, analyzed the reason for admission of individuals from San Francisco to the local asylum. He concluded that "two-thirds of all those persons labeled insane exhibited neither a severely disabling disturbance nor violent or destructive tendencies."[14] To arrive at this figure, Fox specifically excluded as a reason for asylum admission such things as public masturbation, "throwing away money or property," delusions of persecution or grandeur, and other behavior that suggests insanity. Indeed, the actual data in Fox's study appear to directly contradict the conclusions he reaches.

Virtually every other study of admissions to insane asylums in the nineteenth century suggests that it was exceedingly difficult to gain admission and that diagnostic categories became narrower, not broader, with the passing years. Given the exceedingly overcrowded conditions of the asylums, it would be very surprising if it had been otherwise.

In England, for example, a diagnostic breakdown of admissions to all public asylums between 1895 and 1898 reported that 98 percent of the patients were diagnosed with mania, melancholia, dementia, or "congenital insanity." Furthermore, studies that have retrospectively diagnosed nineteenth-century English asylum patients using modern diagnostic criteria have uniformly concluded that almost all patients were severely mentally ill. In Ireland, the percentage of asylum admissions diagnosed as "dangerous lunatics" increased from 37 percent in 1854 to 55 percent in 1880 and 68 percent in 1910. In Canada, admissions to the asylum in New Brunswick were legally restricted in 1881 to "lunatics clearly dangerous and violent." Restrictions on admission to other asylums in the Atlantic provinces similarly dictated that only the most severely affected cases got in, such as the young woman who "threatened to cut her father's head off," who was admitted to the Nova Scotia asylum in 1901. In the United States, according to Gerald Grob, "it was clear that the asylum population was composed overwhelmingly of individuals with a diagnosis of severe mental illness"; Grob cites as an example admission statistics from an asylum in Pennsylvania where "between 1916 and 1925 about 90 percent of all first admissions were in the psychotic (or severely mentally ill) category."[15]

It should be added that asylum statistics from all four countries consistently recorded very few "idiots" (individuals with moderate or severe mental retardation) being admitted to insane asylums unless the individual also had symptoms of insanity. As early as 1837, Amariah Brigham in New York decreed that "idiots should be wholly excluded from hospitals for the insane,"[16] and in most places they were. Most such individuals were kept at home or in local almshouses until public institutions specifically for them began opening at the end of the nineteenth century.

Accumulation and Aged Patients

Almost all adherents of the lumber room thesis accept as a corollary that, once the asylums were opened, they became overcrowded because of an accumulation of chronically ill patients as well as an increasing number of aged patients. The term "accumulation" became, in fact, a virtual litany response among nineteenth-century asylum superintendents when they were asked to explain the reasons for their overcrowded asylums. Even well into the twentieth century, superintendents such as Winfred Overholser at St. Elizabeths Hospital in Washington, D.C, claimed that "the increase in mental hospital population, about which there has been so much popular clamor, is due . . . to the piling-up of long-residence patients" and an increasing length-of-stay of patients.[17]

Accumulation as an explanation for increasing insanity has three parts: a decrease in the cure and discharge rates, a decrease in the death rate of asylum patients, and an increase in the number of aged patients.

Regarding the first, there is some evidence that the cure rate and discharge rate of insane patients from the asylums decreased as the nineteenth century progressed. Reports of decreasing cure rates in several asylums in England were cited in 1890 as proving that "the form of insanity was worse" than it had been earlier in the century. In Ireland the asylum discharge rate decreased from approximately 17 percent per year in 1851 to 9 percent per year in 1901. In Canada the discharge rate at the Nova Scotia Asylum decreased from 17.2 percent per year in 1859–1863 to 11.7 percent per year in 1884–1888. And in the United States, Pliny Earle's 1876 analysis of recovery rates reported that recoveries had been "constantly diminishing during a period of from twenty to fifty years."[18] Thus, there are suggestions that insanity may have become a more severe, and thus more chronic, disease during the nineteenth century; if so, this would help explain the accumulation of patients in the asylums.

Advocates of the lumber room thesis also claim that accumulation of patients in the nineteenth century was caused by falling mortality rates among asylum patients so that they survived longer and thereby filled the wards. The mortality rates in most asylums were, in fact, extraordinarily high by today's standards; at Hanwell Asylum in London in the 1840s, 18 percent of admissions died within the first one and one-half years after entering the hospital.[19] Influenza, cholera, typhus, and tuberculosis spread rapidly among the overcrowded patients, killing as many as one-third of them during some epidemics.

Evidence to support decreasing asylum mortality rates in the nineteenth century is inconsistent. In England there appears to have been a slight decrease, from 10.1 percent annual deaths for 1873–1877 to 9.5 percent for 1893–1897. Similarly, in Ireland the annual asylum mortality rate decreased from 6.8 percent in the mid–nineteenth century to 6.3 percent at the end of the century. In Canada during the same period, the annual mortality rate fell from 13 percent to 11 percent in New Brunswick's asylum, remained unchanged in Nova Scotia, and increased from 7 percent to 9 percent in Newfoundland.[20] Similarly, in the United States annual mortality rates varied widely from state to state and from year to year, but there is no evidence to support any significant decrease in mortality rates until the twentieth century. Thus, if decreasing mortality rates contributed at all to the increase in asylum patients in the nineteenth century, that contribution was relatively minimal.

An alternative way to view mortality rates is the possibility that confining insane persons to asylums during the nineteenth and early twentieth centuries may actually have *decreased* the prevalence of insanity. In 1930 Benjamin Malzberg calculated that the mortality rate for persons ages fifteen to thirty-nine admitted to New York State asylums was more than ten times the mortality rate for the same age groups in the general population.[21] What is not known is how the mortality rate of insane persons admitted to asylums compared with the rate for insane persons not admitted. Given the devastating epidemics that swept through the asylums and the consequent high mortality rates of the confined, it is possible that the increasing institutionalization of insane persons in the nineteenth and early twentieth centuries actually decreased the overall prevalence of insanity by killing more insane individuals than would have died had they remained living in the community.

The third aspect of accumulation as an explanation for the overcrowding of insane asylums is that asylums were required to provide care for an increasing number of aged patients. This is true for the United States after approximately 1900 but does not explain increases in insanity before that time.

In the nineteenth century, there were relatively few people aged sixty and over, and elderly persons who developed senile dementia (which would now be labeled Alzheimer's disease or vascular dementia), with or without insanity, were cared for at home or sent to almshouses rather than to insane asylums. In 1860, for example, only 4.3 percent of the general population was aged sixty or over, and by 1900, the proportion had increased to only 6.4 percent. Elderly patients constituted a very small percentage of admissions to insane asylums, though by 1890 they constituted 40 percent of the almshouse population in Massachusetts.[22]

That situation changed markedly following passage of the State Care Act in 1890 in New York, followed by similar legislation in other states.[23] This act transferred the fiscal onus of supporting insane persons from counties to the state. By rediagnosing senile individuals as insane, counties could transfer them from almshouses, where the county was paying the costs, to state hospitals, where the state was fiscally responsible. The result was a massive transinstitutionalization of senile individuals from almshouses to state hospitals, a transfer that continued until the 1960s, when federal Medicare and Medicaid funding made it fiscally advantageous for states to transinstitutionalize these senile individuals once again, this time from state hospitals to nursing homes.

The transfer of fiscal responsibility for senile individuals from the counties to the state was, according to Gerald Grob, "the conversion of the mental hospital into a surrogate home for elderly and other kinds of chronic cases." Once admitted, the senile patients did not leave the hospitals until they died, so the number of long-stay patients increased rapidly. In 1870 only 14 percent of the patients at Worcester State Hospital had been there five years or longer. By 1904 the proportion had risen to 39 percent, and by 1923 to 54 percent.[24] Similar increases occurred in most other states and account for a substantial percentage of the continuing increase in hospitalized insanity in the United States after 1900.

In summary, then, the lumber room thesis does not appear to adequately explain the rise of insanity in England, Ireland, Canada, or the United States in the nineteenth century. There are suggestions that insanity itself might have become more severe, leading to some accumulation of patients. After 1900, there was a large influx of aged individuals into the asylums in the United States, accounting for some of the increasing prevalence rates of insanity in the twentieth century. But for the vast majority of the increasing number of insane persons from the beginning of the nineteenth century onward, there is no obvious explanation except for one: insanity was truly increasing.

Finally, it should be noted that the lumber room thesis implicitly assumes that nineteenth-century attempts to enumerate insane persons were virtually worthless. It means, for example, that the 1843 census of all insane persons in England, which included the occupants of all public and private asylums, workhouses, and private dwellings and which counted 14,792 insane persons (0.93 per 1,000), failed to count an additional 48,370 insane persons, based on the rate of insanity recorded in 1915 (3.98 per 1,000). It means that the 1851 census in Ireland, which included all insane persons in asylums, almshouses, and jails and which counted 5,345 insane persons (0.82 per 1,000), failed to count an additional 43,295 insane persons, based on the rate of institutionalized insanity in 1956 (7.49 per 1,000). It means that the 1880 census in the United States, which identified insane persons in every asylum, almshouse, jail, and prison and which counted 38,047 institutionalized insane persons (0.76 per 1,000), failed to count an additional 129,360 insane persons, based on the rate of hospitalized insanity in 1955 (3.38 per 1,000). To assume such gross failures for the efforts of our predecessors strains credulity.

Is It Genetic?

Given the limitations of the lumber room thesis, it seems possible that the increase in insanity in the nineteenth and early twentieth centuries was real. And for those who believed that this was so, the most commonly cited cause was consanguineous marriages and other genetic causes. Genetic theories of insanity have waxed and waned for over two hundred years and continue to be prominent today.

It is now clearly established that genetic mechanisms play some role in the cause of insanity. Both schizophrenia and manic-depressive illness, the major forms of insanity, tend to run in families, with the genetic influence being greater for manic-depressive illness than for schizophrenia. Among unselected samples of identical twins, for example, when one twin becomes sick with schizophrenia, the second twin will become sick approximately one-third of the time, but for manic-depressive illness, the second will become sick approximately two-thirds of the time.[25]

To acknowledge that there is a genetic component to schizophrenia and manic-depressive illness is not, however, to say that these are genetic diseases. Most human diseases, including many cancers, have a genetic aspect insofar as people's genes make them more or less predisposed to get the disease if they are exposed to that disease's specific causative agent. Thus, people who smoke heavily may or may not get lung cancer, depending on their genetic predisposition. Conversely, people may carry genes predisposing them to many different diseases, but if they are never exposed to the specific causative agents, they are unlikely to get those diseases.

It is widely accepted that schizophrenia and manic-depressive illness have genetic predispositions, but attempts to prove that they are genetic diseases have so far failed. Inbreeding associated with consanguineous marriages does not appear to increase the prevalence of schizophrenia as shown by studies in Canada, Norway, Saudi Arabia, and the Sudan. Furthermore, an international study of human inbreeding rates identified Japan, Brazil, India, and Israel as having the highest rates of inbreeding, but those countries do not have unusually high rates of schizophrenia or manic-depressive illness.[26]

The most serious criticism of genetic theories of schizophrenia and manic-depressive illness, however, is what Edward Hare labeled "the persistence problem."[27] From the middle of the nineteenth century until the middle of the twentieth century, most individuals with schizophrenia and manic-depressive illness were confined to asylums for the majority of their reproductive years. Their rate of procreation was extraordinarily low, and so the transmission of their genes was infrequent. Yet during these same years, the prevalence of schizophrenia and manic-depressive illness increased rapidly. In short, the less frequently people with insanity reproduced, the more frequently cases of insanity appeared. One can invoke theoretical evolutionary advantages for unaffected carriers of the disease, or posit some recurrent mutation to explain this apparent genetic conundrum, but both seem unlikely. In fact, there is no known genetic disease that is a model for schizophrenia and manic-depressive illness, and the epidemic of insanity that has occurred over the past two centuries is a strong argument against these diseases being primarily genetic in origin.

The Industrial Revolution and Urbanization

If genes cannot explain the increase of insanity, then where should we look? In reviewing the rise of insanity, one of the most striking aspects is its temporal correlation with the industrial revolution. This revolution began in England in the 1760s with the invention of the spinning jenny and the steam engine and with new methods for using coal to make iron. Using improved roads, canals, and, later, railroads, England was gradually transformed from a village-centered, agrarian society to an urban-centered, industrial society. The industrial revolution spread throughout England, to other parts of Europe, including Ireland, and later to the United States and Canada. The rise of insanity in the nineteenth century closely paralleled the rise of the urban, industrialized society.

The correlation of insanity's rise with advancing civilization was noted from the beginning of the epidemic. In 1782 Thomas Arnold attributed England's comparatively high rate of insanity to "an excess of wealth and luxury." In 1816 David Uwins associated England's increase in "nervous and mental affections" with civilization: "In proportion as man emerges from his primaeval state, do the Furies of disease advance upon him and would seem to scourge him back into the paths of nature and simplicity." Ten years later, Sir Alexander Morison stated authoritatively that "the number of insane increases with civilization."[28] The linking of insanity with industrialization, urbanization, or other aspects of civilization continued to be regularly suggested by observers throughout the nineteenth and twentieth centuries.

The correlation of increasing insanity with increasing urbanization, as discussed in chapter 5, is of special interest, since recent studies have definitively established that being born in, or raised in, an urban area significantly increases one's risk of being diagnosed in adulthood with insanity in general and schizophrenia in particular. The urban risk factor, as it is called, was observed as early as 1848 by Dorothea Dix. In 1903 William A. White, utilizing American census data, noted "an almost exact parallel" between the prevalence of insanity and "the greatest density of population."[29]

Longitudinal comparisons of increasing insanity with increasing urbanization and industrialization fit reasonably well for England and the United States, less well for the Atlantic provinces of Canada, and not well at all for Ireland, which was neither industrialized nor urbanized. In 1841, only 20 percent of Ireland's population lived in communities containing twenty or more homes, and urbanization thereafter proceeded very slowly. The lack of correlation between urbanization and rising insanity was noted by Lindsay Prior: "When applied to the sparsely populated lake lands of Fermanagh or to the thinly inhabited townlands of Tyrone, such broad brush hypotheses can, of course, seem a little unconvincing."[30]

On the other hand, it is of interest that Irish immigrants to England, Canada, and the United States had a high prevalence of insanity, since these immigrants settled disproportionately in urban areas. It is a pattern that perhaps foreshadowed the high prevalence of insanity being presently observed among Afro-Caribbean immigrants, who also have settled disproportionately in urban areas in England. If we could understand such relationships, we would then understand more about the causes of insanity.

The Stockings Model of Insanity

What are the concomitants of industrialization and urbanization that might increase one's risk of developing insanity? Stress comes immediately to mind and has been regularly cited by observers for two centuries. For example, in 1828 Sir Andrew Halliday, speculating on why insanity was becoming more prevalent in England, cited an "over exertion of the mind, in overworking its instruments so as to weaken them." A century and a half later, H.B.M. Murphy, speculating on the causes of schizophrenia, said much the same thing: "The feature of civilization most likely to be harmful [for causing schizophrenia] could be its complexity. [The] idea of vulnerable minds being overwhelmed by the extra work needed to handle that complexity remains unrefuted, although also unproven."[31]

Stress theories are attractive for their simplicity but are without supporting evidence, despite many attempts to provide them. There is not a single controlled study showing that stress *causes* any form of insanity, although once a person develops insanity, stress can make the illness worse. One of the strongest arguments against stress as a causative factor in insanity is the absence of any additional increase in insanity during wars or major social upheavals, such as the Great Depression. This was also illustrated in London during World War II, when a committee of psychiatrists organized "a nation-wide mental health service" to handle the anticipated "three to four million acute psychiatric cases" expected to occur due to stress with the onset of the war. No increased cases of severe psychiatric disorders were observed, much to the psychiatrists' surprise.[32]

Besides stress, what other concomitants of industrialization and urbanization might increase one's risk for developing insanity? Industrialization and urbanization bring about many changes in habits, customs, and lifestyles that may be relevant, including changed diets, exposure to toxins, changes in medical care, and exposure to infectious agents. The purpose of the remainder of this chapter is not to convince the reader that any one of these is necessarily a cause of insanity but merely to encourage a spirit of inquiry. Epidemic insanity remains one of the great enigmas of contemporary medicine and demands novel approaches in thinking about its causes.

> 1. *Diet.* Diets have changed markedly during the industrialization
>   and urbanization of Western society. For example, several
>   researchers have theorized that wheat gluten may cause
>   schizophrenia and have shown that its dietary distribution was

compatible with epidemiological aspects of this disease. Another example was the attempt of Amiel Christie to link the dietary intake of potatoes to schizophrenia, theorizing that glycoalkaloid in potatoes may cause damage to the developing nervous system. Furthermore, food intake patterns are dependent on weather conditions, and Christine Miller published a study linking rainfall to the distribution of schizophrenia in two countries.[33]

2. *Alcohol.* The increased availability of commercially made alcoholic beverages and the rise of insanity closely paralleled one another. In England, for example, the consumption of alcohol increased 57 percent between 1801 and 1901. In America it rose 44 percent between 1845 and 1910. It is known that chronic alcohol intake can damage the brain, producing memory loss and a chronic form of insanity. However, chronic alcoholism was cited as the cause of insanity in 10 percent or fewer of asylum admissions in all four countries. Furthermore, this percentage did not appear to increase over time or to vary during periods of less alcohol availability, such as Prohibition.[34]

3. *Toxins.* Organophosphate preparations such as are used in insecticides are known to be toxic to the central nervous system. Attempts have been made to link such toxicity to schizophrenia but so far without success. Another example of research involving toxins was Harold Foster's attempt to link latex allergy, as found in rubber products, to the rise of schizophrenia.[35]

4. *Medical care.* John Cooper, Norman Sartorius, Richard Warner, and other researchers have suggested that the rise of schizophrenia was related to improved obstetrical care; weaker infants were saved and were then more susceptible to developing the disease. Warner has also claimed that this fact explains why insanity rose initially in the higher socioeconomic classes, which would have benefited first from improved medical care, and only later in the lower socioeconomic classes.[36]

5. *Infectious agents.* Several infectious disease hypotheses have been suggested that may be relevant to the rise of insanity.

   a. *The syphilis model:* Syphilis is thought to have been widespread in Europe from the early sixteenth century, yet the brain form of syphilis, known as paresis, was not seen until the end of the eighteenth century. During the latter years of the nineteenth century and the early years of the twentieth century, paresis was responsible for 10 percent or more of asylum admissions, although the rate in Ireland was much lower. It has been theorized that paresis was not seen in earlier years because smallpox and other diseases that cause high fevers protected individuals from paresis by killing the causative spirochete before it caused damage to the brain. Once smallpox vaccinations were introduced in the early nineteenth century, fewer people got smallpox, thereby allowing the spirochete to survive and damage the brain. If this theory is correct, then paresis is a disease of civilization.[37] It therefore presents a model by which an infectious agent could be linked to both insanity and civilization.

b. *The polio model.* Polio is an innocuous infection when contracted by small children, and thereafter they have immunity. The virus is widespread, and under poor sanitary conditions most small children become infected. However, when polio affects older children who have not previously been exposed to it, it may cause paralytic disease. Paralytic polio is thus a disease associated with improved sanitary conditions and is a disease of civilization. The paralytic form of polio was first observed in the late eighteenth century, and the first epidemic was recorded in 1840.[38] The rise of paralytic polio was directly related to improved water supply and sewerage systems in the nineteenth and twentieth centuries and parallels closely the rise of insanity.

c. *The vaccination model.* The prevention of smallpox by inoculating vaccinia virus into the skin of individuals was introduced in 1798 and spread throughout the world. The vaccinia virus used for vaccinations was known to have an affinity for nervous tissue and occasionally to infect the brain. The rise of vaccinations and the rise of insanity closely paralleled each other. In 1855 in the British House of Commons, there was even testimony against making vaccination compulsory; the reason given was a fear that vaccination might be responsible for the rising insanity.

d. *The pet cat model.* Industrialization and urbanization brought about changes in the relationship between humans and some animals. Contact with wild animals and farm animals became less common, but exposure to pets became more common. For example, keeping cats as pets was rare prior to the middle of the eighteenth century but became very popular in the late nineteenth century. The rise of cats as pets, in fact, closely parallels the rise of insanity. Cats are also known to carry many infectious agents that can be transmitted to humans. Two controlled studies have reported that individuals who have schizophrenia and manic-depressive illness have had a greater exposure to cats in childhood compared to matched control subjects without those diseases.[39]

These are examples of how the rise of insanity could be linked to industrialization and urbanization. It is, of course, possible to find correlations between the rise of insanity and an infinite variety of factors. The industrial revolution and urbanization brought many changes, even including such things as the wearing of stockings: "Two centuries ago, not one person in a thousand wore stockings; one century ago, not one person in five hundred wore them; now, not one person in a thousand is without them."[40] The challenge, therefore, is not only to identify correlations but also to prove that they have some causal connection to insanity. If we can do so, we might finally bring to an end this epidemic of insanity, the invisible plague:

> No more war, no more plague, only the dazed silence that follows the ceasing of the heavy guns; noiseless houses with the shades drawn, empty streets, the dead cold light of tomorrow. Now there would be time for everything.[41]

APPENDIX A

What Is Insanity?

The term "insanity," from the Latin *insanus,* unsound in mind, was first used in the early sixteenth century. Until the early twentieth century, insanity was used interchangeably with "madness" and "lunacy" to designate the affliction suffered by individuals who had delusions, hallucinations, disordered thinking, bizarre behavior, excess mood swings, or some combination thereof. For example, Thomas Arnold, in his 1782 *Observations on the Nature, Kinds, Causes, and Prevention of Insanity,* indicated that he was using insanity, madness, and lunacy "as synonymous terms." Similarly, German Berrios, whose *History of Mental Symptoms* is the definitive study in this area, noted that "at the beginning of the 19th century 'insanity' had a clinical, and a legal, meaning and was almost coterminous with madness and named conditions later known as 'psychosis.'"[1]

In the twentieth century, insanity, madness, and lunacy were replaced by the term "psychosis." Based upon knowledge then available, the psychoses were then divided into those said to be "organic," in which a specific cause was known (e.g., syphilis, brain tumor), and those said to be "functional," in which a specific cause was not known. Much effort during the century subsequently went into dividing and subdividing the functional psychoses on the basis of symptoms, with the primary division being into schizophrenia and manic-depressive illness, later renamed bipolar disorder. The introduction of neuroimaging and other techniques for studying the brain in recent years has abolished the traditional dichotomy between organic and functional psychoses and has also cast doubt on whether schizophrenia and bipolar disorder are completely separate diseases rather than being the two ends of a psychosis spectrum. In view of such diagnostic uncertainties about the subtypes of insanity, it seems reasonable to use the term "insanity" to designate all types of psychoses, as was done for most of the historical period under consideration in this book.

Insanity can be defined by what it does not include as well as by what it does. It does not include individuals afflicted only with mental retardation, who have been referred to in history as idiots, natural fools, or born fools. The distinction between insanity and idiocy was defined as early as the thirteenth century in *Prerogativa Regis* and was legally important because idiots could not inherit land, whereas insane persons ("non compos mentis") could, although the land was held for them in a conservatorship until "they come to right mind." Idiocy was congenital, existing since birth or early childhood, whereas insanity afflicted a person "who hath had understanding, but by disease, grief or other accident hath lost the use of his reason."[2]

In early censuses of mentally disordered persons, insane persons and idiots were sometimes combined. In the United States, for example, "insane and idiotic" was a single category in the 1840 census, but the two were separate categories in the 1850 census. In England in the 1871 census, "imbecile or idiot" was a separate category from "lunatic," and enumerators were further instructed to write "from birth" if the person was so afflicted.[3] This additional designation was needed because the terms "idiot" and "imbecile" were also occasionally used for individuals who were in the latter, chronic stages of psychosis.

Very few mentally retarded individuals were admitted to insane asylums unless they also had a secondary diagnosis of insanity. Until the early years of the twentieth century, most individuals with mental retardation either remained at home or, if severely retarded or troublesome, were placed in local workhouses. Since local authorities were responsible for the cost of their care, it was much less expensive to keep the person in a workhouse than in an insane asylum. In the 1880 census of mentally disabled individuals in the United States, fewer than 3 percent of all enumerated "idiots" were in institutions. The first American custodial institution for individuals with mental retardation opened in New York State in 1878; such institutions proliferated after the turn of the century, and by 1923 almost 23,000 individuals with mental retardation were so institutionalized.[4]

The term "insanity" also does not include individuals with nonpsychotic conditions, which in the twentieth century were labeled neuroses or personality disorders. It should be noted that this modern usage of the term "neuroses" differs from its earlier usage; prior to the nineteenth century, the term was used generically to indicate almost all psychiatric and neurological conditions.[5] The distinction between insanity and other "nervous disorders" was relatively clearly demarcated until the twentieth century when, influenced by psychoanalytic theory, insanity came to be viewed by some people as one end of a mental health–mental illness continuum.

Examples of such "nervous disorders" as hysteria, hypochondriasis, and minor depression can be found throughout history, but such individuals were not regarded as insane unless they also had delusions, hallucinations, or other symptoms of insanity. Even Samuel Johnson, the English eighteenth-century critic who apparently had severe obsessive-compulsive disorder, was not regarded as insane by his colleagues despite his strange compulsive behaviors.

In summary, the concept of insanity has changed little for at least five hundred years and is equivalent to the contemporary term "psychosis." It does not include individuals who have only mental retardation or individuals with "nervous disorders," which in modern times have been called neuroses and personality disorders. It was assumed in past centuries that there were subtypes of insanity, just as it is now assumed that there are subtypes of psychosis. Most professional arguments have been, and continue to be, concerned with subdividing psychosis, whereas the boundaries of insanity/psychosis itself appear to be reasonably well established.

Two subtypes of insanity that were used in the past have given rise to confusion. The term "moral insanity" became popular in the nineteenth century, especially in England. Some psychiatric historians have alleged that the term referred to what would now be called psychopathic or sociopathic personality disorders. German Berrios has strongly disputed this, saying that the term was introduced to refer to forms of insanity in which delusions were not present.[6]

The other subtype of insanity that has given rise to confusion is "partial insanity," which was used in the early nineteenth century. According to Berrios, the term was used for cases of intermittent insanity (e.g., with remissions and relapses) and for cases in which the person's insanity consisted only of delusions, usually in a single sphere, with the remainder of the person's thought processes being preserved. Such individuals were thought to have "madness affecting one region of the psyche"[7] and in current parlance would be categorized as having a delusional disorder or paranoid schizophrenia.

The single largest distinction between the use of "psychosis" in the twentieth century and "insanity" in the preceding four centuries is that traditional insanity included neurological disorders in which psychotic symptoms were present. Many neurological disorders may be accompanied by delusions, hallucinations, mania, or disordered behavior. In the past, if the person also had a fever, the condition was called "delirium" or "frenzy" and was not considered to be true insanity.[8] In earlier centuries, when acute infectious diseases were much more common in Western countries and were a frequent cause of death, delirium was a well-known condition. However, if a fever was not present, then the condition was considered to be a form of true insanity. Thus, many cases of encephalitis, brain syphilis, brain tumors, neurointoxications, and the other conditions cited in appendix B were categorized as insanity prior to the twentieth century if a fever was not present. As the medical basis for each of these conditions became known, the condition was removed from the category of insanity and reclassified as a medical or neurological condition. Indeed, it seems increasingly clear that the present category of psychosis merely consists of those conditions for which the medical basis is not yet understood.

For the purposes of comparing the prevalence of insanity over time, this means that insanity in the eighteenth and nineteenth centuries included some individuals who would today be assigned to internists and neurologists. The category of insanity in 1850 was a little broader than the category of functional psychosis in 1950. This difference, although modest, would tend to minimize any real increase in insanity that took place during that time, since more types of insanity were included in 1850 than were included in 1950.

The current definition of insanity, therefore, includes all individuals who are presently categorized as having various forms of psychosis. This includes the various subtypes of schizophrenia, schizoaffective disorder, manic-depressive illness (bipolar disorder), delusional disorder, and major depressive disorder with psychotic features. The only exceptions to this are those cases of manic-depressive illness that do not have psychotic features; for example, mood swings only, without delusions or hallucinations, might not have been classified as insanity in the past. On the other hand, many cases of psychosis with mental retardation and cases in which psychotic symptoms accompany medical and neurological conditions (e.g., epilepsy with psychosis) were often included under insanity in the past but are not included in contemporary studies of the prevalence of psychosis.

Thus, insanity as an entity has been reasonably stable over time and, allowing for the exceptions discussed above, its prevalence can be compared over time. However, when one attempts to compare specific *subtypes* of insanity over time, major problems are encountered. Berrios and other writers on the history of insanity have demonstrated convincingly how terms such as "mania," "melancholia," and "dementia" have changed in meaning in recent centuries. Mania, for example, was originally a type of insanity characterized by excitement, aggression, rage, and lack of control but had no overtones of elation or grandiosity. Melancholia indicated an excess of black bile and was a type of insanity characterized by relatively few delusions, lethargy, and suspicion but did not include sadness until later. Dementia at one time simply indicated longstanding insanity affecting individuals of any age and was thought to be reversible sometimes; it only later acquired cognitive dysfunction as its main characteristic.[9] Because of such changes in terminology, it is virtually impossible to compare subtypes of insanity over time, or even in different countries in the same time period.

The other striking observation one notes when looking at insanity in past centuries is how unsatisfactory all attempts have been to subclassify it. Arguments have been endless regarding whether insanity should be classified by symptom clusters, the relationship of symptom clusters to each other (e.g., mania and melancholia), whether the symptom clusters are discrete entities or part of a continuum, the acuteness or chronicity of symptoms, the course of the illness, the suspected etiology, or the age of onset. German Berrios, in *The History of Mental Symptoms,* documents these arguments and leaves one with the impression that psychiatric nosologists in the 1990s would have felt very much at home in the 1890s, or even the 1790s. The current diagnostic schema, as outlined in the American DSM IV and the European ICD-10, are merely the most recent iterations of attempts to subclassify insanity that have gone on for almost three hundred years.

Behind the many masks of insanity's subtypes, however, insanity itself remains, continuously devastating lives, year after year. By understanding its history, we may enhance our chances of finally unmasking it.

APPENDIX B

The Baseline Rate of Insanity

If the diseases known as schizophrenia and manic-depressive illness did not exist, how many cases of insanity would still be found in the community? The answer to this question establishes the baseline rate of insanity and provides a mark against which to measure the prevalence of insanity at different time periods. The total amount of insanity at any given time is the baseline rate plus the rate of schizophrenia and manic-depressive illness.

A variety of medical conditions sometimes cause delusions, hallucinations, mania, or other symptoms of insanity, and such cases have been described since the time of Hippocrates. Even today, despite modern diagnostic techniques, patients are occasionally admitted to psychiatric wards with diagnoses of schizophrenia or manic-depressive illness, only to find later that their psychiatric symptoms were caused by viral encephalitis, a brain tumor, cerebral syphilis, or another disease. Such diagnostic errors were more frequent in the past, when techniques for diagnosis were less sophisticated.

The following are medical conditions that, at least occasionally, produce symptoms of insanity. Several good reviews of this subject have been published.[1]

1. *Infectious diseases.* As noted in Appendix A, symptoms of insanity sometimes occur as part of the delirium that may accompany virtually any infectious disease, usually in conjunction with a high fever. In cases caused by infection, usually the onset of insanity is sudden and the duration brief.

   In 1904 Dr. William Ireland published a summary of such cases under the title "On Insanity after Acute and Chronic Infectious Diseases." He noted that "typhoid fever appears to head the list as a cause of insanity" but also cited pneumonia, malaria, smallpox, measles, diphtheria, tuberculosis, whooping cough, mumps, cholera, dysentery, leprosy, and gonorrhea. He said that "insanity following infection is generally of short duration" and added that "there are no characteristic symptoms to distinguish insanity following infectious diseases from other forms."[2]

Infectious agents that are known to occasionally cause symptoms of insanity include bacteria (e.g., streptococcus, meningococcus, tubercle bacillus), spirochetes (e.g., syphilis), viruses (e.g., herpes simplex, herpes zoster, Epstein-Barr virus, measles, rubella, mumps, vaccinia, polio, human immunodeficiency virus, influenza), protozoa (e.g., trypanosomiasis, toxoplasmosis), and helminthes (e.g., cysticercosis). Unidentified infectious agents can also cause symptoms of insanity, the most prominent example being the unknown organism that caused the epidemic of encephalitis lethargica in the 1920s.

Cerebral syphilis, in the form of paresis, was in the past an especially important cause of insanity. For example, in the United States in the 1930s, 9 percent of all first admissions to state psychiatric hospitals were diagnosed with paresis. The equivalent figure for English hospitals from 1898 to 1902 was 6 percent.[3]

2. *Alcohol and drug intoxication.* Alcohol is known to cause symptoms of insanity by intoxication delirium, alcohol-induced psychotic or mood disorder, withdrawal (delirium tremens), or alcohol-induced dementia. Except for the last, this insanity is transient and such cases have constituted a very small percentage of individuals in psychiatric hospitals.

Similarly, many prescription medications as well as many illegal drugs produce transient symptoms of insanity. Prescribed medications are now one of the most common causes of psychotic symptoms in the elderly population. In the nineteenth century, excessive doses of bromides were common causes of delirium, delusions, and hallucinations. And the ability of drugs such as LSD, PCP, cocaine, mescaline, amphetamine, and steroids to produce symptoms of insanity is well known to contemporary physicians, as were the effects of opium to physicians in the past.

3. *Neurological diseases.* Of all neurological conditions, temporal lobe epilepsy is probably the most common cause of insanity, with one study reporting symptoms of schizophrenia in 17 percent of cases of this form of epilepsy. Severe head injuries are another frequent cause; a long-term follow-up of men who sustained severe head injuries in the Russo-Finnish War reported that 5 percent of them developed psychotic symptoms.[4] Other neurological conditions that sometimes produce symptoms of insanity include cerebrovascular accidents (strokes), brain tumors (either primary or secondary spread from other sites), Alzheimer's disease, multiple sclerosis,

amyotrophic lateral sclerosis, motor neuron disease, Friedreich's ataxia, Schilder's disease, Sydenham's chorea (rheumatic encephalitis), normal pressure hydrocephalus, and narcolepsy.

4. *Metabolic and toxic disorders.* A variety of metabolic and toxic conditions occasionally cause symptoms of insanity. Liver failure, a consequence of hepatitis or alcoholism, can produce severe psychiatric symptoms (hepatic encephalopathy). Severe nutritional deficiencies of thiamine (vitamin B1), nicotinic acid, and vitamin B12 produce beriberi, pellagra, and megaloblastic (pernicious) anemia. The symptoms of beriberi include delirium; pellagra often includes delirium, dementia, mania, hallucinations, or catatonia; and pernicious anemia can include delirium, dementia, delusions, or hallucinations (sometimes referred to as "megaloblastic madness").

Many toxins also produce symptoms of insanity. The most widely known example is mercury, used in making felt hats and enshrined by Lewis Carroll as "the Mad Hatter." Poisoning by carbon disulfide, which is used in rayon and rubber manufacturing, produces outbursts of rage as well as auditory and visual hallucinations; many such cases were reported in nineteenth-century France. Symptoms of insanity may also be induced by toxic concentrations of manganese (used in the manufacture of batteries and steel), arsenic (used in the glass and fur industries), lead (found in paints and lead pipes), and pesticides containing thallium or organophosphorus compounds.

5. *Genetic disorders.* Genetic disorders that produce symptoms of insanity are rare. The most common is Huntington's disease, which has an incidence of 4–8 per 100,000 population in North America and Europe. One study reported that 23 percent of cases have delusions or hallucinations.[5] Acute intermittent porphyria, phenylketonuria, homocysteinuria, Wilson's disease (hepato-lenticular degeneration), metachromatic leukodystrophy, and Turner's syndrome are other genetic disorders that occasionally exhibit symptoms of insanity.

6. *Endocrine disorders.* The association of thyroid malfunction with psychiatric symptoms is well known, but how often this occurs is less clearly defined. Severe hypofunction of the thyroid sometimes produces delusions and hallucinations (called "myxedema madness"), while severe hyperfunction of the thyroid may produce mania. Similarly, severe hypo- or hyperfunction of the parathyroid or adrenal glands occasionally produces symptoms of insanity.

7. *Other diseases.* Systemic lupus erythematosus, a chronic inflammatory disease of connective tissue, has an incidence of approximately 1 per 1,000 population. Studies of lupus patients have reported that at least 10 percent of them develop hallucinations as a

symptom of their disease; an additional subgroup develops hallucinations as a side effect of their steroid medication.[6] Sarcoidosis is another multiorgan chronic inflammatory disease of unknown origin that occasionally causes psychotic symptoms.

Given this list of conditions that may cause symptoms of insanity, what would the prevalence of such insanity be if schizophrenia and manic-depressive illness did not exist? Such a prevalence would be the baseline rate of insanity.

Estimates of the baseline rate of insanity will vary by both time and place, depending on the prevalence of the specific causes listed above. The prevalence of various infectious diseases, the availability of alcohol and drugs, the prevalence of the various neurological conditions in specific populations, the availability and adulteration of food, and exposure to industrial toxins vary widely in different places and at different times in history. The baseline rate of insanity will also vary demographically, depending on the age distribution of the population. In a population with a high percentage of children, for example, the baseline rate of insanity will be lower than in a population with the opposite age distribution, since many causes of baseline insanity selectively affect adults.

Can we estimate the baseline rate of insanity in seventeenth-century England, Ireland, Canada, and the United States? It is known that infectious diseases were common at that time. Epidemics of plague continued periodically to sweep over Europe, killing 70,000 Londoners in 1665 alone. Other infectious diseases were introduced to England by East India Company crews sent out to explore the Caribbean, India, and the Pacific. Additional evidence suggesting that infectious diseases were common causes of insanity in the seventeenth century was the fact that insanity was popularly associated with death and the fact that "lunacy was regarded as a temporary state and the law decreed that when the madman recovered he should have restored to him all of his property, save the amount the guardians expended for his care."[7]

Syphilis is a type of infection of special interest since it is known that its paretic form often causes insanity. When syphilis first appeared in Europe at the beginning of the sixteenth century, it was known as the "Great Pox," had a high mortality rate, and thus few of those infected would have proceeded to the paretic stage. By the seventeenth century, it had become a milder disease and, like other venereal diseases, was presumably common since official standards of morality were not high; King Charles II, who reigned in England from 1660 to 1685, had thirteen known mistresses and fourteen illegitimate offspring. Paresis, therefore, presumably contributed to the baseline rate of insanity in the seventeenth century, although such cases were time-limited since the infection caused death within a short period of time.

It is also known that some cases of seventeenth-century insanity were caused by alcohol abuse. For example, George Trosse experienced delusions and hallucinations as a young man following periods of alcohol abuse; he was confined in a private asylum, recovered, became a well-known minister, and lived to age eighty-two. Other cases of insanity were caused by neurological conditions. For example, Christoph Haizmann, a German painter, became insane in 1677 following a series of "unnatural convulsions," and Felix Plater, a Swiss physician, described a case of insanity in 1656 subsequently shown to have been caused by a brain tumor.[8] One would also expect to have seen cases of epilepsy caused by birth trauma, which was common at that time. Head trauma caused by injuries was also common; in the English Civil War of 1642–1646, an estimated 100,000 men were killed and presumably many others sustained head injuries.

Nutritional and toxic causes of insanity were also relatively common during the seventeenth century. In the 1590s there was a severe famine in England, with up to 10 percent of the population dying in some regions. The Civil War, subsequent political chaos (e.g., the beheading of King Charles I), and religious insurrections during the century also ensured that the food supply was unpredictable. Under such conditions one would have expected to find deficiencies in thiamine, niacin, and vitamin B_{12} that could have produced symptoms of insanity. Many wines contained high concentrations of lead from the lead piping used in distillation. In addition, many grains grown for consumption were susceptible to ergot and other funguses; "one result was widespread ergotism, a condition manifested in convulsions, hallucinations, and temporary paralysis."[9]

Taking all these possible causes of insanity into consideration, what is a reasonable estimate of the baseline rate of insanity in the seventeenth century? Demographically, the average life expectancy in England at that time was approximately thirty-five years; more than half the population was under age twenty-five, and only 8 to 10 percent was over age sixty.[10]

The largest number of cases of insanity during the seventeenth century were probably caused by infections and toxins, and in most such instances the symptoms of insanity would have been brief. Longer lasting symptoms of insanity would have been caused most commonly by vitamin deficiencies, head trauma, epilepsy, or other neurological conditions. Metabolic (e.g., liver failure), genetic (e.g., Huntington's disease), and endocrine (e.g., thyroid disease) disorders would have contributed an occasional case of insanity.

Given the demographics of the population, and the fact that the majority of people were young, a reasonable estimate of the baseline rate of insanity would appear to be no more than one case per 1,000 adults at any given time, or approximately 0.5 per 1,000 total population. This rate might be higher following wars (head trauma), famines (vitamin deficiencies), or epidemics of encephalitis, such as the encephalitis lethargica-like illness that struck isolated areas of Europe during the seventeenth century.[11] The rate might be lower than 0.5 per 1,000 total population during periods of relative peace, good harvests, and lack of epidemic diseases.

Is there any evidence that can be used to confirm this estimate for the baseline rate of insanity? One approach would be to ascertain how many cases of contemporary insanity are caused by medical conditions such as those listed above. A study in England by Eve Johnstone and her colleagues did exactly that, closely examining 268 individuals referred for first-onset schizophrenia between 1979 and 1981. They found that 15 of the cases were caused by medical conditions, including syphilis, sarcoidosis, alcohol excess, drug abuse, thyroid disease, head injury, lung cancer that had spread to the brain, and a parasitic infection of the brain. Since the rate of schizophrenia in England at that time, as measured by contemporary prevalence studies, was between 3 and 4 cases per 1,000 total population,[12] then the 268 cases of schizophrenia would have been drawn from a population of between 67,000 and 89,000 persons. The 15 cases of medically caused schizophrenia would therefore represent a baseline insanity rate of approximately 0.2 per 1,000 total population. If cases of manic-depressive illness had also been included from this population, the rate would presumably have been approximately 0.3 per 1,000. And since infections and neurointoxications were more common in seventeenth-century England than they are today, the baseline rate of insanity would presumably have been modestly higher.

Given these findings, the estimated rate of one case of insanity per 1,000 adults, or 0.5 per 1,000 total population, seems reasonable. Insanity rates higher than 0.5 per 1,000 therefore suggest either unusual medical conditions (e.g., an epidemic of syphilis) or some other causes of insanity, such as what are now called schizophrenia and manic-depressive illness.

Tables of Insanity Rates

TABLE 1. England and Wales: Insane Persons in Psychiatric Hospitals, Workhouses, and under Care, 1807–1961

Year	Number	Insane Persons per 1,000 Total Population
1807	5,500*	0.67
1829	8,941	0.79
1843	14,792	0.93
1854	30,538	1.61
1859	36,762	1.87
1860	38,058	1.91
1861	39,647	1.97
1862	41,129	2.02
1863	43,118	2.09
1864	44,795	2.15
1865	45,950	2.18
1866	47,648	2.24
1867	49,086	2.29
1868	51,000	2.35
1869	53,177	2.43
1870	54,713	2.47
1871	56,755	2.49
1872	58,640	2.54
1873	60,296	2.58
1874	62,027	2.62
1875	63,793	2.66
1876	64,916	2.69

TABLE 1. (*Continued*)

Year	Number	Insane Persons per 1,000 Total Population
1877	66,636	2.70
1878	68,538	2.74
1879	69,885	2.76
1880	71,191	2.77
1881	73,113	2.81
1882	74,842	2.83
1883	76,765	2.88
1884	78,528	2.92
1885	79,704	2.93
1886	80,156	2.91
1887	80,891	2.91
1888	82,643	2.94
1889	84,340	2.97
1890	86,067	2.99
1891	86,795	2.99
1892	87,848	2.99
1893	89,822	3.02
1894	92,067	3.06
1895	94,081	3.10
1896	96,446	3.14
1897	99,365	3.20
1898	101,972	3.24
1899	105,086	3.30
1900	106,611	3.31
1901	107,944	3.31
1902	110,713	3.36
1903	113,964	3.42
1904	117,199	3.48
1905	119,829	3.53
1906	121,979	3.56
1907	123,988	3.57
1908	126,084	3.60
1909	128,787	3.64
1910	130,553	3.65
1911	133,157	3.68
1912	135,661	3.71
1913	138,377	3.75
1914	140,237	3.76
1915	140,466	3.98
1916	137,188	3.96

TABLE 1. (*Continued*)

Year	Number	Insane Persons per 1,000 Total Population
1917	134,029	3.56
1918	125,841	3.36
1919	116,703	3.12
1920	116,764	3.14
1921	120,344	3.17
1922	123,714	3.25
1923	126,279	3.27
1924	130,334	3.35
1925	131,551	3.38
1926	133,883	3.42
1927	136,626	3.48
1928	138,293	3.50
1929	141,080	3.56
1930	142,387	3.58
1931	144,161	3.61
1932	146,696	3.65
1933	148,775	3.68
1934	150,266	3.71
1935	152,089	3.75
1936	153,771	3.77
1937	155,522	3.79
1938	157,353	3.82
1939	158,723	3.82
1949	144,700	3.34
1954	151,400	3.44
1955	155,000	3.49
1959	133,200	2.90
1961	135,400	3.00

*Identified by county officials.

TABLE 2. Ireland: Insane Persons in Psychiatric Hospitals, Workhouses, and Jails, 1817–1961

Year	Number	Insane Persons per 1,000 Total Population
1817	989	0.15
1828	1,584	0.21
1841	3,622	0.44
1844	4,297	0.53
1851	5,345	0.82
1861	6,821	1.18
1863	8,272	1.45
1865	8,845	1.50
1867	9,086	1.63
1871	10,767	1.85
1876	12,123	2.29
1877	12,380	2.35
1878	12,585	2.40
1879	12,819	2.45
1880	12,982	2.50
1881	13,326	2.59
1882	13,704	2.69
1883	13,981	2.78
1884	14,178	2.85
1885	14,307	2.90
1886	14,590	2.97
1887	15,147	3.12
1888	15,551	3.24
1889	16,026	3.37
1890	16,251	3.44
1891	16,688	3.57
1892	17,124	3.70
1893	17,276	3.75
1894	17,655	3.85
1895	18,357	4.03
1896	18,966	4.18
1897	19,590	4.32
1898	20,304	4.49
1899	20,863	4.63
1900	21,169	4.74
1901	21,630	4.87
1902	22,138	4.99
1903	22,794	5.16
1904	22,996	5.22
1905	23,365	5.32

TABLE 2. (*Continued*)

Year	Number	Insane Persons per 1,000 Total Population
1906	23,554	5.36
1907	23,718	5.41
1908	23,931	5.47
1909	24,144	5.51
1910	24,394	5.57
1911	24,655	5.63
1912	24,839	5.66
1913	25,009	5.71
1914	25,180	5.75
1915	25,103	5.74
1916	24,766	5.68
1917	23,893	5.50
1918	22,868	5.27
1919	22,578	5.22
1923	19,243*	5.91
1924	19,381	6.13
1925	19,539	6.37
1926	19,887	6.69
1927	20,042	6.75
1928	19,753	6.65
1936	20,956	7.07
1940	21,081	7.12
1941	20,826	7.04
1942	20,104	6.80
1943	19,652	6.64
1947	19,541	6.61
1948	19,475	6.58
1949	19,924	6.73
1950	20,079	6.78
1951	20,241	6.84
1952	20,643	6.99
1954	21,242	7.23
1955	21,352	7.32
1956	21,720	7.49
1957	19,808	6.88
1959	19,509	6.86
1960	20,506	7.24
1961	20,099	7.13

*Irish Free State only; Northern Ireland was separated and is not included in subsequent numbers.

TABLE 3. Canadian Atlantic Provinces: Insane Persons in Psychiatric Hospitals, 1847–1960

Year	Number	Insane Persons per 1,000 Total Population
1847*	94	0.28
1855*	180	0.45
1860	403	0.51
1870	642	0.70
1880	963	0.92
1890	1,491	1.38
1900*	952	1.45
1935	3,662	2.72
1945	4,942	3.25
1950	5,098	3.19
1955	6,650	3.83
1960	6,266	3.36

*Data not available for Nova Scotia.

TABLE 4. United States: Insane Persons in Psychiatric Hospitals, 1840–1955

Year	Number	Insane Persons per 1,000 Total Population
1840	2,561	0.15
1850	4,730	0.20
1860	8,500	0.27
1870	17,735	0.46
1880	38,047	0.76
1890	74,028	1.18
1903	150,151	1.86
1910	187,791	2.03
1923	255,245	2.28
1931	318,821	2.57
1940	423,445	3.21
1955	558,922	3.38

NOTES

Preface

1. A. Bradford Hill, "The Environment and Disease: Association or Causation," *Proceedings of the Royal Society of Medicine* 58 (1965): 295–300.
2. Henry David Thoreau, unpublished manuscript in *Miscellanies, Biographical Sketch* 10 (1918): 30.

1. Introduction

1. Lynette Iezzoni, *Influenza 1918* (New York: TV Books, 1999), 16.
2. Anthony S. Fauci, "The AIDS Epidemic," *New England Journal of Medicine* 341 (1999): 1046–1050.
3. David Dean Oberhelman, *Mad Encounters: Nineteenth-Century British Psychological Medicine and the Victorian Novel, 1840–1870* (Ann Arbor, Mich.: University Microfilms International Dissertation Services, 1993), 14, 247.
4. The 1992 cost for schizophrenia alone and total annual cost of insanity are taken from Martin Knapp, "Costs of Schizophrenia," *British Journal of Psychiatry* 171 (1997): 509–518. NHS direct costs are from K. Smith et al., "The Prevalence and Costs of Psychiatric Disorders and Learning Disabilities," *British Journal of Psychiatry* 166 (1995): 9–18.
5. Ron Goeree et al., "The Economic Burden of Schizophrenia in Canada," *Canadian Journal of Psychiatry* 44 (1999): 464–472.
6. Richard Jed Wyatt et al., "An Economic Evaluation of Schizophrenia—1991," *Journal of Social Psychiatry and Psychiatric Epidemiology* 30 (1995): 196–205, and R. J. Wyatt and I. Henter, "An Economic Evaluation of Manic-Depressive Illness—1991," *Journal of Social Psychiatry and Psychiatric Epidemiology* 30 (1995): 213–219.
7. Mary Ann Jimenez, *Changing Faces of Madness: Early American Attitudes and Treatment of the Insane* (Hanover, N.H.: University Press of New England for Brandeis University Press, 1987), 8.

2. The Birth of Bedlam

1. J. R. Whitwell, *Historical Notes on Psychiatry* (London: Lewis, 1936), 22. Nigel M. Bark, "On the History of Schizophrenia: Evidence of Its Existence before 1800," *New York State Journal of Medicine* 88 (1988): 374–383.

2. C. V. Haldipur, "Madness in Ancient India: Concept of Insanity in *Charaka Samhita* (1st Century A.D.)," *Comprehensive Psychiatry* 25 (1984): 335–344.

3. K. A. Menninger, "Appendix," in *The Vital Balance: The Life Process in Mental Health and Illness* (New York: Viking Press, 1963). Joseph Robins, *Fools and Mad: A History of the Insane in Ireland* (Dublin: Institute of Public Administration, 1986), 5. Bennett Simon, *Mind and Madness in Ancient Greece* (Ithaca, N.Y.: Cornell University Press, 1978), 148, 152.

4. Hanafy A. Youssef and Fatma A. Youssef (ed. T. R. Dening), "Evidence for the Existence of Schizophrenia in Medieval Islamic Society," *History of Psychiatry* 7 (1996): 55–62, and Whitwell, *Historical Notes on Psychiatry*, 94.

5. Jerome Kroll and Bernard Bachrach, "Visions and Psychopathology in the Middle Ages," *Journal of Nervous and Mental Disease* 170 (1982): 41–49.

6. Jerome Kroll and Bernard Bachrach, "Sin and Mental Illness in the Middle Ages," *Psychological Medicine* 14 (1984): 507–514.

7. D. V. Jeste et al., "Did Schizophrenia Exist before the Eighteenth Century?" *Comprehensive Psychiatry* 26 (1985): 493–503, and Harry A. Wilmer and Richard E. Scammon, "Neuropsychiatric Patients Reported Cured at St. Bartholomew's Hospital in the Twelfth Century: Selected Cases from the Book of the Foundation of St. Bartholomew's Church in London," *Journal of Nervous and Mental Disease* 119 (1954): 1–22.

8. Basil Clarke, *Mental Disorder in Earlier Britain* (Cardiff: University of Wales Press, 1975), 177.

9. Judith S. Neaman, *Suggestion of the Devil: The Origins of Madness* (New York: Octagon Books, 1978), 122, 123, and B. Clarke, *Mental Disorder*, 138.

10. Patricia Allderidge, "Hospitals, Madhouses and Asylums: Cycles in the Care of the Insane," *British Journal of Psychiatry* 134 (1979): 321–334. Daniel Hack Tuke, *Chapters in the History of the Insane in the British Isles* (London: Kegan Paul, Trench, 1882), 95. Ida Macalpine and Richard Hunter, *Schizophrenia 1677* (London: Dawson, 1956).

11. Allderidge, "Hospitals, Madhouses and Asylums."

12. Michael MacDonald, *Mystical Bedlam: Madness, Anxiety and Healing in Seventeenth-Century England* (Cambridge, U.K.: Cambridge University Press, 1981), 2.

13. A Sussex man: M. MacDonald, *Mystical Bedlam*, 128. Berchet: Cynthia Chermely, "'Nawghtye Mallenchollye': Some Faces of Madness in Tudor England," *Historian* 49, no. 3 (1987): 309–328.

14. David J. Mellett, *The Prerogative of Asylumdom* (New York: Garland, 1982), 86. Joy Wiltenberg, "Madness and Society in the Street Ballads of Early Modern England," *Journal of Popular Culture* 21 (1988): 101–127.

15. Mellett, *The Prerogative of Asylumdom*, 87. Wiltenberg, "Madness and Society."

16. Edward G. O'Donoghue, *The Story of Bethlehem Hospital from Its Foundation in 1247* (London: Unwin, 1914), 139. W. H. Logan, *A Pedlar's Pack of Ballads and Songs* (Edinburgh: William Paterson, 1869).

17. Kathleen Jones, *A History of the Mental Health Services* (London: Routledge and Kegan Paul, 1972), 13. Percy, quoted in Mellett, *The Prerogative of Asylumdom*, 86.

18. J. Thomas Dalby, "Elizabethan Madness: On London's Stage," *Psychological Reports* 81 (1997): 1331–1343.

19. Joseph Collins, "Lunatics of Literature," *North American Review* 218 (1923): 376–387. William Bynum and Michael Neve, "Hamlet on the Couch," *American Scientist* 74 (1986): 390–396.

20. Nigel M. Bark, "Did Shakespeare Know Schizophrenia? The Case of Poor Mad Tom in *King Lear*," *British Journal of Psychiatry* 146 (1985): 436–438.

21. Karin S. Coddon, "*The Duchess of Malfi*: Tyranny and Spectacle in Jacobean Drama," *Madness in Drama* (Cambridge, U.K.: Cambridge University Press, 1993). Dalby, "Elizabethan Madness." M. MacDonald, *Mystical Bedlam*, 122. Robert R. Reed, *Bedlam on the Jacobean Stage* (New York: Octagon Books, 1970), 1.

22. Thomas Kyd, *The First Part of Hieronimo and The Spanish Tragedy*, Act 3, Scene 12, Andrew S. Cairncross (ed.) (Lincoln: University of Nebraska Press, 1967), 140.

23. Jonathan Andrews et al., *The History of Bethlem* (London: Routledge, 1997), 185, 186, 189.

24. The closing quote is taken from O'Donoghue, *The Story of Bethlehem Hospital*, 152. All other quotes in this paragraph are from Andrews et al., *History of Bethlem*, 178, 185–189.

25. Andrews et al., *History of Bethlem*, 134.

26. William Chappell, *The Ballad Literature and Popular Music of the Olden Time*, 2 vols. (New York: Dover Publications, Inc., 1965), 1, 334, quoting Payne Collier.

27. Joan Busfield, *Managing Madness: Changing Ideas and Practice* (London: Hutchinson, 1986), 227.

28. M. MacDonald, *Mystical Bedlam*, 20.

29. M. MacDonald, *Mystical Bedlam*, 20, 21, 148.

30. Michael Shepherd, "Historical Epidemiology and the Functional Psychoses," *Psychological Medicine* 23 (1993): 301–304.

31. M. MacDonald, *Mystical Bedlam*, 20, 148, 281.

32. Richard Neugebauer, "Medieval and Early Modern Theories of Mental Illness," *Archives of General Psychiatry* 36 (1979): 477–483. A. Fessler, "The Management of Lunacy in Seventeenth Century England: An Investigation of Quarter-Sessions Records," *Proceedings of the Royal Society of Medicine* 49 (1956): 901–907; Neugebauer, "Medieval and Early"; Peter Rushton, "Lunatics and Idiots: Mental Disability, the Community, and the Poor Law in North-East England 1600–1800," *Medical History* 32 (1988): 34–50; Akihito Suzuki, "Lunacy in Seventeenth- and Eighteenth-Century England: Analysis of Quarter Sessions Records, Part I," *History of Psychiatry* 2 (1991): 437–456, and "Lunacy in Seventeenth- and Eighteenth-Century England: Analysis of Quarter Sessions Records, Part II," *History of Psychiatry* 3 (1992): 29–44.

33. Richard Neugebauer, "Treatment of the Mentally Ill in Mediaeval and Early Modern England," *Journal of the History of the Behavioral Sciences* 14 (1978): 158–169. Andrew T. Scull, *The Most Solitary of Afflictions: Madness and Society in Britain* (New Haven, Conn.: Yale University Press, 1993), 6, 7. Ibid., quoting Midelfort. Suzuki, "Lunacy, Part II."

34. Suzuki, "Lunacy, Part I." Jeste et al., "Did Schizophrenia Exist?" Edward Hare, "Schizophrenia before 1800? The Case of the Revd George Trosse," *Psychological Medicine* 18 (1988): 279–285.
35. Rushton, "Lunatics and Idiots," 41. Suzuki, "Lunacy, Part II." M. MacDonald, *Mystical Bedlam,* 141, citing Fessler, "Management of Lunacy," 903.
36. Suzuki, "Lunacy, Part II."
37. Neugebauer, "Medieval and Early." Chermely, "'Nawghtye Mallenchollye,'" 313. Andrews, *History of Bethlem,* 330.
38. Bark, "On the History of Schizophrenia."
39. Locke, quoted in Roy Porter, "The Rage of Party: A Glorious Revolution in English Psychiatry?" *Medical History* 27 (1983): 35–50.

3. The "English Malady" Appears

1. James Hey: Millicent Regan, *A Caring Society: A Study of Lunacy in Liverpool and South West Lancashire from 1650 to 1948* (Merseyside, U.K.: St. Helens and Knowsley Health Authority, 1986), 5. Cost of confinement: Richard Hunter and Ida Macalpine, *Three Hundred Years of Psychiatry: A History Presented in Selected English Texts* (London: Oxford University Press, 1963), 299–301.
2. John Strype, quoted in Jonathan Andrews, "The Lot of the 'Incurably' Insane in Enlightenment England," *Eighteenth-Century Life* 12, n.s. 1 (1988): 1–18. Andrews et al., *History of Bethlem,* 126.
3. Hunter and Macalpine, *Three Hundred Years,* 645, quoting William Black's "A Dissertation on Insanity," 1788. Andrews et al., *History of Bethlem,* 323. Andrews, "The Lot of the 'Incurably' Insane."
4. Andrews et al., *History of Bethlem,* 183–184, 186.
5. Andrews et al., *History of Bethlem,* 186.
6. The Prince of Wales: Andrews et al., *History of Bethlem,* 180. Samuel Richardson, *Familiar Letters on Important Occasions* (Norwood, Pa.: Norwood Editions, 1975; first published in 1741), 201.
7. "Webster on the Study of Mental Diseases (review article on John Webster's *Observations on the Admission of Medical Pupils to the Wards of Bethlem Hospital, for the Purpose of Studying Mental Diseases*)," *The Monthly Review* 162, n.s. 3 (1842): 74–88, and Andrews et al., *History of Bethlem,* 186, 190.
8. Andrews et al., *History of Bethlem,* 183, 186. Henry Mackenzie, *The Man of Feeling* (London: Oxford University Press, 1967; originally published in 1771), ch. 20.
9. Mary Chapman: Allderidge, "Hospitals, Madhouses and Asylums." "Reasons for Establishing St. Luke's": Jones, *A History,* 40. St. Luke's statistics: Denis Leigh, *The Historical Development of British Psychiatry,* vol. 1 (Oxford: Pergamon, 1961), 10.
10. Anonymous, *An Account of the Rise, and Present Establishment of the Lunatick Hospital, in Manchester* (Manchester, U.K.: J. Harrop, 1771). Anne Digby, *Madness, Morality and Medicine: A Study of the York Retreat 1796–1914* (Cambridge, U.K.: Cambridge University Press, 1985), 11. Nigel Walker and Sarah McCabe, *Crime and Insanity in England* (Edinburgh: University Press, 1968), 70. Hunter and Macalpine, *Three Hundred Years,* 419.
11. By 1807: Busfield, *Managing Madness,* 172; 1700 advertisement: D. H. Tuke, *Chapters in the History,* 92–93.
12. Louis Simond, *An American in Regency England: The Journal of a Tour in 1810–1811* (London: Robert Maxwell, 1815). Tuke: Digby, *Madness,* 15.

13. Defoe, quoted in Hunter and Macalpine, *Three Hundred Years*, 265–267.

14. Allderidge, "Hospitals, Madhouses and Asylums, 42." William Parry-Jones, *The Trade in Lunacy: A Study of the Private Madhouses in England in the Eighteenth and Nineteenth Centuries* (London: Routledge and Kegan Paul, 1972), 289.

15. Roy Porter, *Disease, Medicine and Society in England, 1550–1860* (Cambridge, U.K.: Cambridge University Press, 1993), 30.

16. Helen Small, *Love's Madness: Medicine, the Novel, and Female Insanity, 1800–1865* (Oxford: Clarendon Press, 1996), 12, 13.

17. George S. Rousseau, "Science and the Discovery of the Imagination in Enlightened England," *Eighteenth-Century Studies* 3 (1969): 117.

18. Samuel Johnson, *Lives of the English Poets* (Oxford: Clarendon Press, 1905), 337–339.

19. Russell Brain, "Christopher Smart: The Flea That Became an Eagle," in *Some Reflections on Genius and Other Essays* (Philadelphia and Montreal: J. B. Lippincott Company, 1960), 113, 117.

20. William R. Benét, *The Reader's Encyclopedia* (New York: Crowell, 1965), 250. Morton D. Paley, "Cowper as Blake's Spectre," *Eighteenth-Century Studies* 1 (1968): 236–249. William Cowper, *Memoir of the Early Life of William Cowper, Esq.*, 1816, quoted in Roy Porter (ed.), *The Faber Book of Madness* (London: Faber and Faber, 1991), 204.

21. Cowper, *Memoir of the Early Life*, 1816, quoted in Porter, *The Faber Book of Madness*, 204.

22. Philip W. Martin, *Mad Women in Romantic Writing* (New York: St. Martin's Press, 1987), 19. Small, *Love's Madness*, 11–12.

23. *American Journal of Insanity* 15 (1858): 47.

24. Kay R. Jamison, *Touched with Fire: Manic-Depressive Illness and the Artistic Temperament* (New York: Simon and Schuster, 1993), 65.

25. Winifred F. Courtney, *Young Charles Lamb, 1775–1802* (New York: New York University Press, 1982), 108, 110, quoting Lamb's letters to Coleridge.

26. Courtney, *Young Charles Lamb*, 114, 115.

27. E. V. Lucas (ed.), *The Letters of Charles Lamb*, vol. 3 (New Haven, Conn.: Yale University Press, 1935), 370, 417.

28. Anonymous, "An Account of the Progress of an Epidemical Madness" (London: J. Roberts, 1735).

29. William Battie, *A Treatise on Madness* (New York: Brunner/Mazel, 1969; originally published in 1758), 1. K. Doerner, *Madness and the Bourgeoisie* (Oxford: Basil Blackwell, 1981), 41, quoting Battie.

30. Kathleen Grange, "Dr. Samuel Johnson's Account of a Schizophrenic Illness in *Rasselas* (1759)," *Medical History* 6 (1962): 162–168.

31. Johnson, quoted in Hunter and Macalpine, *Three Hundred Years*, 417. Anonymous, "Miscellany: Dr. Samuel Johnson on Insanity," *American Journal of Insanity* 3 (1847): 285–287.

32. Boswell, quoted in Judith L. Rapoport, *The Boy Who Couldn't Stop Washing: The Experience and Treatment of Obsessive Compulsive Disorder* (New York: New American Library, 1997), 4. Porter, *The Faber Book of Madness*, 113.

33. Michael Shimer, *Madness and the Muse in Nineteenth-Century English Romantic Poetry* (Ann Arbor, Mich.: University Microfilms International Dissertation Services, 1996), 73.

34. Porter, *The Faber Book of Madness*, 88.

35. Colwyn E. Vulliamy, *James Boswell* (Freeport, N.Y.: Books for Libraries Press, 1932), 269. Charles Ryskamp and Frederick A. Pottle (eds.) *Boswell: The Ominous Years, 1774–1776* (New York: McGraw-Hill, 1963), 44.

36. Thomas Arnold, *Observations on the Nature, Kinds, Causes, and Prevention of Insanity, Lunacy, or Madness* (New York: Arno Press, 1976; originally published in 1782), 14–15, 24.

37. Ida Macalpine and Richard Hunter, *George III and the Mad-Business* (New York: W. W. Norton, 1969), 287–288.

38. Arnold, *Observations,* 23.

39. William Perfect, *Select Cases in the Different Species of Insanity* (Rochester: W. Gillman, 1787), 118. J. Ellard, "Did Schizophrenia Exist before the Eighteenth Century?" *Australian and New Zealand Journal of Psychiatry* 21 (1987): 306–314.

40. William Rowley, *A Treatise of Female, Nervous, Hysterical, Hypochondriacal, Bilious, Convulsive Diseases* (London: C. Nourse, 1788), 253–254. Benjamin Faulkner, quoted in Porter, *The Faber Book of Madness,* 120.

41. William Pargeter, *Observations on Maniacal Disorders* (London: Routledge, 1988; first published in 1792), 1–3.

42. Leigh, *The Historical,* 144. John Haslam, *Observations on Insanity* (London: F. and C. Rivington, 1798), Preface, iii, and Rajendra D. Persaud, "A Comparison of Symptoms Recorded from the Same Patients by an Asylum Doctor and 'A Constant Observer' in 1823: The Implications for Theories about Psychiatric Illness in History," *History of Psychiatry* 3 (1992): 79–94.

43. Harper, quoted in Edward Hare, "Was Insanity on the Increase?" *British Journal of Psychiatry* 142 (1983): 439–455. Peter K. Carpenter, "Descriptions of Schizophrenia in the Psychiatry of Georgian Britain: John Haslam and James Tilly Matthews," *Comprehensive Psychiatry* 30 (1989): 332–338.

44. Leigh, *The Historical,* 122.

45. Leigh, *The Historical,* 84–93.

46. Macalpine and Hunter, *George III,* 291.

47. Macalpine and Hunter, *George III,* 291.

48. Macalpine and Hunter, *George III,* 32, 40. Christopher Reid, "Burke, the Regency Crisis, and the 'Antagonist World of Madness,'" *Eighteenth-Century Life* 16, n.s. 2 (1992): 59–75, quoting *The Morning Chronicle.*

49. Macalpine and Hunter, *George III,* 89. K. Jones, *A History,* 39.

50. C. Reid, "Burke."

4. "The Clap of Tortured Hands"

1. Walker and McCabe, *Crime and Insanity,* 76, and Oberhelman, *Mad Encounters,* 14, 247.

2. Joel Eigen, *Witnessing Insanity: Madness and Mad-Doctors in the English Court* (New Haven, Conn.: Yale University Press, 1995), Appendix 2. Walker and McCabe, *Crime and Insanity,* 70.

3. *Times,* November 4, 1786, 2c.

4. *Times,* September 1, 1787, 3a, June 3, 1788, 2d, and February 26, 1790, 3a.

5. Joseph Cox, *Practical Observations on Insanity* (London: Baldwin, 1804), v. William Stark, *Remarks on the Construction of Public Hospitals for the Cure of Mental Derangement* (Edinburgh: Ballantyne, 1807), v. John Reid, "Report of Diseases," *The Monthly Magazine* 25 (1808): 166, 374.

6. Leonard D. Smith, *'Cure, Comfort and Safe Custody': Public Lunatic Asylums in Early Nineteenth-Century England* (London: Leicester University Press, 1999), 23.

7. House of Commons, *Report of the Select Committee on the State of Criminal and Pauper Lunatics, 1807*. Account of workhouses: K. Jones, *A History*, 18. Suzuki, "Lunacy, Part II." John Howard: Roy Porter, *Mind-Forg'd Manacles: A History of Madness in England from the Restoration to the Regency* (Cambridge, Mass.: Harvard University Press, 1987), 118. *Report, 1807*.

8. L. D. Smith, *Cure, Comfort*, 24. John Crammer, *Asylum History: Buckinghamshire County Pauper Lunatic Asylum—St. John's* (London: Gaskell, Royal College of Psychiatrists, 1990), 15. Vieda Skultans, *English Madness: Ideas on Insanity, 1580–1890* (London: Routledge and Kegan Paul, 1979), 98.

9. L. D. Smith, *Cure, Comfort*, 39.

10. L. D. Smith, *Cure, Comfort*, 40–41.

11. Parry-Jones, *Trade in Lunacy*, 30, 46, 53.

12. Parry-Jones, *Trade in Lunacy*, 240. Skultans, *English Madness*. House of Commons, *Report of the Select Committee on Madhouses, 1815–1816*.

13. Richard Powell, "Observations upon the Comparative Prevalence of Insanity at Different Periods," *Medical Transactions* 4 (1813): 131–159.

14. Crowther, quoted in Hare, "Was Insanity on the Increase?" George Hill, *An Essay on the Prevention and Cure of Insanity* (London: Longman, Hurst, Rees, Orme and Brown, 1814), ix. Simond, *An American in Regency England*, 110, 115.

15. Andrew Scull, *Social Order/Mental Disorder: Anglo-American Psychiatry in Historical Perspective* (Berkeley: University of California Press, 1989), 143–144. Thomas Bakewell, *A Letter Addressed to the Chairman of the Select Committee of the House of Commons* (Stafford, U.K.: Chester, 1815). Uwins, "Insanity and Madhouses," 398.

16. Ann C. Colley, *Tennyson and Madness* (Athens: University of Georgia Press, 1983), 10.

17. Philippe Pinel, *A Treatise on Insanity* (Sheffield, U.K.: Todd, 1806), 113–114. William A. F. Browne, *What Asylums Were, Are, and Ought to Be* (Edinburgh: Black, 1837; New York: Arno Press, 1976), 57.

18. Ian Scott-Kilvert (ed.), *British Writers*, vol. 3 (New York: Charles Scribner's Sons, 1980), 283.

19. Frank Whitehead, *George Crabbe: A Reappraisal* (Selinsgrove, Pa.: Susquehanna University Press, 1995), 50. Arthur Pollard (ed.), *Crabbe: The Critical Heritage* (Boston: Routledge and Kegan Paul, 1972), 53, quoting the *Oxford Review*, January 1808. Whitehead, *George Crabbe*, 143.

20. Shimer, *Madness and the Muse*, 127.

21. Coleridge's discharge and illness: Jamison, *Touched with Fire*, 67, 221. Thomas C. Faulkner (ed.), *Selected Letters and Journals of George Crabbe* (Oxford: Clarendon Press, 1985), 102. Shimer, *Madness and the Muse*, 160–162. Coleridge, in Shimer, 147.

22. Paul Youngquist, *Madness and Blake's Myth* (University Park: Pennsylvania State University Press, 1989), 3, 16, 105–107, 170n.

23. Jamison, *Touched with Fire*, 67. Oberhelman, *Mad Encounters*, 87. Sir Walter Scott, *The Heart of Midlothian* (London: Hawarden Press, 1893), 345. H. Michael Buck, *Insanity, Character Roles, and Authorial Milieu: A Study of Madness in Selected Waverley Novels* (Ann Arbor, Mich.: University Microfilms International Dissertation Services, 1987), 30.

24. Scott, quoted in Jamison, *Touched with Fire*, 179. Byron, quoted in Jamison, *Touched with Fire*, 171. Byron's "The Dream," quoted in John R. Reed, *Victorian Conventions* (Athens: Ohio University Press, 1975), 199.

25. Shelley, quoted in Jamison, *Touched with Fire*, 179, 69.

26. William Blake, "Milton: A Poem in Two Books," preface, in Morris Eaves, Robert N. Essick, and Joseph Viscomi (eds.), *The William Blake Archive*, January 10, 2001 <http://www.blakearchive.org/>.

27. Scull, *Most Solitary*, 182. Andrew Scull, Charlotte MacKenzie, and Nicholas Hervey, *Masters of Bedlam: The Transformation of the Mad-Doctoring Trade* (Princeton, N.J.: Princeton University Press, 1996), 97, and see also Scull, *Most Solitary*, 182, note 28.

28. Robert Willan, *Reports on the Diseases in London* (London: R. Phillips, 1801), 326–327. Thomas Bateman, *Reports on the Diseases of London* (London: Longman, Hurst, Rees, Orme and Brown, 1819), 24–25. *Report from Select Committee, 1808*, 137.

29. George Man Burrows, *An Inquiry into Certain Errors Relative to Insanity* (London: Underwood, 1820), 80, 81, 83.

30. George Man Burrows, *Commentaries on the Causes, Forms, Symptoms, and Treatment, Moral and Medical, of Insanity* (New York: Arno Press, 1976; originally published in 1828), 81.

31. Burrows, *An Inquiry*, 54.

32. Macalpine and Hunter, *George III*, 294.

33. Anonymous, "Inquiries Relative to Insanity," *Quarterly Review* 24 (1821): 181. Anonymous, "Insanity" *Quarterly Review* 42 (1830): 351–377.

34. Geoffrey B.A.M. Finlayson, *The Seventh Earl of Shaftesbury, 1801–1885* (London: Eyre Methuen, 1981), 31, 22, quoting footnote 85. Woodham Smith and Cecil Blanche Fitz Gerald, *Florence Nightingale 1820–1910* (London: Constable, 1950), 589.

35. Finlayson, *Seventh Earl*, 602, 605.

36. "English Evangelicalism," *The Nation* 81 (1905): 196–197. Skultans, *English Madness*.

37. Finlayson, *Seventh Earl*, 461, 209. Nicholas Hervey, "A Slavish Bowing Down: The Lunacy Commission and the Psychiatric Profession 1845–60," in William F. Bynum, Roy Porter, and Michael Shepherd (eds.), *The Anatomy of Madness: Essays in the History of Psychiatry* (London, New York: Tavistock, 1985–1988), 104.

38. Andrew Halliday, "A Report on the Number of Lunatics and Idiots in England and Wales," in *A Letter to Lord Robert Seymour* (London: Underwood, 1829), v.

39. Andrew Halliday, *A General View of the Present State of Lunatics, and Lunatic Asylums* (London: Underwood, 1828), 80.

40. Thomas Beddoes, *Hygeia* (Bristol: Phillips, 1802–1803), vol. 2: 40, cited by Scull, *Most Solitary*, 157. Alexander Morison, *Outlines of Lectures on Mental Diseases* (London: Longman, Rees, Orme, Brown and Green, and Highly, 1826), 61. James Prichard, *A Treatise on Insanity and Other Disorders Affecting the Mind* (London: Sherwood, Gilbert and Piper, 1835), 150. Scull et al., *Masters of Bedlam*, 97. Browne, *What Asylums Were*, 52.

41. *Times*, August 24, 1832, 3b. *Penny Magazine*, September 9, 1837. *New Monthly Magazine* 57 (1839): 364–372. Johann Gaspar Spurzheim, *Observations on the*

Deranged Manifestations of the Mind (Boston: Marsh, Capen and Lyon, 1835), 150.

42. Leonard Manheim, "Dickens' Fools and Madmen," *Dickens Studies Annual* 2 (1972): 69–97. Oberhelman, *Mad Encounters*, 414. Jablow Hershman and Julian Lieb, "Dickens," in *The Key to Genius* (Buffalo, N.Y.: Prometheus Books, 1988), 106.

43. Manheim, "Dickens' Fools," 71–72.

44. Charles Dickens, *The Works of Charles Dickens: Pickwick Papers* (New York: Books, Inc., 1841), 208.

45. Oberhelman, *Mad Encounters*, 381, 393, 389. *The Works of Charles Dickens: Barnaby Rudge* (New York: Books, Inc., 1841), 521.

46. Charles Dickens, "A Curious Dance": *Household Words*, January 17, 1852. Charles Dickens and Wilkie Collins, "The Lazy Tour of Two Idle Apprentices," *Seaside Library*, vol. 19, no. 372 (New York: George Munro, 1857).

47. Gordon Claridge, Ruth Pryor, and GwenWatkins, *Sounds from the Bell Jar* (New York: St. Martin's Press, 1990), 132–133. Hugh Haughton (ed.), *John Clare in Context* (Cambridge, U.K.: Cambridge University Press, 1994), 10. A. T. Quiller-Couch (ed.), *The Oxford Book of English Verse 1250–1900* (Oxford: Clarendon Press, 1907).

48. Colley, *Tennyson and Madness*, 4. Shimer, *Madness and the Muse*, 258.

49. John C. Bucknill, "*Maud and Other Poems*, by Alfred Tennyson," *Asylum Journal of Mental Science* 15 (1855): 94–104. Alfred, Lord Tennyson, *The Works of Tennyson*, vol. 4, *The Princess and Maud* (New York: AMS Press, 1970), 209.

50. Tennyson, *Maud*, 219, 221.

51. Tennyson, *Maud*, 222.

52. Tennyson, *Maud*, 227.

53. Hunter and Macalpine, *Three Hundred Years*, 1039, quoted in Oberhelman, *Mad Encounters*, 205. Colley, *Tennyson and Madness*, 12.

54. K. Jones, *A History*, 227.

55. Lancashire and Wakefield asylums: L. D. Smith, *Cure, Comfort*, 176–177. Hanwell: W. Farr, "Report upon the Mortality."

56. C. Lockhart Robertson, "The Care and Treatment of the Insane Poor," *Journal of Mental Science* 13 (1867): 290.

57. *Report of the Metropolitan Commissioners in Lunacy to the Lord Chancellor* (London: Bradbury and Evans, 1844), Appendix F.

58. Anonymous, "Webster on the Study of Mental Diseases," *The Monthly Review* 162, n.s. 3 (1842): 74–88.

59. Parry-Jones, *Trade in Lunacy*, 159.

60. Eastgate House: Hunter and Macalpine, *Three Hundred Years*, 1000. Dunnington House: Parry-Jones, *Trade in Lunacy*, 56. Haydock Lodge: Parry-Jones, *Trade in Lunacy*, 277–278.

61. Ruth G. Hodgkinson, *The Origins of the National Health Service* (London: Wellcome Historical Medical Library, 1967), 578. Ruth G. Hodgkinson, "Provision for Pauper Lunatics, 1834–1871," *Medical History* 10 (1966): 138–154.

62. Mellett, *The Prerogative of Asylumdom*, 91, quoting J. W. Milligan, 1840. Eigen, *Witnessing Insanity*, and Walker and McCabe, *Crime and Insanity*. Parry-Jones, *Trade in Lunacy*, 65.

63. Charlotte Brontë, *Jane Eyre* (New York: Penguin Books USA, 1982), 295.

64. Small, *Love's Madness*, 165, quoting Brontë's letter of January 4, 1848. Colley, *Tennyson and Madness*, 10.

65. Small, *Love's Madness*, 180–181, quoting Brontë's letter of January 28, 1848.

5. "A Mania for Madness"

1. The Rev. George Clayton, *Sermons on the Great Exhibition* (London: Benjamin L. Green, 1851), 36.

2. Asa Briggs, *A Social History of England* (Harmondsworth: Penguin Books, 1983), 253. Karl Beckson, *London in the 1890s: A Cultural History* (New York: W. W. Norton and Company, 1992), 348.

3. Charles M. Burnett, *Insanity Tested by Science* (London: Highley, 1848), 1. Anonymous, *Familiar Views of Lunacy and Lunatic Life* (London: Parker, 1850), 101–102. Alfred B. Maddox, *Practical Observations on Nervous and Mental Disorders* (London: Simpkin, Marshall, 1854), 13. John Hawkes, "On the Increase of Insanity," *Journal of Psychological Medicine and Mental Pathology* 10 (1857): 508–521.

4. *The Times*, August 6, 1850, 5f. "Horrible Circumstance," *The Times*, October 7, 1844, 4f. Anonymous, "13th Report of the Commission on Lunacy," *Journal of Mental Science* 6 (1860): 141–156.

5. *Report of the Select Committee, 1859*, Appendix 7, 324, quoted in W. J. Corbet, "The Holocaust at Colney Hatch," *Westminster Review* 159 (1903): 383–393.

6. *Report of the Select Committee, 1859*, 7, 9, 33.

7. *Report of the Select Committee, 1859*, 8. Finlayson, *Seventh Earl*, 413, note 44. Hervey, "A Slavish Bowing Down," 104.

8. Finlayson, *Seventh Earl*, 558.

9. John C. Bucknill and Daniel Hack Tuke, *A Manual of Psychological Medicine* (London: Churchill, 1858), 32, 108.

10. C. Lockhart Robertson, "Lunacy in England," *Journal of Psychological Medicine and Mental Pathology* 7 (1881): 185–186. "The Alleged Increase of Lunacy," *Journal of Mental Science* 15 (1869): 1–23.

11. *Journal of Mental Science* 15 (1869): 317–318, 446–447, and *Journal of Mental Science* 16 (1871): 481. *Journal of Mental Science* 16 (1871): 492. C. L. Robertson, "A Further Note on the Alleged Increase in Insanity," *Journal of Mental Science* 16 (1871): 473–497.

12. Trevor Turner, "Henry Maudsley: Psychiatrist, Philosopher, and Entrepreneur," in Bynum et al., *Anatomy of Madness*, 153.

13. Henry Maudsley, "Is Insanity on the Increase?" *British Medical Journal* 1 (1872): 36–39.

14. Henry Maudsley, "The Alleged Increase of Insanity," *Journal of Mental Science* 23 (1877): 45–54. Turner, "Henry Maudsley," 166. Maudsley, *Physiology and Pathology of the Mind* (London: Macmillan, 1867), 206.

15. Scull, *Most Solitary*, 325. William F. Bynum, "Tuke's *Dictionary* and Psychiatry at the Turn of the Century," in German E. Berrios and Hugh Freeman, *150 Years of British Psychiatry, 1841–1991* (London: Royal College of Psychiatrists, 1991), 164. D. H. Tuke, *Chapters in the History*, 261. Tuke, "Alleged Increase of Insanity," *Journal of Mental Science* 40 (1894): 219–231.

16. D. H. Tuke, "Alleged Increase." Tuke, *Chapters in the History*, 260. Tuke, "Alleged Increase." Hare, "Was Insanity on the Increase?"

17. "Psychological Retrospect," *American Journal of Insanity* 30 (1874): 476–477, and Harrington Tuke, "Presidential Address," *Journal of Mental Science* 19 (1873): 327–340 and 479–485. *The Works of Charles Dickens: Our Mutual Friend* (New York: Books, Inc., 1841), 130.

18. Oberhelman, *Mad Encounters*, 7–8.

19. Oberhelman, *Mad Encounters*, 132–133.

20. Oberhelman, *Mad Encounters*, 5.

21. Oberhelman, *Mad Encounters*, 126–127.

22. Wilkie Collins, *The Woman in White* (London: Penguin Books, 1979; first published in 1859), 55.

23. Oberhelman, *Mad Encounters*, 179, 198.

24. David Skilton, *Introduction to* Lady Audley's Secret, *by Mary Elizabeth Braddon* (Oxford: Oxford University Press, 1987). Mary Elizabeth Braddon, *Lady Audley's Secret* (Harmondsworth: Penguin, 1985), 293.

25. Oberhelman, *Mad Encounters*, 139.

26. Scull et al., *Masters of Bedlam*, 76.

27. Scull et al., *Masters of Bedlam*, 76. Charles Reade, *Hard Cash: A Matter-of-Fact Romance* (New York: AMS Press, Inc., 1970; reprinted from 1895 London edition), 586.

28. Oberhelman, *Mad Encounters*, 200, quoting a letter to the *Daily News*. *The Times*, January 2, 1864. Oberhelman, *Mad Encounters*, 200–201.

29. *The Times*, January 11, 1860, 7c. "20th Report," *Journal of Mental Science* 12 (1867), quoting *Scotsman*. *The Times*, August 2, 1868, 4c. Anonymous, "The Increase of Lunacy," *North British Review* 50 (1869): 123. *The Times*, April 5, 1877, 6b.

30. Hervey, "A Slavish Bowing Down," 130. Langford Reed, *The Life of Lewis Carroll* (London: W. and G. Foyle Ltd., 1932), ref. 103. Morton N. Cohen, *Lewis Carroll: A Biography* (New York: Alfred A. Knopf, 1995), 362.

31. Roger B. Henkle, "The Mad Hatter's World," *Virginia Quarterly Review* 49 (Winter 1973): 99–117. *The Dream of Fame:* Cohen, *Lewis Carroll,* 222. *Through the Looking Glass:* Michael G. Myer, "Some Omissions from Martin Gardner's *The Annotated Alice,*" *Notes and Queries* 30 (1983): 302–303.

32. *The Times*, May 30, 1873, 5f. Roger Lancelyn Green (ed.), *The Diaries of Lewis Carroll*, vol. 2 (Westport, Conn.: Greenwood Press, 1971), 322.

33. Cohen, *Lewis Carroll*, 404, 409.

34. John Pudney, *Lewis Carroll and His World* (New York: Charles Scribner's Sons, 1976), 84. Martin Gardner, *The Annotated Snark* (New York: Bramhall House, 1962), 19, and Harold Beaver, "Whale or Boojum: An Agony," in Edward Duilliano (ed.), *Lewis Carroll Observed: A Collection of Unpublished Photographs, Drawings, Poetry, and New Essays* (New York: Clarkson N. Potter, Inc., 1976), 111–131. Gardner, *The Annotated Alice*, 23. Derek Hudson, *Lewis Carroll* (London: Constable, 1954), 221. *Athenaeum* 67 (1876): 495.

35. Lewis Carroll letter of August 18, 1884, quoted in Cohen, *Lewis Carroll*, 409.

36. Mellett, *The Prerogative of Asylumdom*, 225.

37. Hervey, "A Slavish Bowing Down," 130.

38. *The Saturday Review* 41 (1876): 502–503, quoted in Cohen, *Lewis Carroll*, 105.

39. Hare, "Was Insanity on the Increase?" quoting John Arlidge. *The Times*, June 30, 1864, 12b. *Special Report of Commissioners in Lunacy, 1897.*

40. Statistics on asylums: Kathleen Jones, *Lunacy, Law and Conscience 1744–1845* (London: Routledge and Kegan Paul, 1955), 116. Lunacy Commission reports: "Lunacy in England," *The Times*, January 4, 1878, 6f. West Riding Asylum: Alldleridge, "Hospitals, Madhouses and Asylums," 45. Devonshire Asylum: Scull et al., *Masters of Bedlam*, 209.

41. *The Times*, July 4, 1856, 12f, and September 9, 1859, 10c.

42. Hervey, "A Slavish Bowing Down," fn. 92. *The Times*, September 26, 1870, 4f. *Quarterly Review* 101 (1857): 353, quoted in Scull, *Most Solitary*, 278.

43. Andrew Scull, "Psychiatrists and Historical 'Facts': Part Two: Re-Writing the History of Asylumdom," *History of Psychiatry* 6 (1995): 387–394. K. Jones, *A History*, 89. Total expenditures: Mellett, *The Prerogative of Asylumdom*, 169.

44. John K. Walton, "Casting Out and Bringing Back in Victorian England: Pauper Lunatics, 1840–1870," in Bynum et al., *Anatomy of Madness*, vol. 2, 132. Hare, "Was Insanity on the Increase?" quoting John Arlidge. Scull, *Most Solitary*, 268, note 2. Crammer, *Asylum History*, 38–39. Haguch, "Comments on the Report of the Commissioners in Lunacy and the Swing of the Pendulum," *Westminster Review* 148 (1897): 672–681.

45. Cost comparison: Gwendoline M. Ayers, *England's First State Hospitals and the Metropolitan Asylums Board, 1867–1930* (London: Wellcome Institute, 1971), 38. In 1828: K. Jones, *A History*, 124. 12,000 pauper lunatics: Peter McCandless, "'Build! Build!': The Controversy over the Care of the Chronically Insane in England, 1855–1870," *Bulletin of the History of Medicine* 53 (1979): 553–574. By this time: Hodgkinson, "Provision for Pauper Lunatics."

46. Mellett, *The Prerogative of Asylumdom*, 156. St. Luke's and St. Pancras: F. Anstie, "Insane Patients in London Workhouses," *Journal of Mental Science* 11 (1865): 330–333. Mellett, *The Prerogative of Asylumdom*. Dickens: McCandless, "'Build! Build!'"

47. *Report of Commissioners in Lunacy, 1889.*

48. *The Times*, April 21, 1906.

49. D. H. Tuke, *Insanity in Ancient and Modern Life* (London: Macmillan and Co., 1878), 93. John Hawkes, "On the Increase in Insanity," *Journal of Psychological Medicine and Mental Pathology* 10 (1857): 508–521.

50. Kerby Miller, *Emigrants and Exiles: Ireland and the Irish Exodus to North America* (New York: Oxford University Press, 1985), 294–295.

51. Mellett, *The Prerogative of Asylumdom*, 150. "Lunatic Vagrants," *The Times*, April 2, 1870, 5b.

52. M. A. Arieno, *Victorian Lunatics: A Social Epidemiology of Mental Illness in Mid-Nineteenth-Century England* (Selinsgrove, Pa.: Susquehanna University Press, 1989), 87. "26th Lunacy Commission Report," *Journal of Mental Science* 18 (1873): 549–550.

53. Maudsley, *Physiology and Pathology*, 200–201.

54. Burrows, *Commentaries*, 110. Browne, *What Asylums Were*, 59. Scull, *Most Solitary*, 160. Parry-Jones, *Trade in Lunacy*, 22–23.

55. Halliday, "A Report." Rajendra Persaud, "The Reporting of Psychiatric Symptoms in History: The Memorandum Book of Samuel Coates, 1785–1825," *History of Psychiatry* 4 (1993): 499–510. Browne, *What Asylums Were*, 59. An analysis: J. Walton, "Lunacy in the Industrial Revolution: A Study of Asylum Admissions in

Lancashire, 1848–50," *Journal of Social History* 13 (1979): 1–22. Maddox, *Practical Observations,* 13. Bucknill and Tuke, *A Manual,* 40.

56. J. A. Banks, "Population Change and the Victorian City," *Victorian Studies* 11 (1968): 277–289. Scull, *Most Solitary,* 27. Thomas Clouston, "The Local Distribution of Insanity and Its Varieties in England and Wales," *Journal of Mental Science* 19 (1873): 1–19.

57. Noel A. Humphreys, "Statistics of Insanity in England, with Special Reference to Its Alleged Increasing Prevalence," *Journal of the Royal Statistical Society* 53 (1890), 201–252, and *67th Report of the Lunacy Commission,* 1913, 11–12.

58. *59th Report of Lunacy Commission, 1904,* 4. Clouston, "The Local Distribution."

6. "A Great and Progressive Evil"

1. Briggs, *A Social History of England,* 216, 245.

2. James Crichton-Browne, quoted in C. L. Robertson, "A Further Note." P. Martin Duncan, "On Insanity," *Journal of Science* 7 (1870): 165–186. C. L. Robertson, "A Further Note," quoting Arlidge. Harrington Tuke, "Presidential Address." Jamieson, quoted in Hare, "Was Insanity on the Increase?"

3. Ruskin: Jamison, *Touched with Fire,* 96. Weldon: K. Jones, *A History,* 167–169.

4. *The Times,* November 22, 1867, 5b, and May 16, 1876, 11f.

5. *Journal of Mental Science* 30 (1884): 451. W. J. Corbet, "The Increase of Insanity," *Fortnightly Review* 65, n.s. 59 (1896): 431–442. Mellett, *The Prerogative of Asylumdom,* 90, quoting *The Referee,* 1902.

6. Robert Louis Stevenson, *The Strange Case of Dr. Jekyll and Mr. Hyde,* in Charles Neider (ed.), *The Complete Short Stories of Robert Louis Stevenson* (Garden City, N.Y.: Doubleday and Co., 1969), 482, 513–514.

7. Bram Stoker, *Dracula* (New York: Penguin Books, 1993; first published in 1897), 95–96, 143.

8. *Museum of Foreign Literature* 14 (1829): 39–67.

9. Finlayson, *Seventh Earl,* 590, 591. K. Jones, *A History,* 171.

10. *Journal of Mental Science* 39 (1893): 560; 41 (1895): 100; 41 (1896): 140; 45 (1899): 139; and 44 (1898): 113.

11. Humphreys, "Statistics of Insanity."

12. *Special Report, 1897,* 16.

13. C. L. Robertson, "The Care and Treatment."

14. Lancaster: Walton, "Casting Out." Buckingham: Crammer, *Asylum History.* Colney Hatch: Richard Hunter and Ida Macalpine, *Psychiatry for the Poor: 1851 Colney Hatch Asylum–Friern Hospital 1973; A Medical and Social History* (London: Dawsons of Pall Mall, 1974). Hook Norton: Parry-Jones, *Trade in Lunacy,* 207–210. Humphreys, "Statistics of Lunacy." Robert Wilkins, "Hallucinations in Children and Teenagers Admitted to Bethlem Royal Hospital in the Nineteenth Century and Their Possible Relevance to the Incidence of Schizophrenia," *Journal of Child Psychology and Psychiatry* 28 (1987): 569–580. D. H. Tuke, *A Dictionary of Psychological Medicine* (Philadelphia: Blakiston, 1892).

15. Vieda Skultans, *English Madness,* 120.

16. William Farr: Humphreys, "Statistics of Lunacy," 232–235, and A. Mitchell, "Contribution to the Study of Death Rates of Persons in Asylums," *Journal of Mental Science* 25 (1879): 1–4. Lunacy Commission Report: *Journal of Mental Science* 52

(1906): 142–147. 49 percent: John Walton, "The Treatment of Pauper Lunatics in Victorian England: The Case of Lancaster Asylum 1816–70," in Andrew Scull (ed.), *Madhouses, Mad-Doctors, and Madmen: The Social History of Psychiatry in the Victorian Era* (Philadelphia: University of Pennsylvania Press, 1981), 171.

17. John T. Arlidge, *On the State of Lunacy and the Legal Provision for the Insane* (London: Churchill, 1859). Andrew Scull, *Social Order/Mental Disorder*, 231.

18. "Asylum Reports," *Journal of Mental Science* 44 (1898): 195. Charles Williams, *Insanity: Its Causes and Prevention* (London: Ambrose, 1908).

19. *Journal of Mental Science* 47 (1901): 117–126.

20. 11 to 12 percent: Parry-Jones, *Trade in Lunacy*, 216, and "57th Report," *Journal of Mental Science* 50 (1904): 119–124. 7 to 8 percent: Hare, "Was Insanity on the Increase?" Robertson noted: C. L. Robertson, "The Care and Treatment."

21. R. R. Parker et al., "County of Lancaster Asylum, Rainhill: 100 Years Ago and Now," *History of Psychiatry* 4 (1993): 95–105. Trevor Turner, "Rich and Mad in Victorian England," *Psychological Medicine* 19 (1989): 29–44. Edward B. Renvoize and Allan W. Beveridge, "Mental Illness and the Late Victorians: A Study of Patients Admitted to Three Asylums in York, 1880–1884," *Psychological Medicine* 19 (1989): 19–28. Franklin Klaf and John Hamilton, "Schizophrenia—A Hundred Years Ago and Today," *Journal of Mental Science* 107 (1961): 819–827. Parry-Jones, *Trade in Lunacy*, 328–330.

22. *Journal of Mental Science* 44 (1898): 113–126. *Journal of Mental Science* 45 (1899): 139–148.

23. Haguch, "Comments on the Report."

24. Corbet: "Plain Speaking about Lunacy," *Westminster Review* 148 (1897): 117–125; "The Increase of Insanity," 1896; "The Increase of Insanity," *Fortnightly Review* 59, n.s. 53 (1893): 7–19.

25. *The Times*, August 28, 1903, 7f. "56th Report," *Journal of Mental Science* 49 (1903): 126.

26. "Lunacy in 1900," *The Times*, August 5, 1901, 9a. Corbet, "The Holocaust."

27. *The Times*, April 14, 1906, 5a, and April 21, 1906, 4a.

28. *The Times*, March 30, 1907, 4a. Letter to the Editor, *The Times*, April 21, 1906, 4c. Winslow and Allbutt: *The Times*, January 2, 1907, 6c.

29. Maudsley: Janet Saunders, "Quarantining the Weak-Minded: Psychiatric Definitions of Degeneracy and the Late-Victorian Asylum," in Bynum et al., *Anatomy of Madness*, 294. "What can be done": W. J. Corbet, "The Progress of Insanity in Our Time," *Westminster Review* 163 (1905): 198–211. Robert Jones, "The Evolution of Insanity," *Journal of Mental Science* 52 (1906): 629–661. Allan Beveridge, "Thomas Clouston and the Edinburgh School of Psychiatry," in Berrios and Freeman, *150 Years*, 379.

30. T.E.K. Stansfield, "Heredity and Insanity," *Journal of Mental Science* 57 (1911): 55–63. E. Faulks, "The Sterilisation of the Insane," *Journal of Mental Science* 57 (1911): 36–74. Geoffrey Clarke, "Sterilization from the Eugenic Standpoint," *Journal of Mental Science* 58 (1912): 48–49.

31. Crammer, *Asylum History*, 75.

32. Crammer, *Asylum History*, 77.

33. William Ober, *Boswell's Clap and Other Essays: Medical Analyses of Literary Men's Afflictions* (Carbondale: Southern Illinois University Press, 1979), 438.

34. Claridge et al., *Sounds from the Bell Jar*, 183. Nancy Topping Bazin, "Postmortem Diagnoses of Virginia Woolf's 'Madness': The Precarious Quest for Truth," in

Branimir M. Rieger (ed.), *Dionysus in Literature* (Bowling Green, Ohio: Bowling Green State University Popular Press, 1994), 139.

35. Virginia Woolf to Gwen Roverat, May 1, 1925, in Nigel Nicolson and Joanne Trautsmann (eds.), *The Letters of Virginia Woolf: Vol. III: 1923–28* (New York: Harcourt Brace Jovanovich, 1978), 180. Virginia Woolf, *Mrs. Dalloway* (New York: Knopf, 1993), 23.

36. Malcolm I. Ingraham, "Virginia Woolf—Suicide," *Beneath a Rougher Sea: Virginia Woolf's Psychiatric History,* January 8, 2001 <http://ourworld.compuserve.com/homepages/malcolmi/suicide.htm>.

37. Jones, *A History,* 270.

38. H. Freeman and M. Alpert, "Prevalence of Schizophrenia in an Urban Population," *British Journal of Psychiatry* 149 (1986): 603–611.

39. Halliday, "A Report."

40. Michael Shepherd, *A Study of the Major Psychoses in an English County* (London: Chapman and Hall, 1957).

41. N. Takei et al., "Cities, Winter Birth, and Schizophrenia," *Lancet* 340 (1992): 558.

42. Porter, *Mind-Forg'd Manacles,* 83.

43. G. Harrison et al., "Increased Incidence of Psychotic Disorders in Migrants from the Caribbean to the United Kingdom," *Psychological Medicine* 27 (1997): 799–806. Raymond Cochrane and Sukhwant S. Bal, "Migration and Schizophrenia: An Examination of Five Hypotheses," *Social Psychiatry* 221 (1987): 181–191.

44. Geoffrey Der, Sunjai Gupta, and Robin M. Murray, *Lancet* 335 (1990): 513–516. John M. Eagles, *British Journal of Psychiatry* 158 (1991): 834–835.

45. England and Scotland: G. Harrison, J. E. Cooper, and R. Gancarczyk, "Changes in the Administrative Incidence of Schizophrenia," *British Journal of Psychiatry* 159 (1991): 811–816, and J. Allardyce et al., "Schizophrenia Is Not Disappearing in South-West Scotland," *British Journal of Psychiatry* 177 (2000): 38–41. Schizophrenia as a more benign disease: G. Harrison and P. Mason, "Schizophrenia—Falling Incidence and Better Outcome?" *British Journal of Psychiatry* 163 (1993): 535–541.

7. The Road to Grangegorman

1. Jonathan Swift, "Verses on the Death of Dr. Swift, D.S.D.," 1731, quoted in E. Fuller Torrey et al., "Endemic Psychosis in Western Ireland," *American Journal of Psychiatry* 141 (1984): 966–970.

2. Mark Finnane, *Insanity and the Insane in Post-Famine Ireland* (London: Croom Helm, 1981), 13.

3. *1851 Census,* 59.

4. As early as 1684: Robins, *Fools and Mad,* 27. In 1708: Elizabeth Malcolm, *Swift's Hospital: A History of St. Patrick's Hospital, 1746–1989* (Dublin: Gill and Macmillan, 1989), 17.

5. About 1750: Robins, *Fools and Mad,* 11. For the dangerously mad: *1817 Report,* 23.

6. Robins, *Fools and Mad,* 42. Jonathan Swift, "A Digression concerning Madness," in *Tale of a Tub* (Oxford: Clarendon Press, 1958; originally published in 1704). "Even I myself": Swift quoted in Doerner, *Madness and the Bourgeoisie,* 33. Jonathan Swift, "A Character, Panegyric, and Description of the Legion Club," 1736, in Harold Williams (ed.), *The Poems of Jonathan Swift* (Oxford: Clarendon Press, 1937).

7. W. J. Corbet, "On the Increase of Insanity," *American Journal of Insanity* 50 (1893): 224–238.

8. Dublin's workhouse: *1851 Report*, 63. In Cork: Robins, *Fools and Mad*, 57. French visitor and 1787 Act: Robins, *Fools and Mad*, 37, 39.

9. William S. Hallaran, *An Enquiry* (Cork, U.K.: Edwards and Savage, 1810), 2, 24.

10. Robins, *Fools and Mad*, 62.

11. D. H. Tuke, *Chapters in the History*, 401. *1817 Report*, 9.

12. "Report for the Committee of the House of Commons on Mad-Houses," *Pamphleteer* 6 (1815): 257. Burrows, *An Inquiry*, 1820.

13. *Report of the Select Committee on the Lunatic Poor, 1817*.

14. *Report of the Select Committee, 1817*, 12, 14.

15. *Report of the Select Committee, 1817*, 15.

16. Halliday, *A General View, 1828*, 33.

17. Arnold Schrier, *Ireland and the American Emigration, 1850–1900* (New York: Russell and Russell, 1958), 83.

18. Robins, *Fools and Mad*, 33.

19. Census figures: Halliday, *A General View*, 1828; *1851 Census*, 49; and D. H. Tuke, *Chapters in the History*, 414. 1841: "Mental Epidemics," *Dublin Review* 10 (1841): 348–382.

20. Finnane, *Insanity and the Insane*, 18.

21. Finnane, *Insanity and the Insane*, 28. English visitor: Robins, *Fools and Mad*, 76.

22. In 1828: Robins, *Fools and Mad*, 59. In 1838: Finnane, *Insanity and the Insane*, 90.

23. Galway: Alfred J. Bollet, *Plagues and Poxes: The Rise and Fall of Epidemic Disease* (New York: Demos Publications, 1987), 62. Cork and Queens: K. Miller, *Emigrants and Exiles*, 284–291. Connaught and Munster: Schrier, *Ireland and the American Emigration*, 166.

24. 1854: Finnane, *Insanity and the Insane*, 37. Asylum costs: Finnane, *Insanity and the Insane*, 228. 1871: Mark Finnane, "Law and the Social Uses of the Asylum in Nineteenth-Century Ireland," in Dylan R. Tomlinson and John Carrier (eds.), *Asylum in the Community* (London: Routledge, 1996), 91–110.

25. Finnane, *Insanity and the Insane*, 106. "Annual Report," *Journal of Mental Science* 14 (1869): 544.

26. F. MacCabe, "On the Alleged Increase in Lunacy," *Journal of Mental Science* 15 (1869): 363–366.

27. K. Miller, *Emigrants and Exiles*, 37.

28. *1851 Census*. Connaught: K. Miller, *Emigrants and Exiles*, 37.

29. *Report of the Commissioners, 1856*, 2. P. M. Duncan, "On Insanity," 1870. Anonymous, "Increase in Insanity," *American Journal of Insanity* 18 (1861): 95.

30. Annual admissions: Finnane, *Insanity and the Insane*, 232. *Report, 1856*, 22. "34th Report," *Journal of Mental Science* 32 (1886): 78.

31. *Report from Lunacy Inquiry, 1878–79*. "40th Report," *Journal of Mental Science* 38 (1892):103. "45th Report, 1895," *Journal of Mental Science* 43 (1897): 143.

32. Finnane, *Insanity and the Insane*, 180–186.

33. Finnane, *Insanity and the Insane*, 209–210.

34. *Journal of Mental Science* 13 (1868): 470. *Journal of Mental Science* 51 (1905): 162. *Report from Lunacy Inquiry, 1878–79*. Finnane, *Insanity and the Insane*, 71. M. J. Nolan, "The Insane in Workhouses," *Journal of Mental Science* 40 (1894): 621–629.

35. "34th Report," *Journal of Mental Science* 32 (1886): 77. D. H. Tuke, *Chapters in the History*, 424.
36. Finnane, *Insanity and the Insane*, 230.
37. Richmond: *Journal of Mental Science* 10 (1865): 433. Ulster: Finnane, *Insanity and the Insane*, 70. Leitrim and Sligo: "51st Report, 1901," *Journal of Mental Science* 49 (1903): 141. Monaghan: Finnane, *Insanity and the Insane*, 77.
38. I. A. Eames, "Presidential Address," *Journal of Mental Science* 31 (1885): 315–317. J. F. Duncan, "President's Address," *Journal of Mental Science* 21 (1875): 322–339. *Journal of Mental Science* 23 (1878): 585. *40th Report, 1890.*
39. This paragraph and next: *1894 Special Report.*
40. "27th Report," *Journal of Mental Science* 25 (1879): 633.
41. Clouston discussion in D. H. Tuke, "Increase of Insanity in Ireland," *Journal of Mental Science* 40 (1894): 561.
42. Reviews, *Journal of Mental Science* 41 (1895): 325. Robins, *Fools and Mad*, 102.
43. W. J. Corbet, "Is Insanity on the Increase?" *Fortnightly Review* 41 (1884): 482–494.
44. Corbet, "The Increase of Insanity" (1896), and "Is the Increase of Insanity Real or Only 'Apparent'?" *Westminster Review* 147 (1897): 539–550.
45. *47th Report, 1897.*
46. Thomas Drapes, "Is Insanity Increasing?" *Fortnightly Review* 66 (1896): 483–493. "46th Report," *Journal of Mental Science* 44 (1898): 134. "50th Report," *Journal of Mental Science* 48 (1902): 92. "51st Report," *Journal of Mental Science* 49 (1903): 139.
47. "47th Report," *Journal of Mental Science* 45 (1899): 156.
48. *1906 Special Report.*
49. The asylum discharge rates and reports of homicide: Finnane, *Insanity and the Insane*, 154, 234. Irish officials: Thomas Drapes, "On the Alleged Increase of Insanity in Ireland," *Journal of Mental Science* 40 (1894): 519–543.
50. Finnane, *Insanity and the Insane*, 100. Lindsay Prior, "The Appeal to Madness in Ireland," in Tomlinson and Carrier (eds.), *Asylum in the Community*, 84.
51. *1906 Special Report.* Asylum admissions: Finnane, *Insanity and the Insane*, 143.
52. *1906 Special Report*, xxiii.
53. *1906 Special Report*, viii, xix. *40th Report, 1890.* "41st Report, 1891," *Journal of Mental Science* 39 (1893): 83.
54. Tuke, "Increase of Insanity in Ireland." *61st Report, 1911.*
55. *1906 Special Report*, xxv, xxvii.
56. *43rd Report, 1894.*
57. C. A. Cameron, "Consanguineous Marriages in Relation to Deaf-Mutism," *Transactional Academy of Medicine in Ireland*, 1883; S. J. Kilpatrick, J. D. Mathers, and A. C. Stevenson, "The Importance of Population Fertility and Consanguinity Data Being Available in Medico-Social Studies: Some Data on Consanguineous Marriages in Northern Ireland," *Ulster Medical Journal* 24 (1955): 113–122; Newton Freire-Maia, "Inbreeding Levels in Different Countries," *Eugenics Quarterly* 4 (1957): 127–138; and J. G. Masterson, "Consanguinity in Ireland," *Human Heredity* 20 (1970): 371–382. A. H. Ahmed, "Consanguinity and Schizophrenia in Sudan," *British Journal of Psychiatry* 134 (1979): 635–636, and L. Saugsted and O. Odegaard, "Inbreeding and Schizophrenia," *Clinical Genetics* 30 (1986): 261–275.
58. Kenneth S. Kendler et al., "The Roscommon Family Study: I. Methods, Diagnosis

of Probands, and Risk of Schizophrenia in Relatives," *Archives of General Psychiatry* 50 (1993): 527–540.

59. *61st Report, 1911.* "Johnny Jump-Up," no composer listed, from Mudcat Café, April 9, 2001 <http://www.mudcat.org/>.

60. Finnane, *Insanity and the Insane*, 73, 74.

61. David Healy, "Irish Psychiatry, Part 2: Use of Medico-Psychological Association by Its Irish Members—*Plus ça change!*" in Berrios and Freeman, *150 Years*, 286–287.

62. *J. M. Synge: Collected Works*, vol. 2, Alan Frederick Price (ed.) (London: Oxford University Press, 1966), 29, 188.

63. *John Synge: Collected Works*, vol. 2, 209, 216–217.

64. *68th Report, 1918*, 1919.

65. "62nd Report," *Journal of Mental Science* 60 (1914): 307; "an eminent specialist": "59th Report," *Journal of Mental Science* 57 (1911): 134.

66. W. R. Dawson, "The Presidential Address on the Relation between the Geographical Distribution of Insanity and That of Certain Social and Other Conditions in Ireland," *Journal of Mental Science* 57 (1911): 571–597.

67. Robins, *Fools and Mad*, 183.

68. William M. Murphy, *Prodigal Father: The Life of John Butler Yeats (1839–1922)* (Ithaca, N.Y.: Cornell University Press, 1978), 84, 268–269, 373, 382.

69. W. B. Yeats in Peter Allt and Russell K. Alspach (eds.), *The Variorum Edition of the Poems of W. B. Yeats* (New York: Macmillan, 1957).

70. Balachandra Rajan, *W. B. Yeats: A Critical Introduction* (London: Hutchinson University Library, 1965), 148–149.

71. Richard Ellmann, *James Joyce* (New York: Oxford University Press, 1982), 611, 645.

72. Ellmann, *James Joyce*, 650, 663.

73. Ellmann, *James Joyce*, 679, 685.

74. Ellmann, *James Joyce*, 662, 678.

75. N.J.C. Andreason, "James Joyce—A Portrait of the Artist as a Schizoid," *JAMA* 224 (1973): 67–71.

76. Ellmann, *James Joyce*, 649.

77. Samuel Beckett, *Malone Dies* (New York: Grove Press, 1956), 108, 112, 113–114, and *Not I*, in *Collected Shorter Plays* (New York: Grove Press, Inc., 1984), 214–223.

78. Sean O'Casey, *Drums under the Window: Autobiographies*, vol. 1 (London: Macmillan, 1980), 76–77.

79. O'Casey, *Drums under the Window*, 68.

80. Dermot Walsh, "Hospitalized Psychiatric Morbidity in the Republic of Ireland," *British Journal of Psychiatry* 114 (1968): 11–14. Dermot Walsh and Brendan Walsh, "Mental Illness in the Republic of Ireland—First Admissions," *Journal of the Irish Medical Association* 63 (1970): 365–370. Cochrane and Bal, "Migration and Schizophrenia," 1987.

81. M. J. Kelleher and J.R.M. Copeland, "Psychiatric Diagnosis in Cork and London: The Results of a Cross-National Pilot Study," *Journal of the Irish Medical Association* 66 (1973): 553–557, and M. J. Kelleher and J.R.M. Copeland, "Psychiatric Diagnosis in Ireland: A Videotape Study," *Journal of the Irish Medical Association* 67 (1974): 87–92. E. F. Torrey et al., "Endemic Psychosis in Western Ireland," *American Journal of Psychiatry* 141 (1984): 966–970, and Kendler et al., "The Roscommon Family Study: I."

82. Dermot Walsh, *The 1963 Irish Psychiatric Hospital Census* (Dublin: Medico-Social Research Board, 1970).

83. Laffan, *American Journal of Insanity* 53 (1896): 440, originally cited in the *British Medical Journal*. Hanafy A. Youssef, Anthony Kinsella, and John L. Waddington, "Evidence for Geographical Variations in the Prevalence of Schizophrenia in Rural Ireland," *Archives of General Psychiatry* 48 (1991): 254–258. Hanafy A. Youssef et al., "Geographical Variation in Rate of Schizophrenia in Rural Ireland by Place at Birth vs Place at Onset," *Schizophrenia Research* 32 (1999): 233–243. John Waddington, personal communication, January 1995. Torrey et al., "Endemic Psychosis."

84. Roscommon: Torrey et al., "Endemic Psychosis," and Kendler et al., "The Roscommon Family Study: I." Cavan: John L. Waddington and Hanafy A. Youssef, "Evidence for a Gender-Specific Decline in the Rate of Schizophrenia in Rural Ireland over a 50-Year Period," *British Journal of Psychiatry* 164 (1994): 171–176. This decline: Máirin ni Nuállain, Aileen O'Hare, Dermot Walsh, et al., "The Incidence of Mental Illness in Ireland—Patients Contacting Psychiatric Services in Three Irish Counties," *Irish Journal of Psychiatry* 5 (1984): 23–29, and N. Sartorius et al., "Early Manifestations and First-Contact Incidence of Schizophrenia in Different Cultures," *Psychological Medicine* 16 (1986): 909–928.

85. M. R. Cabot, "The Incidence and Prevalence of Schizophrenia in the Republic of Ireland," *Social Psychiatry and Psychiatric Epidemiology* 25 (1990): 210–215. Dermot Walsh and Kenneth Kendler, "The Prevalence of Schizophrenia in Ireland," *Archives of General Psychiatry* 51 (1994): 513–515.

8. "A Constantly Increasing Multitude"

1. Henry Hurd, *The Institutional Care of the Insane in the United States and Canada*, vol. 4 (Baltimore: Johns Hopkins University Press, 1916–1917), 241.

2. Hurd, *The Institutional Care*, vol. 4, 245, 252–254.

3. Hurd, *The Institutional Care*, vol. 4, 37.

4. Daniel Francis, "The Development of the Lunatic Asylum in the Maritime Provinces," in S.E.D. Shortt (ed.) *Medicine in Canadian Society: Historical Perspectives* (Montreal: McGill-Queen's University Press, 1981), 94, 97.

5. Francis, "Development of the Lunatic Asylum," 98. *New Brunswick Journals of the House of Assembly* (*NB JHA*), 1875. Hurd, *The Institutional Care*, vol. 4, 63, 76.

6. The first patients: Francis, "Development of the Lunatic Asylum," 100. Other quotes are from Hurd, *The Institutional Care*, vol. 4, 93, 94.

7. 1836: Hurd, *The Institutional Care*, vol. 4, 97. 1851: Daniel Francis, "That Prison on the Hill: The Historical Origins of the Lunatic Asylum in the Maritime Provinces" (M.A. thesis, Institute of Canadian Studies, Carlton University, Ottawa, 1975), 126. 1849: K. Miller, *Emigrants and Exiles*, 296. 1871: Francis, "That Prison on the Hill," 126. 1885: D. H. Tuke, *The Insane in the United States and Canada* (London: H. K. Lewis, 1885), 240.

8. Francis, "That Prison on the Hill," 63.

9. T.J.W. Burgess, "Presidential Address: The Insane in Canada," *Montreal Medical Journal* 34 (1905): 401. Francis, "That Prison on the Hill," 111.

10. Francis, "That Prison on the Hill," 107.

11. Francis, "That Prison on the Hill," 40, and 25, quoting the *Saint John Daily*

Evening News, October 23, 1882; railroad travel, citing *NB JHA*, 1851, Appendix. *NB JHA*, 1878.

12. Francis, "That Prison on the Hill," 42.
13. Hurd, *The Institutional Care*, vol. 4, 56. *NB JHA*, 1868, 5. Francis, "That Prison on the Hill," 73, quoting the *Saint John Daily Telegraph*, in 1895, 112.
14. *NB JHA*, 1861, 8.
15. Hurd, *The Institutional Care*, vol. 4, 203.
16. Hurd, *The Institutional Care*, vol. 4, 203, 204.
17. Hurd, *The Institutional Care*, vol. 4, 208. Mackieson: Peter E. Rider, "'A Blot upon the Fair Fame of Our Island': The Scandal at the Charlottetown Lunatic Asylum, 1874," *Island Magazine* 39 (1996): 3–9.
18. *Prince Edward Island Journals of the House of Assembly* (*PEI JHA*) asylum reports.
19. *PEI JHA*, 1856, Appendix R. Hurd, *The Institutional Care*, vol. 4, 211. *PEI JHA*, 1871, Appendix CC.
20. *PEI JHA*, 1875, Appendix G.
21. Hurd, *The Institutional Care*, vol. 4, 213. Mackieson: Rider, "'A Blot.'"
22. *Examiner*: Rider, "'A Blot.'" At this time: Wendy Mitchinson, "Reasons for Committal to a Mid-Nineteenth-Century Ontario Insane Asylum: The Case of Toronto," in Wendy Mitchinson and Janice Dickin McGinnis (eds.), *Essays in the History of Canadian Medicine* (Toronto: McClelland and Stewart, 1988), 88–109. "We can lose nothing" and Blanchard: Hurd, *The Institutional Care*, vol. 4, 213, 215.
23. Blanchard: "Report of the Medical Superintendent," *PEI JHA*, 1878, 7. Lunatic asylum: Margaret Atwood, *Alias Grace* (Toronto: Seal Books, 1997), 556.
24. "Superintendent's Report, 1881," *PEI JHA*, 8. "Superintendent's Report, 1885," *PEI JHA*, 10.
25. *PEI JHA*, 1898, 7.
26. William S. MacNutt, *The Atlantic Provinces: The Emergence of Colonial Society 1712–1857* (London: Oxford University Press, 1965), 156.
27. Patricia O'Brien, *Out of Mind, Out of Sight: A History of the Waterford Hospital* (St. John's: Breakwater Books, 1989), 25.
28. 1834 and 1836: Melvin Baker, "Insanity and Politics: The Establishment of a Lunatic Asylum in St. John's, Newfoundland, 1836–1855," *Newfoundland Quarterly* 77, nos. 2–3 (1981): 27–31. The chief justice: O'Brien, *Out of Mind*, 25.
29. Stabb's background and interest: Baker, "Insanity and Politics." Stabb's views on the insane: O'Brien, *Out of Mind*, 8, 27.
30. O'Brien, *Out of Mind*, 31, and *Newfoundland Journals of the House of Assembly* (*Nfld JHA*), 1845, Appendix.
31. O'Brien, *Out of Mind*, 34, 37.
32. *Nfld JHA*, 1849, Appendix 151. O'Brien, *Out of Mind*, 65.
33. O'Brien, *Out of Mind*, 65, 68.
34. "Report of the Physician," *Nfld JHA*, 1849, 154. O'Brien, *Out of Mind*, 79.
35. O'Brien, *Out of Mind*, 90.
36. *Nfld JHA*, 1856, Appendix 232. *Nfld JHA*, 1858, Appendix 520.
37. *Nfld JHA*, 1859, Miscellaneous. O'Brien, *Out of Mind*, 95.
38. O'Brien, *Out of Mind*, 90. *Nfld JHA*, 1870, Appendix, 753.
39. O'Brien, *Out of Mind*, 60.

40. Stabb's family: O'Brien, *Out of Mind*, 74. *Nfld JHA*, 1868, Appendix 559. O'Brien, *Out of Mind*, 71. *Nfld JHA*, 1886, Appendix 771.

41. O'Brien, *Out of Mind*, 116.

42. Judith Fingard, *The Dark Side of Life in Victorian Halifax* (Porters Lake, N.S.: Pottersfield Press, 1989), 17. Relief: MacKay, "Poor Relief and Medicine in Nova Scotia, 1749–1783," *Collections of the Nova Scotia Historical Society* 24 (1938): 33–56. Allan E. Marble, *Surgeons, Smallpox, and the Poor: A History of Medicine and Social Conditions in Nova Scotia, 1749–1799* (Montreal and Kingston: McGill–Queen's University Press, 1993), 79.

43. Francis, "That Prison on the Hill," 49.

44. The Poor's Asylum Admissions Register, 1802–1811, and Public Archives of Nova Scotia, RG 35–102, series 33, #1.

45. *Nova Scotia Journals of the House of Assembly* (*NS JHA*), 1832, Appendix 49. *NS JHA*, March 19, 1830.

46. Much of the increase: Francis, "That Prison on the Hill," 55. That winter: Alexa Bagnell, "Houses of the Insane: Social Influences on the Formation of the Lunatic Asylum in Nova Scotia" (graduate student paper, funded by the Hannah Institute of the History of Medicine, summer 1994).

47. 1844 report: Bagnell, *Houses of the Insane. NS JHA*, 1846, Appendix 32. *NS JLC* (*Journals of Legislative Council*), 1847. Harvey's son: letter from Hugh Bell to Dorothea Dix, August 10, 1850, Dix Papers, file 41, Houghton Library, Harvard University.

48. *NS JHA*, 1847, Appendix 11.

49. *NS JHA*, 1847, Appendix 11.

50. He immediately offered: A. H. MacDonald, *Mount Hope Then and Now: A History of the Nova Scotia Hospital* (Dartmouth, N.S.: Nova Scotia Hospital, 1996), 15. Poor's Asylum: Dorothy M. Grant, "We Shall Conquer Yet!" *Nova Scotia Historical Quarterly* 2 (3) (1972): 243–251. Bell noted: *NS JHA*, 1846, Appendix 32. Bell said: Bagnell, *Houses of the Insane.*

51. Bagnell, *Houses of the Insane*, and *NS JHA*, 1846, Appendix 32.

52. *NS JHA*, 1850, Appendix 18.

53. *NS JHA*, 1850, Appendix 18 (Dix's petition is dated December 10, 1849).

54. A. H. MacDonald, *Mount Hope Then and Now*, 22, and Bell to Dix, June 10, 1850, Dix Papers, file 41, Houghton Library, Harvard. Bagnell, *Houses of the Insane. British Colonist*, June 18, 1853, quoted in A. H. MacDonald, *Mount Hope Then and Now*, 28.

55. Grant, "We Shall Conquer Yet!"

56. Francis, "Development of the Lunatic Asylum," 106. "The Death Penalty," *Nova Scotian*, December 25, 1854, and January 1, 1855. "Horrible Murder on St. Mary's Road," *The Nova Scotian*, August 28, 1854, 3.

57. Hurd, *The Institutional Care*, vol. 4, 119, quoting F. S. Cozzens, "Acadia."

58. A. H. MacDonald, *Mount Hope Then and Now*, 42, and *NS JHA*, 1860, Appendix, 37–372. Hurd, *The Institutional Care*, vol. 4, 119.

59. A. H. MacDonald, *Mount Hope Then and Now*, 56. *NS JHA*, 1864, Appendix 10. *NS JHA*, 1865, Appendix 8.

60. Francis, "Development of the Lunatic Asylum," 106.

61. *NS JHA*, 1876, Appendix 3.

62. *NS JHA*, 1883. *NS JHA*, 1869, Appendix 2.

63. *NS JHA*, 1876, Appendix 3. *NS JHA*, 1899, Appendix 3A.

64. *Census of Nova Scotia, 1861*, 296–297. Helen Creighton, *Songs and Ballads of Nova Scotia*, no. 74, Collected from Ben Henneberry of Devil's Island, Nova Scotia.

65. 1861: Francis, "That Prison on the Hill," 111. 1867: Francis, "Development of the Lunatic Asylum," 109. 1877: Francis, "That Prison on the Hill," 113.

66. *NS JHA*, 1881, Appendix 3A. *NS JHA*, 1883.

67. *NS JHA*, 1894.

68. *NS JHA*, 1897, Appendix 3A. *NS JHA*, 1898.

69. *NS JHA*, 1902.

70. *Fourth Census of Canada, 1901*, Bulletin IX (Ottawa: Census Office, 1902).

71. Burgess, "The Insane in Canada."

72. "Report of the Superintendent of the Provincial Hospital at St. John, NB, for the Year 1912," *Journals of the Proceedings of the House of Assembly, 1912* (Provincial Archives of New Brunswick).

73. O'Brien, *Out of Mind*, 124, 248.

74. *NS JHA*, 1904, Appendix 3. *NS JHA*, 1906. *NS JHA*, 1909.

75. Farnsworth Crowder, "But Is the World Going Mad?" *Survey Graphic* 26 (1937): 219–220.

76. Mental Health Section, Statistics Canada (Dominion Bureau of Statistics).

77. R. C. Bland, "Long-Term Mental Illness in Canada: An Epidemiological Perspective on Schizophrenia and Affective Disorders," *Canadian Journal of Psychiatry* 29 (1984): 242–246.

78. Goeree et al., "The Economic Burden."

79. Hurd, *The Institutional Care*, vol. 4, 254.

9. "The Disease Whose Frequency Has Become Alarming"

1. Richard H. Shryock, "The Beginnings: From Colonial Days to the Foundation of the American Psychiatric Association," in American Psychiatric Association, *One Hundred Years of American Psychiatry* (New York: Columbia University Press, 1944), 28.

2. Albert Deutsch, *The Mentally Ill in America* (New York: Columbia University Press, 1946), 43, cited by Larry D. Eldridge, "'Crazy Brained': Mental Illness in Colonial America," *Bulletin of the History of Medicine* 70 (1996): 361–386. Henry R. Viets, "Some Features of the History of Medicine in Massachusetts during the Colonial Period (1620–1770)," *Isis* 23 (1935): 389–405. Population figures for the colonies are taken from Evarts B. Greene, *American Population before the Federal Census of 1790* (Gloucester, Mass.: Peter Smith, 1966), and U.S. Department of Commerce, *Historical Statistics of the United States* (Washington, D.C.: Government Printing Office, 1975).

3. Gerald Grob, *The Mad among Us: A History of the Care of America's Mentally Ill* (Cambridge, Mass.: Harvard University Press, 1994), 15. Jimenez, *Changing Faces of Madness*, 39.

4. Hurd, *The Institutional Care*, vol. 2, 57.

5. Deutsch, *The Mentally Ill in America*, 37, quoting a 1692 letter.

6. Jimenez, *Changing Faces of Madness*, 38.

7. Mather, quoted in Jimenez, *Changing Faces of Madness*, 15.

8. By 1727: Hurd, *The Institutional Care*, vol. 2, 67–68. Roberts and Humphrey: Deutsch, *The Mentally Ill in America*, 46, 51.

9. Grob, *The Mad among Us,* 17.

10. Deutsch, *The Mentally Ill in America,* 67–68. Hurd, *The Institutional Care,* vol. 2, 58.

11. Jimenez, *Changing Faces of Madness,* 9, 23, 33–34, 41, 157.

12. Jimenez, *Changing Faces of Madness,* 35–36. Jimenez, personal communication, December 23, 1994. Norman Dain, *Concepts of Insanity in the United States, 1789–1865* (New Brunswick, N.J.: Rutgers University Press, 1964), 35, quoting William Tudor, a prominent Boston philanthropist. Waterston, "The Insane in Massachusetts."

13. Deutsch, *The Mentally Ill in America,* 59.

14. Orpheus Everts, "The American System of Public Provision for the Insane, and Despotism in Lunatic Asylums," *American Journal of Insanity* 38 (1881): 113–139. Nancy Tomes, *A Generous Confidence: Thomas Story Kirkbride and the Art of Asylum Keeping, 1840–1883* (Cambridge, U.K.: Cambridge University Press, 1984), 27, 28.

15. Tomes, *A Generous Confidence,* 266. Persaud, "The Reporting of Psychiatric Symptoms."

16. Thomas G. Morton, *A History of the Pennsylvania Hospital* (Philadelphia: Times Printing House, 1895), 131. Gerald Grob, *Mental Institutions in America: Social Policy to 1875* (New York: Free Press, 1973), 20. Morton, *A History of the Pennsylvania Hospital,* 131.

17. Persaud, "The Reporting of Psychiatric Symptoms." Tomes, *A Generous Confidence,* 333–334. David Danbom, *Born in the Country: A History of Rural America* (Baltimore: Johns Hopkins University Press, 1995), 60.

18. Benjamin Rush, *Medical Inquiries and Observations upon the Diseases of the Mind* (Philadelphia: Grigg, 1830), 64. George Hayward, *Some Observations on Dr. Rush's Work, on the Diseases of the Mind,* 1818. Rush's belief: Tomes, *A Generous Confidence,* 29.

19. Norman Dain, *Disordered Minds: The First Century of Eastern State Hospital in Williamsburg, Virginia, 1766–1866* (Williamsburg, Va.: Colonial Williamsburg Foundation, 1971), 7, 8.

20. Danbom, *Born in the Country,* 52–53. Grob, *Mental Institutions in America,* 24.

21. Hurd, *The Institutional Care,* vol. 3, 581. Peter McCandless, *Moonlight, Magnolias and Madness: Insanity in South Carolina from the Colonial Period to the Progressive Era* (Chapel Hill: University of North Carolina Press, 1996), 23.

22. New York City: Hurd, *The Institutional Care,* vol. 3, 110. The proposal: Grob, *Mental Institutions in America,* 30.

23. Edward Cutbush, *An Inaugural Dissertation on Insanity* (Philadelphia: Zachariah Poulson, Jr., 1794), 25.

24. Smith: Charles Brockden Brown, *Three Gothic Novels* (Library of America, 1998), 902. Paul S. Steinberg, *On the Brink of the Precipice: Madness in the Writings of Charles Brockden Brown* (Ann Arbor, Mich.: University Microfilms International Dissertation Services, 1982), 2, quoting Harry Warfel. Lulu Rumsey Wiley, *The Sources and Influence of the Novels of Charles Brockden Brown* (New York: Vantage Press, 1950), 44. Bowdoin papers, no page given. Charles Brockden Brown, *Ormond,* Ernest Marchand (ed.) (New York: Hafner Publishing Company, 1962), xxxviii–xxxix. Nathaniel Hawthorne, *Mosses from an Old Manse* (Columbus: Ohio State University Press, 1974; originally published in 1845, 1846), 380.

374 NOTES TO PAGES 202–212

25. Charles T. Pridgeon, *Insanity in American Fiction from Charles Brockden Brown to Oliver Wendell Holmes* (Ann Arbor, Mich.: University Microfilms International Dissertation Services, 1973), 7, 21, 51.

26. Pridgeon, *Insanity in American Fiction*, 91, 94.

27. Pridgeon, *Insanity in American Fiction*, 87, 161.

28. Steinberg, *On the Brink*, 53, apparently quoting Charles Brockden Brown, *Wieland; or, The Transformation*, in *Charles Brockden Brown's Novels*, vol. 1 (Philadelphia: David McKay, 1887; reprinted., Port Washington, N.Y.: Kennikat Press, 1963), 191.

29. Steinberg, *On the Brink*, 65.

30. Pridgeon, *Insanity in American Fiction*, iii, vi, 3.

31. John B. Chapin, "Insanity in the State of New York," *American Journal of Insanity* 13 (1856): 39–52.

32. Hurd, *The Institutional Care*, vol. 1, 411, and vol. 3, 113.

33. Chapin, "Insanity in the State of New York."

34. Hurd, *The Institutional Care*, vol. 1, 88.

35. Tomes, *A Generous Confidence*, 33. Grob, *Mental Institutions in America*, 353.

36. Morton, *A History*, 153, 156.

37. In 1812: Hurd, *The Institutional Care*, vol. 2, 71.

38. Hurd, *The Institutional Care*, vol. 2, 93–95, 96, 101.

39. Hurd, *The Institutional Care*, vol. 2, 100–101.

40. Gerald Grob, *The State and the Mentally Ill: A History of Worcester State Hospital in Massachusetts, 1830–1920* (Chapel Hill: University of North Carolina Press), 17. Jimenez, *Changing Faces of Madness*, 77.

41. *Second Annual Report of the Boston Prison Discipline Society*, Boston, 1827, quoted in Jimenez, *Changing Faces of Madness*, 104.

42. *Massachusetts House Document no. 50, 1827*, 9, quoted in Jimenez, *Changing Faces of Madness*, 104.

43. Hurd, *The Institutional Care*, vol. 2, 586.

44. Grob, *The Mad among Us*, 44.

45. Amariah Brigham, "Insanity and Insane Hospitals," *North American Review* 4 (1837): 91–121. Over half: Grob, *The State and the Mentally Ill*, 49, 82.

46. 1835: Jimenez, *Changing Faces of Madness*, 121. 1832: Grob, *Mental Institutions in America*, 14.

47. Grob, *The State and the Mentally Ill*, 84.

48. "An Account of the Imprisonment," 1833, 27–28, quoted in Jimenez, *Changing Faces of Madness*, 120. Brigham, "Insanity and Insane Hospitals."

49. Anonymous, "A Retreat for the Sane," *North American Review*, 1817, 324–334.

50. McCandless, *Moonlight, Magnolias*, 24, 171.

51. McCandless, *Moonlight, Magnolias*, 56.

52. McCandless, *Moonlight, Magnolias*, 78.

53. Brigham, "Insanity and Insane Hospitals."

54. Pridgeon, *Insanity in American Fiction*, 27, quoting "Treatment of the Insane," *American Magazine of Useful and Entertaining Knowledge* 3 (January 1837): 150.

55. Pridgeon, *Insanity in American Fiction*, 5, 178. Herman Melville, *Moby-Dick*, vol. 1 (New York: Russell and Russell, 1963; originally published in 1851), 190.

56. Pridgeon, *Insanity in American Fiction*, 308–309.

57. Sir Lionel is depicted: Pridgeon, *Insanity in American Fiction,* 166–167. Lucretia Maria Davidson, "The Fear of Madness," *Poetical Remains of the Late Lucretia Maria Davidson,* electronic text, miscellaneous pieces: University of Michigan Humanities Text Initiative, American Verse Project, April 9, 2001 <http://www.hti.umich.edu/cgi/a/amverse/amverse-idx?type=HTML&rgn=DIV1&byte=8444611>.

58. Pridgeon, *Insanity in American Fiction,* 183.

59. Pridgeon, *Insanity in American Fiction,* 202, 210, and 201, quoting James Kirke Paulding, *Westward Ho!* vol. 2, 50.

60. Pridgeon, *Insanity in American Fiction,* 313–314.

61. Pridgeon, *Insanity in American Fiction,* 212.

10. An Apostle for Asylums

1. Shryock, "The Beginnings," 25, and Pridgeon, *Insanity in American Fiction,* 41.

2. Hurd, *The Institutional Care,* vol. 1, 412.

3. Edward Jarvis, "Statistics of Insanity in the United States," *Boston Medical and Surgical Journal* 27 (1843): 281–282. Amariah Brigham, "Brief Notice of the New York State Lunatic Asylum, at Utica,—and of the appropriations by the state, for the benefit of the insane," *American Journal of Insanity* 1 (1844): 1–8.

4. Dr. Kurt Gorwitz utilized the insane : idiot ratio from the 1850 census, then applied it retrospectively to the 1840 combined insane and idiot figures (Kurt Gorwitz, "Census Enumeration of the Mentally Ill and the Mentally Retarded in the Nineteenth Century," *Health Services Report* 89 (1974): 180–187.

5. Brigham, "Insanity and Insane Hospitals."

6. "Statistics of Population: Table of Lunacy in the United States," *Merchants' Magazine* 8 (1843): 290. C. B. Hayden, "On the Distribution of Insanity in the United States," *Southern Literary Messenger* 10 (1844): 178–181, and Deutsch, *The Mentally Ill in America,* 473.

7. Deutsch, *The Mentally Ill in America,* 473, and Lynn Gamwell and Nancy Tomes, *Madness in America: Medical Perceptions of Mental Illness before 1914* (Ithaca, N.Y.: Cornell University Press, 1995), 101. Calhoun knew: McCandless, *Moonlight, Magnolias,* 146.

8. Edward Jarvis, "Insanity among the Colored Population of the Free States," *American Journal of Insanity* 8 (1852): 268–282.

9. Jarvis, "Insanity among the Colored Population." Deutsch, *The Mentally Ill in America,* 476–477.

10. Dain, *Concepts of Insanity,* 239. "Mistaken Sympathy, or Mistaken Figures," *Land We Love* 5 (1866): 349–360. Hurd, *The Institutional Care,* vol. 1, 414.

11. Dorothea Dix, *On Behalf of the Insane Poor: Selected Reports* (New York: Arno Press and the New York Times, 1971), 3, 25.

12. Waterston, R. C. "The Insane in Massachusetts," *Christian Examiner* 33(1843): 338–352. Samuel Gridley Howe, 1843, quoted in Jarvis, "Statistics of Insanity."

13. Grob, *The State and the Mentally Ill,* 83. Jimenez, *Changing Faces of Madness,* 134, quoting the 1848 Report of the Board of Visitors. Jimenez, *Changing Faces of Madness,* 188–189, and Waterston, "The Insane in Massachusetts." Grob, *The State and the Mentally Ill,* 156.

14. Dix, quoted in Francis Tiffany, *Life of Dorothea Lynde Dix* (Ann Arbor, Mich.: Plutarch Press, 1971; originally published in 1918), 105.

15. Dorothea L. Dix, "Memorial. To the Honorable the Legislature of the State of New York, 1844," in Dorothea L. Dix, *On Behalf of the Insane Poor*, 7–8.

16. Utica Asylum: Grob, *Mental Institutions in America*, 353. Ellen Dwyer, *Homes for the Mad: Life inside Two Nineteenth-Century Asylums* (New Brunswick, N.J.: Rutgers University Press, 1987), 38.

17. Charles Dickens, *American Notes for General Circulation* (New York: Harper and Brothers, 1842), 106–107.

18. Dix, "Memorial," in *On Behalf of the Insane Poor*, 56.

19. Hurd, *The Institutional Care*, vol. 3, 115. One superintendent: Chapin, "Insanity in the State of New York." Another county: ibid. Counties considered: Ellen Dwyer, "Civil Commitment Laws in Nineteenth-Century New York," *Behavioral Sciences and the Law* 6 (1988): 79–98.

20. John C. Bucknill, *Notes on Asylums for the Insane in America* (London: Churchill, 1876), 21, quoting an Ohio official.

21. McCandless, *Moonlight, Magnolias*, 67. Grob, *Mental Institutions in America*, 364. Georgia Lunatic Asylum: Grob, *The Mad among Us*, 48.

22. Bucknill, *Notes on Asylums*, 22.

23. Forbes Winslow, "The Plea of Insanity in Criminal Cases," *Southern Literary Messenger* 10 (1844): 667–671, cited in Pridgeon, *Insanity in American Fiction*. "Editor's Drawer: The Mathematical Monomaniac," *Harper's Monthly* 4 (1851): 135–136. Anonymous, "Visit to a Private Asylum for the Insane of the Higher Classes," *Chambers' Journal*, reprinted in *Littell's Living Age* 9 (1846): 367–370. "Re: *A Treatise on the Medical Jurisprudence of Insanity*, by I. Ray," *North American Review* 60 (1845): 1–37. Anonymous, "'The Ruined Mind,'" *Home Journal*, 1850, reprinted in *Littell's Living Age* 26 (1850): 306.

24. "A Day in a Lunatic Asylum," *Harper's Monthly* 9 (1854): 653–659.

25. Hurd, *The Institutional Care*, vol. 2, 72, and vol. 1, 95. Maine: Edward Jarvis, *Insanity and Idiocy in Massachusetts: Report of the Commission on Lunacy, 1855* (Cambridge, Mass.: Harvard University Press, 1855).

26. John M. Hunter, Gary W. Shannon, and Stephanie L. Sambrook, "Rings of Madness: Service Areas of 19th Century Asylums in North America," *Social Science and Medicine* 23 (1986): 1033–1050. E. Bruce Thompson, "Reforms in the Care of the Insane in Tennessee, 1830–1850," *Tennessee Historical Quarterly* 3 (1944): 319–334.

27. Deutsch, *The Mentally Ill in America*, 132. Tomes, *A Generous Confidence*, 32.

28. Andrew Scull, "The Discovery of the Asylum Revisited: Lunacy Reform in the New American Republic," in Scull (ed.), *Madhouses*, 154. William Awl: Pliny Earle, "The Curability of Insanity," *American Journal of Insanity* 33 (1877): 483–533.

29. Waterston, "The Insane in Massachusetts."

30. Pridgeon, *Insanity in American Fiction*, 256–257.

31. In John W. Ostrom (ed.), *The Letters of Edgar Allan Poe* (Cambridge, Mass.: Harvard University Press, 1948), 452.

32. Robert Louis Stevenson, "[Review of] *The Works of Edgar Allan Poe*," *Academy* 7 (January 2, 1875), reprinted in C. C. Bigelow and Temple Scott (eds.), *The Works of Robert Louis Stevenson*, 10 vols. (New York: Greenock Press, 1906), vol. 9, 255–262. Pridgeon, *Insanity in American Fiction*, 234, 246.

33. Frederick S. Frank and Anthony Magistrale, *The Poe Encyclopedia* (Westport, Conn.: Greenwood Press, 1997), 53.

34. Edward Wagenknecht, *Edgar Allan Poe: The Man behind the Legend* (New York: Oxford University Press, 1963), 60. Edgar Allan Poe, "Berenice," 1835, in G. R. Thompson (ed.), *Great Short Works of Edgar Allan Poe* (New York: Harper and Row, 1970), 152–161.

35. Edgar Allan Poe, "The Fall of the House of Usher," 1839, in G. R. Thompson, *Great Short Works*, 216–238. Jamison, *Touched with Fire*, 192, and Pridgeon, *Insanity in American Fiction*, 289.

36. "The Tell-Tale Heart," 1843, in G. R. Thompson, *Great Short Works*, 384–389.

37. Pamela Moore, "The System of Doctor Tarr and Professor Fether," Hippocrates Project, New York University School of Medicine, Medical Humanities, Literature, Arts and Medicine, April 9, 2001 <http://endeavor.med.nyu.edu/lit-med/lit-med-db/webdocs/webdescrips/poe285-des-.html>.

38. James C. Wilson (ed.), *The Hawthorne and Melville Friendship: An Annotated Bibliography, Biographical and Critical Essays, and Correspondence between the Two* (Jefferson, N.C.: McFarland and Co., 1991), citing William Dean Howells, *Literary Friends and Acquaintances* (Bloomington: Indiana University Press, 1968), 37. Letter to J. T. Fields, in Thomas Woodson, L. Neal Smith, and Norman Holmes Pearson (eds.), *The Letters, 1843–1853/Nathaniel Hawthorne* (Columbus: Ohio State University Press, 1984), 378. Nathaniel Hawthorne, *The American Notebooks*, C. M. Simpson (ed.) (Columbus: Ohio State University Press, 1932–1972), 244.

39. Pridgeon, *Insanity in American Fiction*, 330. Hawthorne, *American Notebooks*, 169–170, 181.

40. Nathaniel Hawthorne, "The Hollow of the Three Hills," in *Tales and Sketches; A Wonder Book for Girls and Boys; Tanglewood Tales for Girls and Boys* (New York: Library of America, 1996).

41. Nathaniel Hawthorne, "Egotism; or, The Bosom-Serpent," 1842, in *Mosses from an Old Manse*.

42. Nathaniel Hawthorne, "P's Correspondence," in *Mosses from an Old Manse*, 379.

43. Julian Hawthorne, *Hawthorne and His Circle* (Hamden, Conn.: Archon Books, 1968), 33, and see also Jamison, *Touched with Fire*, 216–217.

44. Jamison, *Touched with Fire*, 217. Paul McCarthy, *"The Twisted Mind": Madness in Herman Melville's Fiction* (Iowa City: University of Iowa Press, 1990), 7–8. Benjamin D. Riess, "Madness and Mastery in Melville's 'Benito Cereno,'" *Criticism* 38 (1996): 115–150.

45. McCarthy, *Twisted*, 24, 53. Dan McCall, *The Silence of Bartleby* (Ithaca, N.Y.: Cornell University Press, 1989), 53.

46. Pridgeon, *Insanity in American Fiction*, 382–383. Henry Nash Smith, "The Madness of Ahab," *Yale Review* 66 (1976): 14–32. Pridgeon, *Insanity in American Fiction*, 389.

47. Herman Melville, *Pierre; or, The Ambiguities* (Evanston and Chicago: Northwestern University Press and Newberry College, 1971), 119–121. *Philadelphia Graham's Magazine*, October 1852, *The Life and Works of Herman Melville*, April 9, 2001 <http://www.melville.org/hmpierre.htm>.

48. *Bartleby the Scrivener*, in *Herman Melville: Four Short Novels* (New York: Bantam Books, 1959), 40. [no first name] Leary, in M. Thomas Inge (ed.), *Bartleby the*

Inscrutable: A Collection of Commentary on Herman Melville's Tale "Bartleby the Scrivener" (Hamden, Conn.: Archon Books, 1979), 15–16, and Dan McCall, *The Silence of Bartleby,* 52. Laurie Robertson-Lorant, *Melville: A Biography* (New York: Clarkson Potter, 1996), 269.

49. Edgar Allan Poe, "Eleanora," in *Edgar Allan Poe,* Philip Van Doren Stern (ed.) (New York: Viking Press, 1945), 95.

50. Melville, *Pierre,* quoted in Jamison, *Touched with Fire,* 216.

51. *Seventh Census of the United States* (Washington, D.C.: Robert Armstrong, Public Printer, 1853). Gorwitz, "Census Enumeration."

52. Grob, *Mental Institutions in America,* 371–372.

53. Edward Jarvis, "On the Supposed Increase of Insanity," *American Journal of Insanity* 8 (1852): 333–364.

54. Howe, 1843, quoted in Jarvis, "Statistics of Insanity."

55. Jarvis, *Insanity and Idiocy,* 9.

56. Jarvis, *Insanity and Idiocy,* 9. Isaac Ray, "Statistics of Insanity in Massachusetts: Report on Insanity and Idiocy in Massachusetts, by the Commission on Lunacy, under Resolve of the Legislature of 1854," *North American Review* 82 (1856): 78–100.

57. Jarvis, *Insanity and Idiocy,* 79.

58. Ray, "Statistics of Insanity." "Insanity in Massachusetts," *American Journal of Insanity* 18 (1861): 94–95.

59. Jarvis, *Insanity and Idiocy,* 57, 59.

60. Browne, *What Asylums Were,* 65. Isaac Ray, "The Statistics of Insane Hospitals," *American Journal of Insanity* 6 (1849): 23–52. Grob, *The State and the Mentally Ill,* 177, quoting Massachusetts official reports from 1860 and 1863.

61. Grob, *Mental Institutions in America,* 238. Boston Lunatic Hospital: Dorothea Dix, "Memorial Soliciting Enlarged and Improved Accommodations for the Insane of the State of Tennessee by the Establishment of a New Hospital, November, 1847," in Dorothea L. Dix, *On Behalf of the Insane Poor;* Jimenez, *Changing Faces of Madness,* 188; and Jarvis, "On the Supposed Increase of Insanity."

62. Jarvis, *Insanity and Idiocy,* 62. George Chandler: Gerald Grob, Introduction to Jarvis, *Insanity and Idiocy,* 20.

63. Blackwell's Island: Grob, *Mental Institutions in America,* 231. Furthermore: Grob, Introduction to Jarvis, *Insanity and Idiocy,* 20. Maine: Ray, "Statistics of Insanity," 1856.

64. Jimenez, *Changing Faces of Madness,* 133, 186, 187.

65. In the 1820s: Marjorie Fallows, *Irish Americans: Identity and Assimilation* (Englewood Cliffs, N.J.: Prentice Hall, Inc., 1979), 48. Dingle men: K. Miller, *Emigrants and Exiles,* 521.

66. K. Miller, *Emigrants and Exiles,* 103, 227.

67. K. Miller, *Emigrants and Exiles,* 197, 240, 280, 319.

68. Jarvis, *Insanity and Idiocy,* 53, 55.

69. Ray, "Statistics of Insanity." John Chapin, "Insanity in the State of New York."

70. Ray, "Statistics of Insanity."

71. Dorothea Dix, *Memorial D. L. Dix, Praying a Grant of Land for the Relief and Support of the Indigent and Incurable Insane in the United States, June 23, 1848,* in Porter, *The Faber Book of Madness,* 8–9.

72. Walt Whitman: Gunther Barth, *City People: The Rise of Modern City Culture in*

Nineteenth-Century America (New York: Oxford University Press, 1980), 42. Oscar Handlin, *The Uprooted* (Boston: Little, Brown and Co., 1951), 136–137.

73. "Insanity and Treatment of the Insane," *National Magazine* 11 (December 1857): 518.

11. "A Very Startling Increase"

1. McCandless, *Moonlight, Magnolias,* 215.
2. McCandless, *Moonlight, Magnolias,* 216–217.
3. J. M. Hunter et al., "Rings of Madness." Statistics: Grob, *Mental Institutions in America,* 371.
4. P. M. Duncan, "On Insanity."
5. "Review of Annual Report of the Hartford Retreat," *American Journal of Insanity* 24 (1867): 216–230. "Conference of Boards of Public Charities," *Journal of Social Science* 6 (1874): 60–99. McCandless, *Moonlight, Magnolias,* 255.
6. "The Cadmean Madness," *Atlantic Monthly* 83 (1864): 265.
7. Donald A. Treffert, "The MacArthur Coercion Studies: A Wisconsin Perspective," *Marquette Law Review* 82 (1999): 759–785, quoting *First Annual Report,* Wisconsin State Board of Charity and Reform, 1873.
8. Treffert, "The MacArthur Coercion Studies," 761.
9. Hurd, *The Institutional Care,* vol. 3, 116. Greene County and Delaware County: P. M. Duncan, "On Insanity."
10. Deutsch, *The Mentally Ill in America,* 252, 253. 1880 survey: Grob, *The Mad among Us,* 119.
11. Deutsch, *The Mentally Ill in America,* 232.
12. Dwyer, *Homes for the Mad,* 38.
13. Statistics on insanity rates in California: Gorwitz, "Census Enumeration." Californians: Richard W. Fox, *So Far Disordered in Mind: Insanity in California, 1870–1930* (Berkeley: University of California Press, 1978), 18.
14. Stuart A. Brody, "Hospitalization of the Mentally Ill during California's Early Years: 1849–1853," *Psychiatric Quarterly Supplement* 38 (1964): 262–272. Henry Harris, *California's Medical Story* (Springfield, Ill.: Thomas, 1932). San Francisco Hospital: Brody, "Hospitalization of the Mentally Ill during California's Early Years."
15. Fox, *So Far Disordered,* 21. John W. Robertson, "Prevalence of Insanity in California," *American Journal of Insanity* 60 (1903): 75–88.
16. Fox, *So Far Disordered,* 19.
17. J. W. Robertson, "Prevalence of Insanity in California." William A. White, "The Geographical Distribution of Insanity in the United States," *National Geographic Magazine* 14 (1903): 361–378. Paula M. Marks, *Precious Dust: The American Gold Rush Era: 1848–1900* (New York: William Morrow, 1994), 235. Brody, "Hospitalization of the Mentally Ill," 268.
18. Fox, *So Far Disordered,* 21, quoting Dr. George Shurtleff, 1875. Chinese: Marks, *Precious Dust,* 299, and Fox, *So Far Disordered,* 21.
19. Fox, *So Far Disordered,* 42, quoting Dr. George Shurtleff. Brody, "Hospitalization of the Mentally Ill," 270.
20. E. T. Wilkins, *Insanity and Insane Asylums* (Sacramento, Calif.: T. A. Springer, 1872), 200–201.
21. John M. Faragher, "Great Migrations: The Pioneer in the American West," in

Geoffrey C. Ward, *The West: An Illustrated History* (Boston: Little, Brown and Co., 1996), 285–289.

22. Brody, "Hospitalization of the Mentally Ill," 271.

23. Dain, *Concepts of Insanity,* 254.

24. Pridgeon, *Insanity in American Fiction,* 453, 460.

25. Charlotte Perkins Gilman, *The Yellow Wallpaper* (New York: Pantheon Books, 1980; originally published in *New England Magazine,* 1891).

26. Grob, *The Mad among Us,* 84. 1849: Dain, *Concepts of Insanity.* 1852: Gamwell and Tomes, *Madness in America,* 62.

27. Deutsch, *The Mentally Ill in America,* 424.

28. Tomes, *A Generous Confidence,* 276.

29. Details of the two cases: Dwyer, "Civil Commitment Laws." "It seems": Deutsch, *The Mentally Ill in America,* 426.

30. New York City Lunatic Asylum: Grob, *The Mad among Us,* 85. An official: Grob, *The Mad among Us,* 94. *New York Tribune:* Tomes, *A Generous Confidence,* 259. "Ten Days": Deutsch, *The Mentally Ill in America,* 307. Civil War onward: Tomes, *A Generous Confidence,* 261.

31. Tomes, *A Generous Confidence,* 226–233, 267.

32. Tomes, *A Generous Confidence,* 277, 279.

33. Earle, "The Curability of Insanity."

34. Webb Haymaker, *The Founders of Neurology* (Springfield, Ill.: C. C. Thomas, 1953), 448. Hammond's court-martial: David S. Werman, "True and False Experts: A Second Look," *American Journal of Psychiatry* 130 (1973): 1351–1354. Hammond's fees: Bonnie Ellen Blustein, "New York Neurologists and the Specialization of American Medicine," *Bulletin of the History of Medicine* 53 (1979): 170–183.

35. Edward C. Spitzka, "Merits and Motives of the Movement for Asylum Reform," *Journal of Nervous and Mental Disease* 5 (1878): 694–714.

36. Charles E. Rosenberg, *The Trial of the Assassin Guiteau* (Chicago: University of Chicago Press, 1968), 63, 73, 190, and Dwyer, *Homes for the Mad,* 66.

37. M. G. Echeverria, "Criminal Responsibility of Epileptics as Illustrated by the Case of David Montgomery," *American Journal of Insanity* 29 (1873): 341–425.

38. Tomes, *A Generous Confidence,* 293.

39. Bonnie Ellen Blustein, "'A Hollow Square of Psychological Science,'" in Scull, *Madhouses,* 244 (Spitzka's paper was published as "Reform in the Scientific Study of Psychiatry," *Journal of Nervous and Mental Disease* 5 [1878]: 201–228), and Rosenberg, *The Trial,* 72.

40. Spitzka, "Reform."

41. Blustein, "'A Hollow Square,'" 247.

42. Eugene Grissom, "True and False Experts," *American Journal of Insanity* 35 (1878): 1–36.

43. Grissom, "True and False Experts." Spitzka, "Merits and Motives."

44. Blustein, "New York Neurologists."

45. Spitzka, "Merits and Motives."

46. Spitzka, "Merits and Motives." *New York Times,* October 8, 1878, p. 2, col. 5.

47. Blustein, "'A Hollow Square,'" 248–249.

48. Blustein, "'A Hollow Square,'" 252. Michigan: Leland V. Bell, "From the Asylum to the Community in U.S. Mental Health Care: A Historical Overview," in David A.

Rochefort (ed.), *Handbook on Mental Health Policy in the United States* (New York: Greenwood Press, 1989), 101. "Treatment of the Insane," *New York Times,* November 14, 1879, p. 3, col. 1.

49. Blustein, "'A Hollow Square,'" 254.

50. Dwyer, "Civil Commitment Laws." "[If he] does not die": Blustein, "'A Hollow Square,'" 257, 269.

51. L. A. Tourtellot, "Utica Asylum Investigation," *American Psychological Journal* 2 (1884): 31–40, and see also Deutsch, *The Mentally Ill in America,* 311–314. Samuel Ayres, "Our Asylums and Our Insane," *American Psychological Journal* 1 (1884): 341–347. Everts, "The American System."

52. "The Care of the Insane," *New York Times,* December 8, 1880, p. 2, cols. 2 and 3. "Insane Asylum Methods," *New York Times,* December 2, 1880, p. 8, col. 1. "The Care of the Insane," *New York Times,* December 8, 1880, p. 2, cols. 2 and 3. Blustein, "'A Hollow Square,'" 261.

53. D. B. Eaton, "Despotism in Lunatic Asylums."

54. Everts, "The American System."

55. Rosenberg, *The Trial,* 90; this book is an excellent account of the trial.

56. Rosenberg, *The Trial,* 158. John Gray, "The Guiteau Trial," *American Journal of Insanity* 38 (1882): 303–448.

57. Rosenberg, *The Trial,* 240.

58. Editorial, *New York Times,* November 18, 1879, p. 4, col. 6.

59. "A la Guiteau," *Utica Daily Press,* March 17, 1882, 2. Werman, "True and False Experts."

60. Barbara Miller Solomon, *Ancestors and Immigrants: A Changing New England Tradition* (Boston: Northeastern University Press, 1956), 71.

61. *Report on the 1880 Census,* ix and x.

62. *Report on the 1880 Census,* xli.

63. Judson B. Andrews, "The Distribution and Care of the Insane in the United States," *American Journal of Insanity* 44 (1887): 192–209.

64. "Insanity in the United States," *Times* (London), August 16, 1883, 10e.

65. Foster Pratt, "The Increase of Insanity in the United States: Its Causes and Its Sources" (Concord, N.H., 1884; reprinted from *Public Health Papers and Reports,* vol. 9, 1883), in Gerald Grob, *Immigrants and Insanity: Dissenting Views, 1883–1914* (New York: Arno Press, 1980), 334. Pliny Earle, "Popular Fallacies in Regard to Insanity and the Insane," *Journal of Social Science* 26 (1890): 107–117.

66. "The Increase of Insanity," *American Journal of Insanity* 40 (1883): 214–215, reprinted from *Lancet,* July 21, 1883. William W. Godding, "Progress in Provision for the Insane," *American Journal of Insanity* (1884): 129–150.

67. D. H. Tuke, "The Curability of Insanity," *Journal of Mental Science* (1887): 148–152. Anonymous, "The Increase of Insanity," *Boston Medical and Surgical Journal* 113 (1885): 259–260. *Eighth Annual Report of the State Board of Lunacy and Charity* (Boston, 1887).

68. *Report of the Insane, 11th Census, 1890,* 4.

69. *1890 Census,* 12, 13.

70. *1890 Census,* 72. Anonymous, "Insanity and Civilization," *The Nation* 41 (1885): 356–357. Editorial, "Sewer Gas and Insanity," *American Psychological Journal* 1 (1884): 310, and Henry Putnam Stearns, *Insanity: Its Causes and Prevention* (New York: G. P. Putnam's Sons, 1883), 13.

12. "The Apocalyptic Beast"

1. Godding, "Progress in Provision."

2. S. Weir Mitchell, "Address before the Fiftieth Annual Meeting of the American Medico-Psychological Association," *Journal of Nervous and Mental Disease* 21 (1894): 413–437.

3. Abraham Jacobi, in S. W. Mitchell, "Address."

4. Walter Channing, "Some Remarks on the Address Delivered to the American Medico-Psychological Association, by S. Weir Mitchell, M.D., May 16, 1894," *American Journal of Insanity* 51 (1895): 171–184.

5. Franklin B. Sanborn, "Is American Insanity Increasing? A Study," *Journal of Mental Science* 40 (1894): 214–219.

6. *Insane and Feeble-Minded in Hospitals and Institutions, 1904* (Washington, D.C.: Government Printing Office, 1906), 3.

7. Bureau of the Census, *Insane and Feeble-Minded in Institutions, 1910* (Washington, D.C.: Government Printing Office, 1914), 4, 6.

8. Hurd, *The Institutional Care*, vol. 1, 401–410.

9. William Seton, "Is Insanity Increasing?" *Catholic World* 70 (1899): 321–327. Anonymous, "A Disease of Civilization," *The Nation* 81 (1905): 196. G. Harvey, "The Race Not Going Mad," *North American Review* 204 (1916): 16–20.

10. E. Jarvis, "Causes of Mental Disease: Report of the Trustees of the Massachusetts General Hospital for the Year 1858," *North American Review* 89 (1859): 316–339. "Insanity and Civilization," *Nation* 41 (1885): 356–357. J. S. Jewell, "Influence of Our Present Civilization in the Production of Nervous and Mental Diseases," *Journal of Nervous and Mental Disease* 8 (1881): 1–24.

11. Stearns, *Insanity,* 34.

12. J. W. Robertson, "Prevalence of Insanity in California."

13. For similar state reports, see, for example, the 1875 report of Dr. Nathan Allen, summarized in Grob, *The State and the Mentally Ill,* 241. Pratt, "The Increase of Insanity," 330–332.

14. Samuel P. Hays, *The Response to Industrialization, 1885–1914* (Chicago: University of Chicago Press, 1957), 104. Watson, quoted in Richard Hofstadter, *The Age of Reform: From Bryan to F.D.R.* (New York: Vintage Books, 1955), 83.

15. Francis A. Walker, "Restriction of Immigration," *Atlantic Monthly,* June 1896, 822–829.

16. Solomon, *Ancestors and Immigrants,* 149–150. Scandinavians, 160. Jews, 169. Irish: [no first name given] Bannister, "Progress in Psychiatry in 1903: United States," *Journal of Mental Science* 50 (1904): 139–142. William Godding, quoted in Jarvis, "Causes of Mental Disease."

17. Thaddeus S. Dayton, "Importing Our Insane," *Harper's Weekly* 56 (1912): 9.

18. E. Fuller Torrey, *Freudian Fraud: The Malignant Effect of Freud's Theory on American Thought and Culture* (New York: HarperCollins, 1992; reprinted by Lucas Books, 1999), 48.

19. *1910 Census,* 26.

20. H. L. Reed, "Immigration and Insanity," *Journal of Political Economy* 21 (1913): 954–956. Aaron J. Rosanoff, "Some Neglected Phases of Immigration in Relation to Insanity," *American Journal of Insanity* 72 (1915): 45–58.

21. Fox, *So Far Disordered,* 30.

22. Allan Chase, *The Legacy of Malthus* (Urbana: University of Illinois Press, 1980), 16, 135.

23. Grob, *Mental Institutions in America*, 173. Fox, *So Far Disordered*, 28, quoting a 1922 California state report.

24. Nathan Hale, *Freud and the Americans* (New York: Oxford University Press, 1971–1995), 80. Barbara Sicherman, *The Quest for Mental Health in America, 1880–1917* (Ann Arbor, Mich.: University Microfilms International Dissertation Services, 1967), 347. Ian Dowbiggin, "'An Exodus of Enthusiasm': G. Alder Blumer, Eugenics and U.S. Psychiatry, 1890–1920," *Medical History* 36 (1992): 379–402. Meyer: Sicherman, *The Quest*, 351.

25. Dowbiggin, "Exodus of Enthusiasm."

26. Grob, *The Mad among Us*, 161.

27. Robert H. Wiebe, *The Search for Order, 1877–1920* (New York: Hill and Wang, 1967), 11–12.

28. *Action for Mental Health: Final Report of the Joint Commission on Mental Illness and Health* (New York: John Wiley and Sons, 1961), 69.

29. Sicherman, *The Quest*.

30. Henry Farrand Griffin, "The Mental Hygiene Movement: A National Campaign against Insanity," *The Outlook* 103 (1913): 311–316.

31. William F. Ogburn and Ellen Winston, "The Frequency and Probability of Insanity," *American Journal of Sociology* 34 (1929): 822–831. The influenza pandemic: *Annual Reports*, New York State Hospital Commission, 1918–1923.

32. Kenneth L. Roberts, "Ports of Embarkation," *Saturday Evening Post*, May 7, 1921. Cornelia J. Cannon, "American Misgivings," *Atlantic Monthly*, February 1922, 145–157. Calvin Coolidge, "Whose Country Is This?" *Good Housekeeping* 72 (1921): 13–107.

33. Harlan D. Unrau, *Historic Resource Study*, vol. 1 (National Park Service, U.S. Department of the Interior, 1984), 201, quoting the *Annual Report of the Commissioner General of Immigration, 1931*.

34. Grob, *The Mad among Us*, 170. Carney Landis and James D. Page, *Modern Society and Mental Disease* (New York: Arno Press, 1980; original publication: New York: Farrar and Rinehart, Inc., 1938), 24. "The Problem of Mental Disease in the United States," *Hygiea* 17 (1939): 6. Landis and Page, *Modern Society*, 26.

35. Henry A. Cotton, "The Physical Causes of Mental Disorders," *American Mercury* 29 (1933): 221–225.

36. Henry B. Elkind, "The Epidemiology of Mental Disease," *American Journal of Psychiatry* 6 (1927): 623–640.

37. Henry B. Elkind and Maurice Taylor, "The Alleged Increase in the Incidence of the Major Psychoses," *American Journal of Psychiatry* 92 (1936): 817–826. Ellen Winston, "The Assumed Increase of Mental Disease," *American Journal of Sociology* 40 (1935): 427–439.

38. R. L. Duffus, "Is Civilization Driving Us Crazy?" *Scribner's Magazine* 91 (1932): 350–352. Leslie C. Barber, "The Age of Schizophrenia," *Harper's Monthly* 176 (1937): 70–78. Crowder, "But *Is* the World Going Mad?"

39. *1910 Census*, 49–50.

40. Horatio M. Pollock and William J. Nolan, "Mental Disease in Cities, Villages and Rural Districts of New York State, 1915–1920," *State Hospital Quarterly* 7 (1921): 38–65. Robert E. L. Faris and H. Warren Dunham, *Mental Disorders in Urban*

Areas: An Ecological Study of Schizophrenia and Other Psychoses (New York: Hafner Publishing Co., 1960; originally published in 1939). "Insanity Zones," *Time* 40 (1942): 58–61. H. Warren Dunham, "Mental Disorders in Urban Areas: A Retrospective View," in M. M. Weissman, J. K. Myers, and C. E. Ross (eds.), *Community Surveys of Psychiatric Disorders* (New Brunswick, N.J.: Rutgers University Press, 1986), 65–76.

41. Jacqueline O'Connor, *Dramatizing Dementia: Madness in the Plays of Tennessee Williams* (Bowling Green, Ohio: Bowling Green State University Popular Press, 1997), 17.

42. Zelda Fitzgerald, *Save Me the Waltz* (New York: New American Library, 1968), 186.

43. F. Scott Fitzgerald, *Tender Is the Night* (New York: Charles Scribner's Sons, 1933, 1934), 192.

44. Fitzgerald, *Tender*, 191–192. Letter, Fitzgerald to Dr. Slocum, *New York Times Magazine*, December 1, 1996.

45. O'Connor, *Dramatizing Dementia*, 4–6.

46. Edward Butscher, *Conrad Aiken, Poet of White Horse Vale* (Athens: University of Georgia Press, 1988), 38. Catharine S. Siegel, *The Fictive World of Conrad Aiken: A Celebration of Consciousness* (Dekalb: Northern Illinois University Press, 1992), 110. Conrad Aiken, "Silent Snow, Secret Snow," in Mary Louise Atwell (ed.), *The World Within: Fiction Illuminating Neuroses of Our Time* (New York: McGraw-Hill, 1947), 237–260.

47. Gen. Lewis Hershey, Hearings on the National Neuropsychiatric Institute Act, Subcommittee on Health and Education of the Committee on Education and Labor, United States Senate, March 6–8, 1946, 55. Harry S Truman, "Compulsory Medical Insurance: The National Health Program," Message to the U.S. Congress, November 19, 1945.

48. The background of this study was described by Mr. Andrew Marshall in an interview with the senior author, July 21, 1999. Herbert Goldhamer and Andrew W. Marshall, *Psychosis and Civilization: Two Studies in the Frequency of Mental Disease* (Glencoe, Ill.: Free Press, 1953). Fredrick C. Redlich and Daniel X. Freedman, *The Theory and Practice of Psychiatry* (New York: Basic Books, 1966), 186, and H. E. Lehmann, "Schizophrenia. I. Introduction and History," in A. M. Freedman and H. I. Kaplan (eds.), *Comprehensive Textbook of Psychiatry* (Baltimore: Williams and Wilkins, 1967), 593–598. Grob, *The Mad among Us*, 324, note 5, Grob, *The State and the Mentally Ill*, 96, and Rothman, *Discovery*, 127.

49. Goldhamer and Marshall, *Psychosis and Civilization*, 40, 29, and 75.

50. William W. Eaton, *The Sociology of Mental Disorders* (New York: Praeger, 1980), 174–176.

51. Goldhamer and Marshall, *Psychosis and Civilization*, 92, 96.

52. Grob, *The Mad among Us*, 167, 170.

53. M. Kramer et al., "State and County Mental Hospitals, 1946–66," in *Mental Disorders/Suicide* (Cambridge, Mass.: Harvard University Press, 1972), 48. William F. Roth, Jr., and Frank H. Luton, "The Mental Health Program in Tennessee," *American Journal of Psychiatry* 99 (1943): 662–675. August B. Hollingshead and Fredrick C. Redlich, *Social Class and Mental Illness* (New York: John Wiley, 1958).

54. *Action for Mental Health*. Grob, *The Mad among Us*, 2, 202.

55. D. A. Regier et al., "The De Facto U.S. Mental and Addictive Disorders Service Sys-

tem," *Archives of General Psychiatry* 50 (1993): 85–94, and "Health Care Reform for Americans with Severe Mental Illnesses: Report of the National Advisory Mental Health Council," *American Journal of Psychiatry* 150 (1993):1447–1465. The 2.2 percent is an unduplicated count of individuals with schizophrenia and manic-depressive illness (bipolar disorder) (personal communication from Dr. Darrel Regier, National Institute of Mental Health, December 1999).

56. *Annual Statistical Supplement, 1998, to the Social Security Bulletin* (Washington, D.C.: Social Security Administration, 1998).

13. Why Is the Epidemic Forgotten?

1. Heinz E. Lehmann, "Schizophrenia," 593. Rothman, *Discovery,* 127, and see also Grob, *The State and the Mentally Ill,* 96. Macalpine and Hunter, *George III,* 294.
2. Carlin Romano, "The Philosopher of Madness and Punishment," *Washington Post Book World,* January 5, 1992, 11–12.
3. Michel Foucault, *Madness and Civilization* (New York: Random House, 1965), 61.
4. Scull, *Most Solitary of Afflictions,* 5, and *Social Order,* 252. Berrios and Freeman, *150 Years,* Introduction. Foucault, quoted by Scull, *Social Order,* 14.
5. Arieno, *Victorian Lunatics,* 2. Lawrence Stone, "Madness," *New York Review of Books,* December 16, 1982, 28–36. Scull, *Most Solitary,* 5. Foucault, *Madness and Civilization,* 33.
6. Thomas Szasz, *Schizophrenia: The Sacred Symbol of Psychiatry* (New York: Basic Books, 1976), 67, 191.
7. Thomas Szasz, "New Ideas, Not Old Institutions, for the Homeless," *Wall Street Journal,* June 7, 1985, 24; *Cruel Compassion: Psychiatric Control of Society's Unwanted* (New York: Wiley, 1994), 98; and "The Origin of Psychiatry: The Alienist as Nanny for Troublesome Adults," *History of Psychiatry* 6 (1995): 1–19.
8. Erving Goffman, *Asylums: Essays on the Social Situation of Mental Patients and Other Inmates* (New York: Anchor Books, 1961), 354.
9. Laing, quoted by Nick Crossley, "R. D. Laing and the British Anti-Psychiatry Movement: A Socio-Historical Analysis," *Social Science and Medicine* 47 (1998): 877–889.
10. Mary Barnes and Joseph Berke, *Two Accounts of a Journey through Madness* (New York: Ballantine Books, 1971), 83. Adrian Laing, *R. D. Laing: A Biography* (London: Peter Owen, 1994), 133, 194. "Britain's Offbeat Psychoanalyst," *Newsweek,* November 1, 1982, 16.
11. Rothman, *Discovery,* xiii–xix, 121.
12. Jacques Quen, "David Rothman's *Discovery of the Asylum,*" *Journal of Psychiatry and the Law* 2 (1974): 105–120. Norman Dain, "From Colonial Times to Bicentennial America: Two Centuries of Vicissitudes in the Institutional Care of Mental Patients," *Bulletin of the New York Academy of Medicine* 52 (1976): 1179–1196. Scull, *Social Order,* 259. David J. Rothman, "Decarcerating Prisoners and Patients," *Civil Liberties Review* 1 (1973): 830.
13. Scull, *Social Order,* 7.
14. Scull, *Most Solitary,* 1, 29, and *Social Order,* 217.
15. Scull, *Most Solitary,* 35.
16. Andrew Scull, "Madness and Segregative Control: The Rise of the Insane Asylum," *Social Problems* 24 (1977): 338–351, and *Social Order,* 230, quoting Andrew Wyn-

ter, "Non-Restraint in the Treatment of the Insane," *Edinburgh Review* 131 (1870): 221.

17. Scull, *Most Solitary*, 35, and "Was Insanity Increasing? A Response to Edward Hare," *British Journal of Psychiatry* 144 (1984): 432–436.

18. Scull, *Social Order*, 121, 125; *Most Solitary*, 41, 289; "Psychiatry and Social Control in the Nineteenth and Twentieth Centuries," *History of Psychiatry* 2 (1991), 155; and *Social Order*, 8.

19. M. MacDonald, *Mystical Bedlam*, 1981. Harold Merskey, "Somatic Treatments, Ignorance, and the Historiography of Psychiatry," *History of Psychiatry* 5 (1994): 387–391. Edward Shorter, *A History of Psychiatry: From the Era of the Asylum to the Age of Prozac* (New York: Wiley, 1997). Kathleen Jones, "Scull's Dilemma," *British Journal of Psychiatry* 141 (1982): 221–226. Andrew Scull, "Asylums: Utopias and Realities," in D. Tomlinson and J. Carrier (eds.), *Asylum in the Community* (London: Routledge, 1996), 7–17.

20. Grob, *Mental Institutions in America*, 109, 342.

21. Grob, *The State and the Mentally Ill*, 96; *The Mad among Us*, 48; and "Institutional Origins and Early Transformations, 1830–1855," in J. P. Morrissey, H. H. Goldman, and L. V. Klerman (eds.), *The Enduring Asylum: Cycles of Institutional Reform at Worcester State Hospital* (New York: Grune and Stratton, 1980), 44.

22. Grob, *Mental Institutions in America*, 342.

23. Scull, *Social Order*, 38, 41.

24. Porter, *Mind-Forg'd Manacles*, 164 .

25. Porter, *Mind-Forg'd Manacles*, 167.

26. Roy Porter, "Being Mad in Georgian England," *History Today* (December 1981): 42–48. Claridge et al., *Sounds from the Bell Jar*, 132–133. Roy Porter, "'All Madness for Writing': John Clare and the Asylum," in Hugh Haughton (ed.), *John Clare in Context* (Cambridge, U.K.: Cambridge University Press, 1994): 259–278.

27. Elaine Showalter, *The Female Malady: Women, Madness and English Culture, 1830–1980* (New York: Pantheon, 1985), 3.

28. Joan Busfield, "The Female Malady? Men, Women and Madness in 19th Century Britain," *Sociology* 28 (1994): 259–277, and Andrew Scull, *Most Solitary*, 160.

29. E. Fuller Torrey, *Schizophrenia and Civilization* (New York: Jason Aronson, Inc., 1980), 41.

30. Hare, "Was Insanity on the Increase?" Scull, "Was Insanity Increasing? A Response."

14. Possible Causes of Epidemic Insanity

1. Wynter, "Non-Restraint."

2. Andrew Scull, *Museums of Madness: The Social Organization of Insanity in Nineteenth-Century England* (London: Allen Lane, 1979), quoted by Hare, "Was Insanity Increasing?" (no page number given). Turner, "Rich and Mad."

3. Kathleen Jones, "The Culture of the Mental Hospital," in Berrios and Freeman, *150 Years*, 17. Grob, *The Mad among Us*, 50.

4. L. D. Smith, *Cure, Comfort*, 40–41. Scull, *Most Solitary*, 268, note 2. Scull, *Most Solitary*, citing Crammer, *Asylum History*. Finnane, *Insanity and the Insane*, 70; the *51st Report, 1901;* and *Journal of Mental Science* 49 (1903): 141. Gerald Grob, *Mental Illness and American Society* (Princeton, N.J.: Princeton University Press, 1983), 226.

5. Foucault, *Madness and Civilization*, 61. Goffman, *Asylums*, 354. Rothman, *Discovery*, xiii. Scull, *Most Solitary*, 35.

6. Walton, "Casting Out." L. D. Smith, *Cure, Comfort*, 94.

7. Prior, "The Appeal to Madness," 75, 86. Canada: O'Brien, *Out of Mind*, 10. Chapin, "Insanity in the State of New York." Shorter, *A History of Psychiatry*, 48.

8. John R. Sutton, "The Political Economy of Madness: The Expansion of the Asylum in Progressive America," *American Sociological Review* 56 (1991): 665–678. In Ireland: Finnane, *Insanity and the Insane*, 73.

9. J. A. Campbell, "Discussion," *Journal of Mental Science* 40 (1894): 231. Robins, *Fools and Mad*, 110. Skultans, *English Madness*, 124.

10. Tomes, *A Generous Confidence*, 127.

11. Charlotte MacKenzie, "Social Factors in the Admission, Discharge and Continuing Stay of Patients at Ticehurst Asylum, 1845–1917," in Bynum et al., *Anatomy of Madness, Vol. II: Institutions and Society*, 153. Walton, "Casting Out." Samuel Thielman, *Madness and Medicine: The Medical Approach to Madness in Antebellum America, with Particular Reference to the Eastern Lunatic Asylum of Virginia and the South Carolina Lunatic Asylum* (Ann Arbor, Mich.: University Microfilms International Dissertation Services, 1988), 196. Grob, *Mental Illness*, 9.

12. Carl N. Degler, *At Odds: Women and the Family in America from the Revolution to the Present* (New York: Oxford University Press, 1980), 384.

13. Scull, "Was Insanity Increasing? A Response."

14. Jimenez, *Changing Faces of Madness*, 124. Fox, *So Far Disordered*, 144.

15. "54th Report," *Journal of Mental Science* 47 (1901): 117–126. Parker et al., "County of Lancaster Asylum"; Turner, "Rich and Mad"; Renvoize and Beveridge, "Mental Illness and the Late Victorians"; and Klaf and Hamilton, "Schizophrenia." Finnane, *Insanity and the Insane*, 100. Hurd, *The Institutional Care*, vol. 4, 56. *NS JHA, 1904–1905*, 6. Grob, *The Mad among Us*, 166.

16. Brigham, "Insanity and Insane Hospitals."

17. Winfred Overholser, "Are Mental Disorders Increasing?" *Scientific Monthly* 50 (1940): 559–561.

18. Humphreys, "Statistics of Insanity." Finnane, *Insanity and the Insane* 234. M. MacDonald, *Mystical Bedlam*. Earle, "The Curability of Insanity."

19. Farr, "Report upon the Mortality."

20. Skultans, *English Madness*, 120. Finnane, *Insanity and the Insane* 234. *NB JHA, 1900*, 52, and O'Brien, *Out of Mind*, 95.

21. Grob, *Mental Illness*, 194, and Landis and Page, *Modern Society*, 134.

22. Grob, *Mental Illness*, 10, 180.

23. Grob, *The Mad among Us*, 121.

24. Grob, *The Mad among Us*, 120; and *The Inner World of American Psychiatry, 1890–1940: Selected Correspondence* (New Brunswick, N.J.: Rutgers University Press, 1985), 11–12.

25. E. Fuller Torrey, "Are We Overestimating the Genetic Contribution to Schizophrenia?" *Schizophrenia Bulletin* 18 (1992): 159–170.

26. A. J. Prasad, "First Cousin Marriages and Psychiatric Morbidity," *Canadian Journal of Psychiatry* 30 (1985): 69–70, and O. Odegaard, "Inbreeding and Schizophrenia," *Clinical Genetics* 30 (1986): 261–275. Kutaiba Chaleby and T. A. Tuma, "Cousin Marriages and Schizophrenia in Saudi Arabia," *British Journal of*

Psychiatry 150 (1987): 547–549, and Ahmed, "Consanguinity and Schizophrenia." Freire-Maia, "Inbreeding Levels."

27. Hare, "Schizophrenia before 1800?"

28. Arnold, *Observations on the Nature,* 23. Uwins, "Insanity and Madhouses." Morison, *Outlines of Lectures,* 61.

29. Glyn Lewis et al., "Schizophrenia and City Life," *Lancet* 340 (1992): 137–140; Noriyoshi Takei et al., "Schizophrenia: Increased Risk Associated with Winter and City Birth—A Case-Control Study in 12 Regions within England and Wales," *Journal of Epidemiology and Community Health* 49 (1995): 106–109; E. F. Torrey, A. E. Bowler, and K. Clark, "Urban Birth and Residence as Risk Factors for Psychoses: An Analysis of 1880 Data," *Schizophrenia Research* 25 (1997): 169–176; Hélène Verdoux et al., "Seasonality of Birth in Schizophrenia: The Effect of Regional Population Density," *Schizophrenia Research* 23 (1997): 175–180; M. Marcelis et al., "Urbanization and Psychosis: A Study of 1942–1978 Birth Cohorts in the Netherlands," *Psychological Medicine* 28 (1998): 871–879; and Preben Bo Mortensen et al., "Effects of Family History and Place and Season of Birth on the Risk of Schizophrenia," *New England Journal of Medicine* 340 (1999): 603–608. White, "The Geographic Distribution."

30. K. Miller, *Emigrants and Exiles,* 35. Prior, "The Appeal to Madness," 69.

31. Halliday, *A General View,* 80. H.B.M. Murphy, "Diseases of Civilization?" *Psychological Medicine* 14 (1984): 487–490.

32. Jones, *A History,* 271.

33. F. C. Dohan, "Cereals and Schizophrenia: Data and Hypothesis," *Acta Psychiatrica Scandinavica* 42 (1966): 125–152; Man Mohan Singh and Stanley R. Kay, "Wheat Gluten as a Pathogenic Factor in Schizophrenia," *Science* 191 (1976): 401–402; and David S. King, "Statistical Power of the Controlled Research on Wheat Gluten and Schizophrenia," *Biological Psychiatry* 20 (1985): 785–787. A. C. Christie, "Schizophrenia: Is the Potato the Environmental Culprit?" *Medical Hypotheses* 53 (1999): 80–86. Christine L. Miller, "Rates of Schizophrenia Correlate with Mean Rainfall in Two European Countries," *Schizophrenia Research* 24 (1997): 254.

34. Shorter, *A History of Psychiatry,* 59.

35. Linda Rosenstock et al., "Chronic Central Nervous System Effects of Acute Organophosphate Pesticide Intoxication," *Lancet* 338 (1991): 223–227; S. Gershon and F. H. Shaw, "Psychiatric Sequelae of Chronic Exposure to Organophosphorus Insecticides," *Lancet* (June 24, 1961): 1371–1374; and A. Stoller et al., "Organophosphorus Insecticides and Major Mental Illness: An Epidemiological Investigation," *Lancet* (June 26, 1965): 1387–1388. Harold D. Foster, "Schizophrenia: The Latex Allergy Hypothesis," *Journal of Orthomolecular Medicine* 14 (1999): 83–90.

36. John Cooper and Norman Sartorius, "Cultural and Temporal Variations in Schizophrenia: A Speculation on the Importance of Industrialization," *British Journal of Psychiatry* 130 (1977): 50–55; Richard Warner, "Time Trends in Schizophrenia: Changes in Obstetric Risk Factors with Industrialization," *Schizophrenia Bulletin* 21 (1995): 483–500.

37. Irwin C. Sutton, "A Concise History of Syphilis," *American Journal of Syphilis* 8 (1924): 155–161, and Bernhard Jacobowsky, "General Paresis and Civilization," *Acta Psychiatrica Scandinavica* 41 (1965): 267–273.

38. Arno Karlen, *Man and Microbes* (New York: Simon and Schuster, 1996), 150, and

Hans Zinsser, *Rats, Lice and History: A Bacteriologist's Classic History of Mankind's Epic Struggle to Conquer the Scourge of Typhus* (Boston: Little, Brown and Co., 1934, 1935), 78.

39. E. F. Torrey and R. H. Yolken, "Could Schizophrenia Be a Viral Zoonosis Transmitted from House Cats?" *Schizophrenia Research* 21 (1995): 167–171, and E. F. Torrey, R. Rawlings, R. H. Yolken, "The Antecedents of Psychoses: A Case-Control Study of Selected Risk Factors," *Schizophrenia Research* 46 (2000): 17–23.

40. "Industrial Revolution," *Encyclopaedia Britannica*, 1954, vol. 12, 309, quoting *The Results of Machinery*.

41. Katherine Anne Porter, *Pale Horse, Pale Rider* (New York: New American Library, 1962; first published in 1936), 165.

Appendix A

1. Dalby, "Elizabethan Madness." Arnold, *Observations*, 13. G. E. Berrios, "Historical Aspects of Psychoses: 19th Century Issues," *British Medical Bulletin* 43 (1987): 484–498.

2. Neugebauer, "Treatment of the Mentally Ill." Gwendoline M. Ayers, *England's First State Hospitals*, 44.

3. Humphreys, "Statistics of Insanity," 206.

4. *1880 Census*. James W. Trent Jr., *Inventing the Feeble Mind: A History of Mental Retardation in the United States* (Berkeley: University of California Press, 1994), 68, 188.

5. Berrios, "Historical Aspects."

6. German E. Berrios, *The History of Mental Symptoms: Descriptive Psychopathology since the Nineteenth Century* (Cambridge, U.K.: Cambridge University Press, 1996), 426.

7. Berrios, *The History of Mental Symptoms*, 243.

8. G. E. Berrios, "Depressive and Manic States during the Nineteenth Century," in Anastosios Georgotas and Robert Cancro (eds.), *Depression and Mania* (New York: Elsevier, 1988), 18.

9. Mania: Berrios, "Depressive and Manic States," 14. Melancholia: L. Babb, *The Elizabethan Malady: A Study of Melancholia in English Literature from 1580 to 1640* (East Lansing: Michigan State College Press, 1951), 30, and Berrios in German E. Berrios and Roy Porter, *A History of Clinical Psychiatry* (New York: New York University Press, 1995), 385. Dementia: Berrios, "Historical Aspects."

Appendix B

1. K. Davison and C. R. Bagley, "Schizophrenia-like Psychoses Associated with Organic Disorders of the Central Nervous System: A Review of the Literature," in R. N. Herrington (ed.), *Current Problems in Neuropsychiatry* (Ashford, Kent, U.K.: Hedley, 1969), 113–184; C. Krauthammer and G. L. Klerman, "Secondary Mania: Manic Syndromes Associated with Antecedent Physical Illness or Drugs," *Archives of General Psychiatry* 35 (1978): 1333–1339; K. Davison, "Schizophrenia-like Psychoses Associated with Organic Cerebral Disorders: A Review," *Psychiatric Developments* 1 (1983): 1–34; and P. Propping, "Genetic Disorders Presenting as 'Schizophrenia.' Karl Bonhoeffer's Early View of the Psychoses in the Light of Medical Genetics," *Human Genetics* 65 (1983): 1–10.

2. William Ireland, "On Insanity after Acute and Chronic Infectious Diseases," *Journal of Mental Science* 50 (1904): 772–773.

3. Joel T. Braslow, "The Influence of a Biological Therapy on Physicians' Narratives and Interrogations: The Case of General Paralysis of the Insane and Malaria Fever Therapy, 1910–1950," *Bulletin of the History of Medicine* 70 (1996): 577–608. Robert Jones, "Presidential Address on the Evolution of Insanity," *Journal of Mental Science* 52 (1906): 446.

4. G. D. Shukla et al., "Psychiatric Manifestations in Temporal Lobe Epilepsy: A Controlled Study," *British Journal of Psychiatry* 135 (1979): 411–417. K. A. Achté, E. Hillbom, and V. Aalbreg, "Psychoses following War Brain Injuries," *Acta Psychiatrica Scandinavica* 45 (1969): 1–18.

5. Eric D. Caine and Ira Shoulson, "Psychiatric Syndromes in Huntington's Disease," *American Journal of Psychiatry* 140 (1983): 728–733.

6. R.C.W. Hall, S. K. Stickney, and E. R. Gardner, "Psychiatric Symptoms in Systemic Lupus Erythematosus," *Psychosomatics* 22 (1981): 15–24.

7. Michael MacDonald, "Psychiatric Disorders in Early Modern England," in Paul Williams, Greg Wilkinson, and Kenneth Rawnsley (eds.), *The Scope of Epidemiological Psychiatry: Essays in Honour of Michael Shepherd* (London: Routledge, 1989), 153. M. MacDonald, *Mystical Bedlam*, 5.

8. Trosse: Hare, "Schizophrenia before 1800?" Haizmann: D. Petersen, *A Mad People's History of Madness* (Pittsburgh: University of Pittsburgh Press, 1982), 19. Plater : Whitwell, *Historical Notes on Psychiatry*.

9. David B. Danbom, *Born in the Country*, 7.

10. Briggs, *A Social History of England*, 131–132.

11. Hans Zinsser, *Rats, Lice and History*, 78.

12. E. C. Johnstone, J. F. Macmillan, and T. J. Crow, "The Occurrence of Organic Disease of Possible or Probable Aetiological Significance in a Population of 268 Cases of First Episode Schizophrenia," *Psychological Medicine* 17 (1987): 371–379. E. F. Torrey, "Prevalence Studies in Schizophrenia," *British Journal of Psychiatry* 150 (1987): 598–608.

SELECTED REFERENCES

The following is a selected reference list of the most useful books, papers, and theses on the issue of increasing insanity.

ALLDERIDGE, PATRICIA. "Hospitals, Madhouses and Asylums," *British Journal of Psychiatry* 134 (1979): 321–334.

BARK, NIGEL M. "On the History of Schizophrenia: Evidence of Its Existence before 1800," *New York State Journal of Medicine* 88 (1988): 374–383.

BERRIOS, GERMAN E. *The History of Mental Symptoms* (Cambridge, U.K.: Cambridge University Press, 1996).

BERRIOS, GERMAN E., AND HUGH FREEMAN. *150 Years of British Psychiatry, 1841–1991* (London: Royal College of Psychiatrists, 1991).

BEVERIDGE, ALLAN. "Madness in Victorian Edinburgh," *History of Psychiatry* 6 (1995): 133–156.

BURGESS, T.J.W. "A Historical Sketch of Our Canadian Institutions for the Insane," *Transactions of the Royal Society of Canada* 4 (1898): 3–47.

BYNUM, WILLIAM F., ROY PORTER, AND MICHAEL SHEPHERD (eds.). *The Anatomy of Madness* (London, New York: Tavistock, 1985–1988).

CARPENTER, PETER K. "Schizophrenia before 1800," *British Journal of Psychiatry* 154 (1989): 411–412.

CLARKE, BASIL. *Mental Disorder in Earlier Britain* (Cardiff, U.K.: University of Wales Press, 1975).

CLOUSTON, THOMAS. "The Local Distribution of Insanity and Its Varieties in England and Wales," *Journal of Mental Science* 19 (1873): 1–19.

COOPER, JOHN, AND NORMAN SARTORIUS. "Cultural and Temporal Variations in Schizophrenia," *British Journal of Psychiatry* 130 (1977): 50–55.

CORBET, W. J. "Is Insanity on the Increase?" *Fortnightly Review* 41 (1884): 482–494.

———. "On the Increase of Insanity," *American Journal of Insanity* 50 (1893): 224–238.

————. "The Increase of Insanity," *Fortnightly Review* 59 (n.s. 53) (1893): 7–19.

————. "The Increase of Insanity," *Fortnightly Review* 65 (n.s. 59) (1896): 431–442.

————. "Is the Increase of Insanity Real or Only 'Apparent'?" *Westminster Review* 147 (1897): 539–550.

————. "The Progress of Insanity in Our Time," *Westminster Review* 163 (1905): 198–211.

DAIN, NORMAN. *Concepts of Insanity in the United States, 1789–1865* (New Brunswick, N.J.: Rutgers University Press, 1964).

————. *Disordered Minds: The First Century of Eastern State Hospital in Williamsburg, Virginia, 1766–1866* (Williamsburg, Va.: Colonial Williamsburg Foundation, 1971).

DAWSON, W. R. "The Presidential Address on the Relation between the Geographical Distribution of Insanity and That of Certain Social and Other Conditions in Ireland," *Journal of Mental Science* 57 (1911): 571–597.

DEUTSCH, ALBERT. *The Mentally Ill in America* (New York: Columbia University Press, 1946).

DIGBY, ANNE. *Madness, Morality and Medicine: A Study of the York Retreat 1796–1914* (Cambridge, U.K.: Cambridge University Press, 1985).

DOODY, G. A., A. BEVERIDGE, AND E. C. JOHNSTONE. "Poor and Mad," *Psychological Medicine* 26 (1996): 887–897.

DRAPES, THOMAS. "On the Alleged Increase of Insanity in Ireland," *Journal of Mental Science* 40 (1894): 519–543.

————. "Is Insanity Increasing?" *Fortnightly Review* 66 (1896): 483–493.

DWYER, ELLEN. *Homes for the Mad* (New Brunswick, N.J.: Rutgers University Press, 1987).

EARLE, PLINY. "The Curability of Insanity," *American Journal of Insanity* 33 (1877): 483–533.

ELDRIDGE, LARRY D. "'Crazy Brained': Mental Illness in Colonial America," *Bulletin of the History of Medicine* 70 (1996): 361–386.

ELLARD, J. "Did Schizophrenia Exist before the Eighteenth Century?" *Australian and New Zealand Journal of Psychiatry* 21 (1987): 306–314.

FESSLER, A. "The Management of Lunacy in Seventeenth-Century England: An Investigation of Quarter-Sessions Records," *Proceedings of the Royal Society of Medicine* 49 (1956): 901–907.

FINNANE, MARK. *Insanity and the Insane in Post-Famine Ireland* (London: Croom Helm, 1981).

FOUCAULT, MICHEL. *Madness and Civilization* (New York: Random House, 1965).

FOX, RICHARD W. *So Far Disordered in Mind: Insanity in California, 1870–1930* (Berkeley: University of California Press, 1978).

FRANCIS, DANIEL. "That Prison on the Hill: The Historical Origins of the Lunatic Asylum in the Maritime Provinces" (M.A. thesis, Institute of Canadian Studies, Carlton University, Ottawa, 1975).

GAMWELL, LYNN, AND NANCY TOMES. *Madness in America* (Ithaca, N.Y.: Cornell University Press, 1995).

GOLDHAMER, HERBERT, AND ANDREW W. MARSHALL. *Psychosis and Civilization* (Glencoe, Ill.: Free Press, 1953).

GORWITZ, KURT, "Census Enumeration of the Mentally Ill and the Mentally Retarded in the Nineteenth Century," *Health Services Report* 89 (1974): 180–187.

GROB, GERALD. *The State and the Mentally Ill* (Chapel Hill: University of North Carolina Press, 1966).

———. *Mental Institutions in America* (New York: Free Press, 1973).

———. *Mental Illness and American Society* (Princeton, N.J.: Princeton University Press, 1983).

———. *The Mad among Us* (Cambridge, Mass.: Harvard University Press, 1994).

HALLIDAY, ANDREW. "A Report on the Number of Lunatics and Idiots in England and Wales," in *A Letter to Lord Robert Seymour* (London: Underwood, 1829).

HARE, EDWARD. "Was Insanity on the Increase?" *British Journal of Psychiatry* 142 (1983): 439–455.

HASLAM, JOHN. *Illustrations of Madness* (London: G. Hayden, 1810).

HAWKES, JOHN. "On the Increase in Insanity," *Journal of Psychological Medicine and Mental Pathology* 10 (1857): 508–521.

HODGKINSON, RUTH G. "Provision for Pauper Lunatics, 1834–1871," *Medical History* 10 (1966): 138–154.

———. *The Origins of the National Health Service* (London: Wellcome Historical Medical Library, 1967).

HOOD, WILLIAM C. *Statistics of Insanity* (London: Batten, 1862).

HUMPHREYS, NOEL A. "Statistics of Insanity in England, with Special Reference to Its Alleged Increasing Prevalence," *Journal of the Royal Statistical Society* 53 (1890): 201–252.

HUNTER, JOHN M., GARY W. SHANNON, AND STEPHANIE L. SAMBROOK. "Rings of Madness: Service Areas of 19th Century Asylums in North America," *Social Science and Medicine* 23 (1986): 1033–1050.

HUNTER, RICHARD, AND IDA MACALPINE. *Three Hundred Years of Psychiatry* (London: Oxford University Press, 1963).

HURD, HENRY. *The Institutional Care of the Insane in the United States and Canada*, vol. 4 (Baltimore: Johns Hopkins University Press, 1916–1917).

JARVIS, EDWARD. "Statistics of Insanity in the United States," *Boston Medical and Surgical Journal* 27 (1843): 281–282.

———. "Insanity among the Colored Population of the Free States," *American Journal of Insanity* 8 (1852): 268–282.

———. "On the Supposed Increase of Insanity," *American Journal of Insanity* 8 (1852): 333–364.

———. *Insanity and Idiocy in Massachusetts* (Cambridge, Mass.: Harvard University Press, 1855).

JESTE, D. V., et al. "Did Schizophrenia Exist before the Eighteenth Century?" *Comprehensive Psychiatry* 26 (1985): 493–503.

JIMENEZ, MARY ANN. *Changing Faces of Madness* (Hanover, N.H.: University Press of New England for Brandeis University Press, 1987).

JONES, KATHLEEN. *Lunacy, Law and Conscience 1744–1845* (London: Routledge and Kegan Paul, 1955).

KROLL, JEROME, AND BERNARD BACHRACH. "Sin and Mental Illness in the Middle Ages," *Psychological Medicine* 14 (1984): 507–514.

LEIGH, DENIS. *The Historical Development of British Psychiatry*, vol. 1 (Oxford: Pergamon, 1961).

MACALPINE, IDA, AND RICHARD HUNTER. *George III and the Mad-Business* (New York: W. W. Norton, 1969).

MACCABE, F. "On the Alleged Increase in Lunacy," *Journal of Mental Science* 15 (1869): 363–366.

MACDONALD, MICHAEL. *Mystical Bedlam* (Cambridge, U.K.: Cambridge University Press, 1981).

MACKENZIE, CHARLOTTE. "Social Factors in the Admission, Discharge and Continuing Stay of Patients at Ticehurst Asylum, 1845–1917," in Bynum et al., *Anatomy of Madness*, vol. 2.

MACKENZIE, CHARLOTTE. "Psychiatry for the Rich," *Psychological Medicine* 18 (1988): 545–549.

MAUDSLEY, HENRY. "Is Insanity on the Increase?" *British Medical Journal* 1 (1872): 36–39.

MAUDSLEY, HENRY. "The Alleged Increase of Insanity," *Journal of Mental Science* 23 (1877): 45–54.

MCCANDLESS, PETER. "'Build! Build!': The Controversy over the Care of the Chronically Insane in England, 1855–1870," *Bulletin of the History of Medicine* 53 (1979): 553–574.

———. *Moonlight, Magnolias and Madness: Insanity in South Carolina from the Colonial Period to the Progressive Era* (Chapel Hill: University of North Carolina Press, 1996).

MELLETT, DAVID J. *The Prerogative of Asylumdom* (New York: Garland, 1982).

MORRISSEY, J. P., H. H. GOLDMAN, AND L. V. KLERMAN (eds.). *The Enduring Asylum* (New York: Grune and Stratton, 1980).

NEUGEBAUER, RICHARD. "Treatment of the Mentally Ill in Mediaeval and Early Modern England," *Journal of the History of the Behavioral Sciences* 14 (1978): 158–169.

———. "Medieval and Early Modern Theories of Mental Illness," *Archives of General Psychiatry* 36 (1979): 477–483.

OBERHELMAN, DAVID DEAN. *Mad Encounters: Nineteenth-Century British Psychological Medicine and the Victorian Novel, 1840–1870* (Ann Arbor, Mich.: University Microfilms International, 1993).

PARRY-JONES, WILLIAM. *The Trade in Lunacy* (London: Routledge and Kegan Paul, 1972).

PERSAUD, RAJENDRA D. "A Comparison of Symptoms Recorded from the Same Patients by an Asylum Doctor and 'A Constant Observer' in 1823," *History of Psychiatry* 3 (1992): 79–94.

———. "The Reporting of Psychiatric Symptoms in History," *History of Psychiatry* 4 (1993): 499–510.

PORTER, ROY. "Being Mad in Georgian England," *History Today* (December 1981): 42–48.

————. *Mind-Forg'd Manacles: A History of Madness in England from the Restoration to the Regency* (Cambridge, Mass.: Harvard University Press, 1987).

POWELL, RICHARD, "Observations upon the Comparative Prevalence of Insanity at Different Periods," *Medical Transactions* 4 (1813): 131–159.

PRIDGEON, CHARLES T. *Insanity in American Fiction from Charles Brockden Brown to Oliver Wendell Holmes* (Ann Arbor, Mich.: University Microfilms International, 1973).

RAY, ISAAC. "Statistics of Insanity in Massachusetts," *North American Review* 82 (1856): 78–100.

REID, JOHN. "Report of Diseases," *Monthly Magazine* 25 (1808): 166, 374.

RENVOIZE, EDWARD B., AND ALLAN W. BEVERIDGE. "Mental Illness and the Late Victorians," *Psychological Medicine* 19 (1989): 19–28.

ROBERTSON, C. LOCKHART. "The Alleged Increase of Lunacy," *Journal of Mental Science* 15 (1869): 1–23.

————. "A Further Note on the Alleged Increase in Insanity," *Journal of Mental Science* 16 (1871): 473–497.

ROBINS, JOSEPH. *Fools and Mad: A History of the Insane in Ireland* (Dublin: Institute of Public Administration, 1986).

ROTHMAN, DAVID J. *The Discovery of the Asylum* (Boston: Little, Brown, 1971).

RUSHTON, PETER. "Lunatics and Idiots: Mental Disability, the Community, and the Poor Law in North-East England 1600–1800," *Medical History* 32 (1988): 34–50.

SANBORN, FRANKLIN B. "Is American Insanity Increasing?" *Journal of Mental Science* 40 (1894): 214–219.

SCULL, ANDREW. "Was Insanity Increasing? A Response to Edward Hare," *British Journal of Psychiatry* 144 (1984): 432–436.

————. *Social Order/Mental Disorder* (Berkeley: University of California Press, 1989).

————. *The Most Solitary of Afflictions* (New Haven: Yale University Press, 1993).

SCULL, ANDREW (ed.). *Madhouses, Mad-Doctors, and Madmen: The Social History of Psychiatry in the Victorian Era* (Philadelphia: University of Pennsylvania Press, 1981).

SHEPHERD, MICHAEL. *A Study of the Major Psychoses in an English County* (London: Chapman and Hall, 1957).

SKULTANS, VIEDA. *English Madness* (London: Routledge and Kegan Paul, 1979).

SMITH, LEONARD D. *"Cure, Comfort and Safe Custody": Public Lunatic Asylums in Early Nineteenth-Century England* (London: Leicester University Press, 1999).

STEARNS, HENRY P. "The Relations of Insanity to Modern Civilization," *Scribner's Monthly* 17 (1878): 582–586.

STROUP, ATLEE L., AND RONALD W. MANDERSCHEID. "The Development of the State Mental Hospital System in the United States: 1840–1980," *Journal of the Washington Academy of Sciences* 78 (1988): 59–68.

SUZUKI, AKIHITO. "Lunacy in Seventeenth- and Eighteenth-Century England: Analysis of Quarter Sessions Records, Part I," *History of Psychiatry* 2 (1991): 437–456, and "Part II," *History of Psychiatry* 3 (1992): 29–44.

THURMAN, JOHN. *Observations and Essays on the Statistics of Insanity* (New York: Arno Press, 1976; originally published in 1845).

TOMES, NANCY. *A Generous Confidence: Thomas Story Kirkbride and the Art of Asylum Keeping, 1840–1883* (Cambridge, U.K.: Cambridge University Press, 1984).

TOMLINSON, DYLAN R., AND JOHN CARRIER (eds.). *Asylum in the Community* (London: Routledge, 1996).

TORREY, E. FULLER. *Schizophrenia and Civilization* (New York: Jason Aronson, Inc., 1980).

TUKE, DANIEL HACK. *Insanity in Ancient and Modern Life* (London: Macmillan, 1878).

Chapters in the History of the Insane in the British Isles (London: Kegan Paul, Trench, 1882).

———. *The Insane in the United States and Canada* (London: H. K. Lewis, 1885).

———. "Alleged Increase of Insanity," *Journal of Mental Science* 40 (1894): 219–231.

———. "Increase of Insanity in Ireland," *Journal of Mental Science* 40 (1894): 561.

TURNER, T. H. "Schizophrenia as a Permanent Problem," *History of Psychiatry* 3 (1992): 413–429.

TURNER, TREVOR. "Rich and Mad in Victorian England," *Psychological Medicine* 19 (1989): 29–44.

WALKER, NIGEL, AND SARAH McCABE. *Crime and Insanity in England* (Edinburgh: University Press, 1968).

WALSH, DERMOT. *The 1963 Irish Psychiatric Hospital Census* (Dublin: The Medico-Social Research Board, 1970).

WALTON, JOHN. "Lunacy in the Industrial Revolution," *Journal of Social History* 13 (1979): 1–22.

WARNER, RICHARD. "Time Trends in Schizophrenia: Changes in Obstetric Risk Factors with Industrialization," *Schizophrenia Bulletin* 21 (1995): 483–500.

WHITE, WILLIAM A. "The Geographical Distribution of Insanity in the United States," *National Geographic Magazine* 14 (1903): 361–378.

WINSTON, ELLEN. "The Assumed Increase of Mental Disease," *American Journal of Sociology* 40 (1935): 427–439.

Act for Regulating Madhouses (1774), 28–30
Act of Union (1800), 128, 130–131
Acts of Parliament. *See* insanity legislation
AIDS, 2–3, 299
Aiken, Conrad, 294
Alabama, 210, 216
alcohol abuse: among asylum staff, 258; among writers, 155, 228, 294, 305; as diagnostic category, 97, 112–113, 168, 270; as explanation for "apparent" increase in insanity, 315; as explanation for real increase in insanity, 76–77, 79, 97, 107, 148, 331; as medical condition that can cause psychiatric symptoms, 8, 20, 40, 128, 331, 340, 342, 344; as suggested cause of insanity: in California, 251; in Canada, 165, 185; among the Irish, 128, 139, 145, 148–149, 239
alienists. *See* psychiatrists
Allbutt, Clifford, 116
Allderidge, Patricia, 29
Allen, Matthew, 65–66
almshouses. *See* poorhouses; workhouses
Alzheimer's disease, 4, 113, 291, 297, 325, 340

amentia, 174. *See also* mental retardation
American Journal of Insanity, 263
American Medico-Psychological Association, 281, 284, 285
American Neurological Association, 259
American Psychiatric Association, 223. *See also* Association of Medical Superintendents of American Institutions for the Insane
American Psychological Journal, 265
Andreasen, Nancy, 156
Andrews, Jonathan, 25
anti-vagrancy laws, 11, 23–24
antipsychiatry, 304, 307, 309
Antrim, 152
Apothecaries Act (1815), 57
Ariano, Marlene, 303
Arizona, 271
Arlidge, John, 93, 104, 112
Armagh: asylum, 130, 144; county, 135
Arnold, Thomas, 36–38, 328, 335
art, depictions of insanity in, 9, 25, 30, 33
Ashley, Lord. *See* Cooper, Anthony Ashley
Association of Medical Officers of Asylums and Hospitals for the Insane, 78. *See also* British Medico-Psychological Association

Association of Medical Superintendents of American Institutions for the Insane (AMSAII), 223, 227, 259, 262, 273

asylum doctors. *See* psychiatrists

asylums. *See* confinement of the insane; private asylums; public asylums

Austen, Jane, 50

Awl, William ("Dr. Cure-Awl"), 222, 227, 258

Ayurvedic medicine, 7

Bachrach, Bernard, 8

"baile," 125

Bakewell, Thomas, 49

ballads, 11–12, 54, 149, 185

Ballinasloe Asylum, 130, 137, 149

Ballymena Workhouse, 138

Bard, Samuel, 201

Bark, Nigel, 13

baseline rate of insanity, 6–7, 19, 47, 315, 339–344. *See also* medical conditions that can cause psychiatric symptoms

Bateman, Thomas, 58

Battie, William, 35

Beard, George, 259

Beckett, Samuel, 156

Beddoes, Thomas, 62

Bedfordshire: asylum, 47, 69; county, 17, 121

Bedlam. *See* Bethlem Hospital

Beers, Clifford, 286

Belfast Asylum, 130, 138, 151

Bell, Hugh, 179–180, 181

Bell, Luther, 223

Bellingham, John, 71

Bemis, Merrick, 258

Benedict, Nathan, 260

Berchet, Peter, 10

Berke, Joseph, 305

Berkshire County, 69, 100, 102

Berrios, German, 303, 335, 337, 338

Bethlem Hospital ("Bedlam"): analyses of admissions, discharges, 21, 25, 114; as model asylum, 172, 197; as tourist attraction, 14–16, 25–26; "bedlam" as diagnosis, 18; Bedlam Beggars, 11–12, 16; building and renovations, 10, 15,

24; escapees, 45–46; for the violent insane, 20, 45; John Haslam, 39–40; in art, 25; in ballads, 11–12; in literature, 13–14, 25–26, 30, 54, 64, 126; patient abuse, 48; the Prince of Wales, 25; Jonathan Swift, 127; Toms o' Bedlam, 12, 13, 71; violence in, 45; waiting list, 58; young patients, 111

Beveridge, Allan, 114

bipolar disorder. *See* manic-depressive illness

Bird, Robert Montgomery, 213, 214

Blackwell Asylum. *See under* New York

Blake, William, 53, 57

Blanchard, Edward, 169–170

Bland, Roger, 191

Bloomfield Retreat, 131

Blumer, Alder, 285, 287

Blundell, Nicholas, 25

Bly, Nellie, 257

Bond, Thomas, 197

Boswell, James, 35–36, 37

Braddon, Mary Elizabeth, 85

Brain, Russell, 31

brain disease, insanity as, 2, 3, 4, 304, 335

brain tumors/trauma. *See* medical conditions that can cause psychiatric symptoms

Brigham, Amariah, 13, 209, 211, 223, 323

Brislington House, 114

British Journal of Psychiatry, 78, 122, 158

British Medico-Psychological Association, 78–80, 85, 104, 112, 117, 140

Brontë, Charlotte, 72

Brown, Charles Brockden, 202–203, 229

Brown, D. T., 258

Browne, William A. F., 50, 62, 99–100, 239

Bruckshaw, Samuel, 29

bubonic plague, 16, 342

Buckinghamshire: asylum, 111, 118; county, 17–18, 96, 121, 318

Bucknill, John, 12–13, 78, 82, 94, 100, 224, 260

Burgess, Thomas, 189

Burke, Edmund, 42

Burnett, Charles M., 74

Burrows, George Man, 57–59, 99, 129
Burton, Robert, 21, 63, 232
Busfield, Joan, 313
Butler, John, 223
Bynum, William, 81
Byron, Lord, 54–55, 65, 232, 312

Calhoun, John C., 217–218
California: asylum admissions, 322; asylum building, 223, 250–252; early provisions for the insane, 250; prevalence of insanity, 249–252, 270–271, 272 (map), 275, 298; sterilization of the insane, 284; Stockton State Hospital, 246, 250, 251, 283
carbon disulfide poisoning, 341
Carlow: asylum, 130; county, 159
Carroll, Lewis (Charles Lutwidge Dodgson), 87–93, 341
catatonic behavior, 9, 156, 341
cats, exposure to, as a risk factor for insanity, 332–333
Cavan, 135, 159
censuses of the insane: Canada, 162, 165, 167, 170, 179, 183–184, 185, 187–188, 188 (graph); England, 46, 61–62, 69, 74, 75, 87, 93, 107, 118, 326, 336; Ireland, 125, 129, 131, 133, 134–136, 140, 142–143, 151–152, 326; United States, 216–218, 222, 235–236, 248–249, 251, 269–275, 278–280, 283, 287–289, 326, 336; lack of, after World War II, 120, 191–192, 298, 316. See also Salford case register; and see Connecticut; Massachusetts; New York
Chandler, George, 239
Channing, Walter, 278
Chapin, John, 242, 319
Chapman, Mary, 27
Charles I, King of England, 65, 343
Charles II, King of England, 342
Charles VI, King of France, 9
Chatterton, Thomas, 31, 33, 51
Cheshire County, 69, 100
Cheyne, George, 38, 122
childbirth, insanity following, 7, 9, 40, 50, 174, 254–255
cholera, 132; as cause of asylum deaths,

69, 111, 132, 222, 324; as cause of psychiatric symptoms, 339
Christie, Amiel, 331
Citizen's Commission on Human Rights, Church of Scientology, 304
civil libertarian movement, 4, 304, 307
Civil War (English), 16, 343
Civil War (U.S.), 244–245, 255, 268, 315
Clare, John, 65–66, 312
Clare (Ireland), 159
Clarke, Geoffrey, 117
Clonmel Asylum, 130, 153
Clouston, Thomas, 100, 102, 116, 117, 141
Cockton, Henry, 83
Coddon, Karin, 13
Coleridge, Samuel Taylor, 34, 53
"Collegium Insanorum," 32
Colley, Ann, 50, 68, 72
Collins, Joseph, 12
Collins, Michael, 153
Collins, Wilkie, 65, 82–85
Collins, William, 31
Colney Hatch, 76, 111, 115
Colorado, 271
Commissioners in Lunacy. See Lunacy Commission/Commissioners (England)
confinement of the insane: as advantageous to psychiatrists, 308–309; as last resort of family members, 112, 320–321; as means of social control, 305–313; as portrayed in popular journals, 225; as tourist attraction, 64, 170, 198, 205–206, 210, 225, 317; boarding homes, 175; commitment laws, 255–257; early accommodations for the insane, 8, 10, 16, 162, 194; effects of confinement on the prevalence of insanity, 111, 324–325, 328; failure of, 310–311; foreign observers, 48; funding, 24, 27, 47, 95–96, 130, 138, 198, 204, 207, 209, 318, 325; the "great confinement," 302–303, 304–311, 317, 319–320; linked to social unrest, 306, 317; Packard Laws, 256; patient abuse, 29–30, 48, 70, 83, 164, 169, 179, 186, 256, 263–264; pa-

confinement of the insane (*continued*)
per lunatics, 16, 24, 28, 59–60, 70, 76,
95–96, 110; public's fear of violence,
19–20, 128, 197, 200, 224; wrongful
confinement, 29–30, 85, 256–257. *See
also* Bethlem Hospital; home care;
hospitals; jails/prisons; literature;
poorhouses; private asylums; public
asylums; workhouses
congenital insanity, 322
Connaught, 133, 135
Connecticut: asylum admissions, 246;
asylum building/resistance to building, 207, 245, 318; censuses of the
insane, 206–207; early case findings,
197; early provisions for the insane,
194, 195–196, 201; Hartford Retreat,
207, 210, 211, 227; immigration
restrictions, 283; Irish immigrants,
147; prevalence of insanity, 216, 271,
297, 298
Connecticut Hospital for the Insane at
Middletown, 226
Connecticut Medical Society, 206, 264
Conolly, John, 12, 63–64, 80, 85–86
consanguineous marriage, 139, 148, 315,
327
conservatorship, 336
Coolidge, Calvin, 288
Cooper, Anthony Ashley, 1st Earl of
Shaftesbury, 59–61, 70, 71, 76–79, 87,
88, 90, 95, 97, 107
Cooper, James Fenimore, 202, 212
Cooper, John, 331
Corbet, W. J., 114, 142, 148
Cork: asylums and workhouses,
127–128, 129, 133; emigration to
Canada, 147, 171; famine, 133; vio-
lence and insanity, 132
Cornwall, 69, 100
Cotton, Henry, 290
Cotton, Nathaniel, 32
Coué, Emil, 288
County Asylum Acts (1808, 1828), 47,
61
Cowper, William, 31, 32–33, 52
Cox, Joseph, 45
Crabbe, George, 50–51, 53

Crammer, John L., 47
Crazy Jane, 154–155
Crazy Kate, 33, 52, 154
creativity and insanity, 31, 34, 50, 235.
See also specific individuals
Crichton-Browne, James, 104
criminal lunatics. *See* literature: the
criminally insane; violence and insan-
ity
Criminal Lunatics Act (1800), 45
Crowther, Bryan, 49
Cruden, Alexander, 29
"cult of curability," 226. *See also* insanity,
treatment of: curability of insanity
Cutbush, Edward, 201
cyclothymia, 60

Dadd, Richard, 71
Dain, Norman, 306–307
Dalby, Thomas, 12, 13
Dana, Richard Henry, 212
Darwin, Charles, 81, 117, 202
Darwin, Erasmus, 202
Davidson, Lucretia Maria, 213
Dawson, William R., 152
decarceration, 307. *See also* deinstitutionalization
Defoe, Daniel, 29
deinstitutionalization, 4, 15, 94, 118, 120,
157–158, 191, 295–299, 307, 316
Dekker, Thomas, 14
delirium, 7, 18, 337, 339, 340, 341
delirium tremens, 163, 340
delusional disorder, 338
delusions: among poets, writers, 32, 34,
65, 119, 228, 312; among royalty, 9, 41;
as hallmark of insanity, 2, 22, 35, 126,
322, 336; as not present in "moral
insanity," 337; case studies, 7, 8, 17–19,
202; caused by other medical conditions, 315, 337, 340–342; in literature,
35, 67, 119, 212, 213–214, 231–232;
monomania, 213, 214, 216, 224, 229,
233–234, 270
dementia: caused by alcohol, 112, 148,
340; caused by vitamin deficiency,
341; defined, 338; in literature, 13;
senile dementia, 4, 13, 121, 190, 291,

325. *See also* Alzheimer's disease; insanity, diagnostic categories of

Depression, the Great, 289, 316, 330

depression/melancholy: among poets, 31, 32, 51, 53, 65; among other writers, 34, 38, 53, 55, 228, 254–255, 293, 294; as the "English malady," 38; case studies, 7, 8, 194, 198; changes in definition, 338; in literature, 10, 151, 229, 230; "moody melancholy," 206. *See also* insanity, diagnostic categories of; manic-depressive illness

Derbyshire County, 69, 100, 102

Derry Asylum, 130, 131, 137, 138, 318

Deutsch, Albert, 226, 295

Devonshire: asylum, 78, 94; county, 69

DeWolf, James, 182–186

Diagnostic and Statistical Manual of Mental Disorders, Fourth Edition (DSM-IV), 338

diagnostic boundaries, broadening of. *See* insanity, explanations for "apparent" increase in

diagnostic categories of insanity. *See* insanity, diagnostic categories of

Dialectics of Liberation Congress, 305

Diamond, Hugh, 88

Dickens, Charles: friendships, 64, 85; interest in insanity, 63, 85; "A Madman's Manuscript," 63, 64, 229, 232; novels, 64–65, 82; visits to asylums and workhouses, 63, 65, 97, 221, 229; visits to the United States, 65, 221

Dickie, Susan, 257, 265

Dickinson, Emily, 253–254

dipsomania, 168, 270. *See also* alcohol abuse

disordered thinking/behavior, 2, 312, 315, 337

Disraeli, Benjamin, 96, 104, 318

Dix, Dorothea: advocacy in Canada, 173, 180–181, 318; advocacy in the United States, 219, 220–222, 224, 318; as Union Army nurse, 268; belief in the curability of insanity, 227, 258; belief in the urban risk factor, 242, 329; visit to England, 219

Dodgson, Charles Lutwidge (Lewis Carroll), 87–93, 341

Donegal, 148

Donizetti, Gaetano, 54

Dorset County, 17, 69, 102

Dowbiggin, Ian, 284–285

Down, 152

Drapes, Thomas, 143

drug use/abuse. *See* medical conditions that can cause psychiatric symptoms: prescription or illegal drug use

Drummond, Edward, 71

DSM-IV (Diagnostic and Statistical Manual of Mental Disorders, Fourth Edition), 338

Dublin: asylums and workhouses, 124–125, 127, 129, 131, 132; in literature, 156–157; prevalence of insanity, 135, 152, 159

Duddeston Hall, 114

Duncan, Martin, 104

Dundrum Asylum, 132, 142

Dunham, Warren, 292

Dunnington House, 70

Durham (England), 100, 102

Durham (North Carolina), 298

Dwyer, Ellen, 221

Earle, Pliny, 223, 227, 258–259, 261, 273, 324

East European immigrants, prejudice against, 3, 288

Eastgate House, 70

Eaton, Dorman, 266

Eaton, William, 296

Edward VII, King of England, 116

Eigen, Joel, 44

Eldridge, Larry, 194

Elkind, Henry, 290

Ellmann, Richard, 155–156

emigration, as a risk factor. *See* insanity, explanations for "apparent" increase in: emigration; *specific immigrant groups under* immigration: prevalence of insanity among

encephalitis. *See under* medical conditions that can cause psychiatric symptoms

encephalitis lethargica, 340, 343
endocrine disorders. *See* medical conditions that can cause psychiatric symptoms
English Civil War, 16, 343
"English malady," 23, 38, 45. *See also* Cheyne, George; insanity, prevalence of: as an English malady
epidemic insanity, 2–5, 34–35, 68, 85, 299, 300–302, 314–315
epidemics: as cause of death in asylums, 69, 111, 118, 151, 222, 288, 316, 324–325. *See also* AIDS; bubonic plague; cholera; encephalitis lethargica; influenza; syphilis; tuberculosis; typhus
Epidemiologic Catchment Area (ECA) study, 298
epilepsy: as diagnostic category, 97, 112–113, 145, 270, 298; as hereditary disease, 285; as insanity defense, 260; as medical condition that can cause psychiatric symptoms, 7, 9, 340, 343; caused by birth trauma, 343; early descriptions of, 7
ergotism, 343
Esquirol, Jean, 213
Essex County, 65
eugenics movement, 3, 116–117, 184, 280–286
Evangelical Christianity, 60–61, 76, 88
Everts, Orpheus, 266

famine, 160, 171, 343. *See also* Irish Famine
Faris, Robert, 292
Farquhar, George, 25
Farr, William, 99, 111
Faulkner, Benjamin, 38
Faulks, E., 117
Fauquier, Francis, 199
feigned insanity, 12, 13, 16, 304
Fessler, A., 19
fever, high. *See* medical conditions that can cause psychiatric symptoms
Fielding, Henry, 30
Fitzgerald, F. Scott, 293–294
Fitzgerald, Zelda, 293

Fleming, May Agnes, 165
Fletcher, John, 14
Florida, 210
Fly, Eli James Murdock, 234
folk songs. *See* ballads
Forster, John, 64, 91
Foster, Harold, 331
Foucault, Michel, 4, 19, 95, 112, 302–305, 306, 307, 312, 316–317, 319, 322
Fox, Richard, 251, 322
Franklin, Benjamin, 197
Freeman, Hugh, 303
frenzy, 18, 337
Freud, Sigmund/Freudian theory, 13, 119, 286–287, 297, 301
Fuller, Robert, 256
functional psychosis, 335
Fuseli, Henry, 33

Galton, Francis, 117
Galway: emigration, 147, 240; famine, 133; prevalence of insanity, 135, 148–149, 158
Garfield, James, 267
genetic disorders. *See* medical conditions that can cause psychiatric symptoms
genetic predisposition to insanity, 97, 99, 116–117, 148, 184, 189, 211, 281, 285, 302, 327–328
geographic variation in the prevalence of insanity, 315; England, 69, 100–102; Ireland, 135–136, 152, 153 (map), 158–159; United States, 210–211, 216, 235–236, 249, 271–272, 272 (map), 292
George III, King of England, 23, 40–42, 44
Georgia, 210, 216, 223, 224, 226
Gidley, Richard, 169
Gilman, Charlotte Perkins, 254–255
Glennagalt, 125
Gloucestershire: asylum, 47–48; county, 69, 100, 102
Godding, William, 273, 276–277, 282
Goffman, Irving, 302–305, 316, 319
Goldhamer, Herbert, 296–297, 301, 306, 310
Goodman, Paul, 305

Gordon, Lord George (M.P.), 45, 64
Gordon, Lord George (poet). *See* Lord
    Byron
Gorwitz, Kurt, 235
Gosling, Abraham, 265
Government Hospital for the Insane/St.
    Elizabeths Hospital, 258, 273, 287, 323
"Grangegorman." *See* Richmond Asylum
Grant, Madison, 282–283, 285
Gray, John, 260–269
Gray, Thomas, 30–31
Great Depression, 289, 316, 330
"Great Pox," 342. *See also* syphilis
Greek mythology, 7
Grissom, Eugene, 262–264, 268
Grob, Gerald, 208, 209, 301, 306,
    310–311, 318, 321, 322, 325–326
Grosley, Pierre J., 36–37
Guiteau, Charles, 267–269
Guy, Thomas/Guy's Hospital, 27

Hadfield, James, 44–45
Haizmann, Christoph, 342
Haldipur, C. V., 7
Hale, Nathan, 284
Hallaran, William S., 128
Halliday, Sir Andrew, 46, 61–62, 63, 99,
    121, 130, 330
hallucinations: among poets, writers, 32,
    55, 65, 104, 119, 155; among royalty, 9,
    41; as hallmark of insanity, 2, 336;
    case studies, 8, 9, 111, 198, 202; caused
    by alcohol, 8, 340, 342; caused by
    other medical conditions, 6, 8, 315,
    337, 339–342; caused by stress, 8; hyp-
    nagogic hallucinations, 8; in the Bible,
    7; in literature, 50, 66–67, 119, 156,
    212, 229–230, 232, 294–295; in opera,
    54
Hamilton, Allan, 265
Hamilton, John, 114
Hamlin, Oscar, 243
Hammond, William, 259–269
Hampshire County, 69
Hancock, Thomas, 196
Hanwell Asylum, 69, 85, 172, 324
Hare, Edward, 20, 82, 313, 328
Harper, Andrew, 39

Hartford Retreat, 207, 210, 211, 227
Harvey, Sir John, 178
Haslam, John, 39–40
Hattie, William, 187
Haverfordwest Asylum, 95
Hawkes, John, 75, 98
Hawkins, Sir John, 10
Hawthorne, Nathaniel, 197, 202,
    230–232, 233
Haydock Lodge, 70
Hayward, George, 199
head injuries. *See* medical conditions
    that can cause psychiatric
    symptoms
Healy, David, 150
Hebrew Bible, 7
Henry VI, King of England, 9
Henry VIII, King of England, 10, 16
hepatic encephalopathy, 341
hepatitis, 341
heredity. *See* genetic predisposition to
    insanity
Herefordshire County, 100, 102
Hershey, Gen. Lewis, 295
Hervey, Nicholas, 77
Hey, James, 24
High Beech, asylum at, 65
Hill, George, 49
Hippocrates, 7, 339
*Histoire de la Folie/Madness and Civiliza-
    tion* (Foucault), 19, 95, 302–303
Hogarth, William, 25
Hollingshead, August B., 297
Holmes, Oliver Wendell, 202, 230–231,
    252–253
home care, 15, 19, 20, 62, 87, 175, 194,
    206, 323
homeless mentally ill, the, 4, 15, 299,
    304, 316
Hood, W. C., 63
Hook Norton Asylum, 70, 111
hospitals, 10, 125, 171, 250–251. *See also*
    private asylums; public asylums
House of Industry, 129
Howard, John, 46
Howe, Samuel Gridley, 219, 237
Humphreys, Noel, 109
Hunt, Isaac, 256

Hunter, Richard, 40, 59, 301
"The Hunting of the Snark" (Carroll), 89–93
Huntington's disease, 341, 343
Hurd, Henry, 218
hypnagogic hallucinations, 8
hypochondriasis, 336
hysteria, 336

ICD (International Classification of Diseases), 113, 338
Idaho, 271, 274
idiocy. See mental retardation
Illinois, 223, 245, 256, 258, 292
immigration: as suggested cause of insanity, 98, 122, 238–240, 251, 280–281, 315; discrimination against immigrants, 3, 240–241; Immigration Act (1921), 288; Immigration Commission, 282; Immigration Restriction League, 281; Johnson-Reed Act (1924), 288; prevalence of insanity among: African-Caribbean immigrants, 122, 329; Chinese immigrants, 251; immigrants in general, 251, 270–273, 274, 280–286; Irish immigrants in Canada, 147, 163, 167, 174, 185, 329; Irish immigrants in England, 98, 147, 329; Irish immigrants in the United States, 240–241, 280, 282, 329; Jewish immigrants, 281–282; Scandinavian immigrants, 281. See also eugenics movement
inbreeding. See consanguineous marriage
Indiana, 223, 284
industrialization, 242, 328–329. See also urban risk factor
infectious agents/diseases. See medical conditions that can cause psychiatric symptoms
inflammatory disease. See medical conditions that can cause psychiatric symptoms
influenza, 2; as cause of asylum deaths, 69, 118, 151, 288, 316, 324; as cause of psychiatric symptoms, 340
insanity, cost of, 4–5, 152, 192, 238, 282,

287, 289, 299. See also Massachusetts; public asylums (England); public asylums (Ireland); workhouses; individual disorders
insanity, definition of, 335–338
insanity, descriptions of, 7, 39–40. See also individual disorders, symptoms
insanity, diagnostic categories of, 97, 112–113, 120–121, 163, 167, 168, 174, 270, 297, 322. See also alcohol abuse; epilepsy; mental retardation; syphilis; insanity, explanations for "apparent" increase in: broadening of diagnostic boundaries
insanity, explanations for "apparent" increase in: accessibility of asylums, 144, 191, 308–310, 316–326; accumulation of chronic cases, 77, 79, 80, 139, 141, 144–145, 323–330; backlog of cases, 109–110, 114; broadening of diagnostic boundaries, 24, 112–114, 132, 144–145, 191, 308, 313, 321–322; confinement of nonproductive members of society, 302–311, 317, 319–320; declining asylum cure/discharge rates, 110–111, 141, 144–145, 323; declining asylum death rates, 110–111, 114, 116, 141, 144, 175, 323, 324; decreased stigma, 144–145, 320–321; emergence of market economy, 307–312, 316–317; emigration, 146–147, 160; financial benefits for counties, 80; financial benefits for psychiatrists, 308–309, 311; improved case-finding, 77, 79, 80, 191; increased care for elderly, 160, 291, 323, 325–326; lumber room thesis, 308–310, 316–326; returning emigrants, 144, 146; transfers from workhouses to asylums, 144, 146; true increase in the numbers of the insane, 313, 326. See also alcohol abuse
insanity, fear of: fear of others' insanity, 63, 64, 68, 71–72, 84; fear of own insanity, 36, 55, 126, 213, 232, 253, 294; Salem witchcraft trials, 3, 194–195. See also confinement of the insane: wrongful confinement and

public's fear of violence; eugenics movement; immigration: discrimination against immigrants; sterilization

insanity, feigned, 12, 13, 16, 304

insanity, increase in severity of, 16, 114, 323–324, 326

insanity, moral, 119, 167, 252–253, 337 (defined)

insanity, possible decrease in, 159

insanity, prevalence of: among Californians, 249–252; among free colored persons, 217–218; among males, 313; among military personnel, 295; among Quakers, 28; among the educated/wealthy, 50, 99, 125, 136, 197, 199, 331; among the poor, 102, 241–242; among writers, 119; among young people, 39–40, 250; as a female malady, 312–313; as an English malady, 12, 23, 35, 37–39, 45, 49, 58, 63, 70, 75; as an Irish malady, 125, 141, 143, 147, 150, 154, 158; as nonexistent, 302–305, 312; as rare before 1700, 17–19, 20, 161, 193–194, 196, 315; as unvarying, 301; comparisons over time, 3, 16, 301, 316, 337–338, 339; effects of rainfall, 331; in Canada, 188 (graph), 191–192, 315, 350 (table); in England and Wales, 94 (graph), 101 (map), 120–123, 313, 315, 345–347 (table); in Ireland, 152 (graph), 153 (map), 158, 160, 313, 315, 348–349 (table); in the United States, 271 (graph), 272 (map), 297–299, 301, 313, 315, 350 (table); in Third World countries, 5; linked to industrialization, 242, 328–329; possible decrease in, due to confinement, 111, 324–325, 328; World Health Organization reports, 158, 159. See also specific immigrant groups under immigration: prevalence of insanity among; baseline rate of insanity; censuses of the insane; creativity and insanity; geographic variation in the prevalence of insanity; urban risk factor

insanity, prevention of, 286–290. See also eugenics movement; sterilization

insanity, romanticization of, 235, 280, 303, 304–307

insanity, suggested causes of, 97-102: abnormal blood flow, 199, 233; air pollution, 275, 279; cats, 332–333; childhood experiences, 301; civilization, 38, 49, 62–63, 79, 99, 165, 184–185, 189, 236–237, 279, 290, 328–329, 332; "desocialization," 304; diet, 8, 139, 330; divine retribution, 7, 8, 9; English rule in Ireland, 149; freedom from slavery, 217–218; frontier living, 243; grief, 8; household crowding, 102, 243; humoral imbalance, 8; immorality, 98, 195, 251; improved obstetrical care, 331; incest, 293; irritable temperament, 239; isolation, 151; love/unrequited love, 11, 37; miscellaneous causes, 98; natural selection, 81; newspapers, 211; noise, 275; overwork, 8; parental pressure, 305; poverty, 100, 102, 147, 153, 241–242; premature passion, 78, 184; psychological causes, 128; rabies, 8; railway travel, 98, 165; religious sentiment, 37, 77; repression, 291; reversals of fortune, 251; stress, 63, 285, 330; tobacco, 36, 252; vaccinations, 332; wealth, 37–39, 49, 199, 328–329. See also alcohol abuse; consanguineous marriage; genetic predisposition; immigration; medical conditions that can cause psychiatric symptoms; postpartum psychosis; urban risk factor

insanity, symptoms of, 2, 322; as coming from God, 7, 9–10; as temporary in early cases, 6, 21, 339, 342; attachment to royalty, 45, 105, 166; command hallucinations, 8; organic lesions, 128; suicide, 2, 59. See also insanity, treatment of: curability of insanity; violence and insanity; individual symptoms

insanity, treatment of: curability of insanity, 6, 21, 207, 211, 226–227, 237–238, 258, 278, 310, 321, 323; diet, 8; early treatments, 8, 9; mental hygiene, 286–292; moral therapy/

insanity, treatment of (*continued*)
treatment, 65, 226; need for research on, 4; prayer, 9; psychotherapy, 260, 287; restraints/lack of restraints, 65, 261; surgery, 289; swinging chair, 45; workshops, 211. *See also* confinement of the insane; eugenics movement; sterilization
insanity as a brain disease, 2, 3, 4, 304, 335
insanity as nonexistent, 302–305, 312
insanity defense, 44, 72, 224, 232–233
insanity legislation: Canada, 163, 177, 183; England, 11, 23–24, 28–30, 45, 47, 57, 61, 70, 120; Ireland, 128, 132, 154; United States, 194, 195, 204–205, 210, 248, 256, 265, 266, 284, 285, 325
intermittent insanity, 337
International Classification of Diseases (ICD), 113, 338
intoxication delirium, 340
Iowa, 245, 256, 281, 284
Ireland, William, 339
Irish Famine, 98, 132–135, 240, 241, 315
Irish immigrants. *See* immigration
Irish Inspectors of Lunatics/Lunacy Commissioners, 136–137, 139–148, 149, 151
Irish Lunacy Department, 114–115, 142
Irish nationalism, 128, 140, 149–150, 153, 316
Irish Royal Society, 142
Irving, Washington, 203
Islamic medicine, 8, 10

Jacobi, Abraham, 278
jails/prisons: conditions in, 163, 207, 219, 220, 247; confinement of the insane, 24, 46, 87, 131, 140, 163, 177, 216, 250, 317; confinement of social deviants, 307–308, 320; confinement of the violent insane, 20, 132, 208, 219; for overflow from the asylums, 140, 166, 168, 208, 219; modern-day confinement of the insane, 4, 299, 316; numbers of insane patients in, 204, 238; violence in, 46
James, William, 286
Jamieson, Robert, 104
Jamison, Kay, 33, 55, 232
Jarvis, Edward, 218, 227, 236–238, 252
Jeste, D. V., 9
Jewell, J. S., 280
Jimenez, Mary Ann, 5, 196–197
Johnson, Samuel, 31, 35–36, 50, 336
Johnson-Reed Act (1924), 288
Johnstone, Eve, 343
Joint Commission on Mental Illness and Health, 298
Jones, Ernest, 13
Jones, Kathleen, 12, 309, 318
Jones, Robert, 117
Jonson, Ben, 14
Journal of Mental Science, 78–81, 98, 107, 140–141, 143, 152
journals. *See* newspapers and periodicals
Joyce, James, 155–156
Jung, Carl, 155
justices of the peace, 19, 20, 24, 30

Kansas, 245, 284
Kempe, Margery, 9
Kempster, Walter, 247
Kendler, Kenneth, 148
Kent: asylum, 75, 95; county, 38
Kentucky, 223, 245
Kerry, 125, 147, 148, 158, 240
Kesey, Ken, 304
Kilkenny: asylum, 133, 139; county, 152
King of Hearts (film), 305
Kirkbride, Thomas, 223, 258
Klaf, Franklin, 114
Kroll, Jerome, 8
Kyd, Thomas, 14

Laing, Ronald, 4, 305, 312, 316
Lamb, Charles, 31, 34, 53
Lamb, Mary, 34
Lancashire: asylum admissions, 100; Haydock Lodge, 70; James Hey, 24; prevalence rates, 69, 100, 120–121; public asylum, 47, 69, 111; Rainhill Asylum, 98, 113
Lancaster Asylum, 319, 321

Lawless, George, 144
Le Fanu, Sheridan, 131
lead poisoning, 343
Legislative Council of Lower Canada, 162
Leicestershire County, 37
Leigh, Denis, 39, 40
Leinster, 135
Leitrim, 135, 139, 318
Limerick: asylum, 130; county, 147; workhouse, 129–130
Lincoln, Levi, 237
Lincolnshire County, 70
literature: asylum doctors, 83, 84–85, 86, 230, 304; asylum inmates, 30, 50–51, 55–56, 64, 65, 67–68, 126, 156–157, 232; asylums/madhouses, 30, 50–51, 55–56, 86, 151, 156–157, 225, 230, 231, 233–234, 304; commercial appeal of, 228; Crazy Jane, 154–155; Crazy Kate, 33, 52, 154; the criminally insane, 214; Elizabethan and Jacobean theater, 12–14, 15; fear of insanity, 203; feigned insanity, 13; insanity in general, 7, 10, 30, 41, 51, 54, 88–93, 202, 203–204, 293–294; Maria, 30; monomania, 213, 214, 229, 233–234; postpartum depression, 254–255; psychotic thinking, 31, 293; Richmond Asylum, 151, 157; senile dementia, 13; suicide, 10; syphilis, 157; violence and insanity, 64, 72, 105–106, 203, 214; wrongful confinement, 29, 83–86, 257. See also ballads; opera; individual works and authors; and see Bethlem Hospital; suicide/attempted suicide; syphilis; individual disorders
liver failure, 341, 343
Liverpool Asylum, 27
Locke, John, 22, 35
Lodge, Henry Cabot, 281
London: rapid growth, 16; sharp increase in asylum admissions, 49. See also Bethlem Hospital; Colney Hatch; Hanwell Asylum; St. Luke's Hospital/Asylum; St. Mary's priory
London County Asylum at Bexley, 115

Lord Ashley/Lord Shaftesbury. See Cooper, Anthony Ashley
Louisiana, 223
Louth, 159
lumber room thesis, 308–310, 316–326
Lunacy Commission/Commissioners (England): 1871 prevalence study, 121; 1897 Special Report, 109–116, 141; as national body, 70; commissioners, 64, 87, 115; madhouse inspections, 64; Metropolitan Commissioners in Lunacy, 61, 87; official position on "apparent" increase, 77; portrayal in "The Hunting of the Snark," 90–93
Lunacy Commission/Commissioners (Ireland). See Irish Inspectors of Lunatics/Lunacy Commissioners
Lunatic Asylum West of the Allegheny Mountains, 245
Lunatics Act/"Ashley's Act" (1845), 70
lupus, 341
Lutwidge, Robert Wilfred Skeffington, 87–93

Macalpine, Ida, 40, 59, 301
MacCabe, Frederick, 134–135
MacDonald, Michael, 10, 13, 17–19, 309
MacKenzie, Charlotte, 321
Mackenzie, Henry, 26, 30
MacKenzie, Kenneth, 176
Mackieson, John, 167, 169
mad-doctors. See psychiatrists
Maddox, Alfred, 75, 100
Madhouse and County Asylum Acts (1828), 61
"A Madman's Manuscript" (Dickens), 63, 64, 229, 232
Madness and Civilization/Histoire de la Folie (Foucault), 19, 95, 302–303
magazines. See newspapers and periodicals
magnetic resonance imaging (MRI), 304
Maine, 216, 217, 218, 223, 226, 240, 256
Malin, William, 205–206
Malzberg, Benjamin, 324
Manchester Lunatic Hospital, 27

mania: among poets, writers, 32, 34; case studies, 7, 8; caused by neurological disorder, 337; caused by other medical conditions, 8, 337, 339, 341; defined, 338; in literature, 119, 213, 229; King George III, 41; "mania mitis," 167; rabies, 8; "reasoning mania," 267; religious mania, 32, 119, 213; Victorian views of, 119. *See also* insanity, diagnostic categories of; manic-depressive illness

manic-depressive illness: among immigrants, 122; among novelists, 63, 119, 293; among poets, 31, 33, 34, 53, 55, 228; analyses of admissions, 290, 292; as a brain disease, 3, 304, 335; as part of baseline rate of insanity, 339, 342, 344; case studies, 17–19, 38, 40, 198; cost of, 4–5; exposure to cats as risk factor, 333; genetic predisposition, 148, 302, 327–328; geographic distribution, 158–159, 292; in the Bible, 7; in literature, 229–230; prevalence rates, 191, 298; relationship to schizophrenia, 335; symptoms of, caused by other medical conditions, 339. *See also* depression/melancholy; insanity, diagnostic categories of; mania

Mann, Horace, 208, 231
Marcuse, Herbert, 305
Marlowe, Christopher, 14
Marshall, Andrew, 296–297, 301, 306, 310
Martin, Jonathan, 71
Martin, Philip, 32
Maryborough Asylum, 130, 137
Maryland, 216, 298
Massachusetts: asylum building/resistance to building, 209, 223, 245, 318; Asylum for Chronic Insane at Tewksbury, 246; Boston Lunatic Hospital, 209, 239; Boston Prison Discipline Society, 207; Boston Sanitary Association, 238; censuses of the insane, 208, 237–238, 273–274; Charles Dickens, 221, 229; cost of insanity, 238; Danvers State Lunatic Hospital, 274; Department of Mental Diseases, 318;

Dorothea Dix, 219, 227; early case findings, 194, 196–197, 209; early provisions for the insane, 194, 196, 201, 207; immigrants and insanity, 147, 238–240; Northampton State Lunatic Asylum, 220, 257; prevalence of insanity, 216–217, 236, 270–271, 272 (map), 275, 288, 289, 290; State Board of Lunacy and Charity, 274; Taunton Asylum, 220; Worcester, 275; Worcester State Lunatic Hospital, 208–209, 211, 219–220, 227, 231, 237, 239, 240, 258, 326

Massachusetts Commission on Lunacy, 237–242, 280
Massachusetts General Hospital and McLean Asylum, 207, 208, 209, 256, 322
Massachusetts Medical Society, 252
Massachusetts Society for Mental Hygiene, 290
Massinger, Philip, 14
Mather, Cotton, 3, 195
Maudsley, Henry, 13, 78–79, 80–81, 82, 99, 116–117
Maxwell, John, 85
Mayo, 132, 135, 146, 147, 158–159
McCabe, Sarah, 28, 44
McCarthy, Paul, 232
McFarland, Andrew, 256, 258
Meath, 152, 159
medical conditions that can cause psychiatric symptoms, 6–9, 21, 293, 339–344; brain tumors/trauma, 228, 337, 339, 340, 343, 344; encephalitis, 38, 40, 228, 337, 339, 343; endocrine disorders, 341, 343; genetic disorders, 341, 343; head injuries, 18, 44, 214, 340, 343–344; high fever ("phrenitis"), 7, 8, 18, 339; infectious agents/diseases, 8, 18, 100, 290, 331–332, 339–340, 342, 343, 344; inflammatory disease, 341–342; metabolic disorders, 341, 343; neurological disorders, 337, 340, 342, 343; poor nutrition, 8, 330–331, 341, 342, 343; porphyria, 41–42, 341; prescription or illegal drug use, 113, 228, 340, 342, 344; thy-

roid malfunction, 341, 343, 344; toxic disorders, 38, 341, 342, 343, 344. *See also* alcohol abuse; baseline rate of insanity; epilepsy; syphilis
Medicare/Medicaid, 325
Medico-Psychological Association. *See* American Medico-Psychological Association; British Medico-Psychological Association
"megaloblastic madness," 341
"melancholia tranquilla," 167
melancholy. *See* depression/melancholy
Mellett, David, 12
Melville, Herman, 212, 232–235
Mental Health Act (1959), 120
Mental Health Law Project, 307
mental hygiene movement, 3
mental retardation ("amentia," "idiocy"): as diagnosis, 97, 113, 134, 163, 168, 174, 297, 322; as unaffected by urban risk factor, 275; case studies, 194; efforts at preventing, 117, 281–284; in East European immigrants, 288; *versus* insanity, 22, 270, 336; prevalence of, in asylums, 110, 113, 145, 323, 336; with psychosis, 338
Mental Treatment Act (Ireland, 1945), 154
mercury poisoning, 38, 341
Merskey, Harold, 309
metabolic disorders. *See under* medical conditions that can cause psychiatric symptoms
Metropolitan Commissioners in Lunacy, 61, 87
Metropolitan Life Insurance Company, 289
Meyer, Adolf, 284, 286
Michigan, 223, 257, 264, 272, 284, 285, 292
Middlesex County, 48. *See also* Hanwell Asylum
Middleton, Thomas, 14
Midelfort, Eric, 19
Miller, Christine, 331
Miller, Kerby, 98
Minnesota, 245, 292
Mississippi, 216, 223

Missouri, 223, 245, 284, 298
Mitchell, S. Weir, 254, 277–278
M'Kave, 89, 92
M'Naghten, Daniel, 71
Monaghan: asylum, 133, 138, 153; county, 139, 159
monasteries, 10, 16
monomania. *See under* delusions
Montgomery, David, 260
mood swings, 2, 315, 335, 338
Moody, Joseph, 231
Moore, Rev. Jedidiah, 207
moral insanity, 119, 167, 252–253, 337 (defined)
moral therapy/treatment, 65, 226
Morison, Sir Alexander, 62, 329
Mullingar Asylum, 133, 137
Munster, 133
Murphy, H. B. M., 330
Myles, William, 139
"myxedema madness," 341

Napier, Richard, 17–19, 121
National Association for the Protection of the Insane and the Prevention of Insanity (NAPIPI), 265
National Committee for Mental Hygiene, 286, 287
National Health Service (England), 4, 120
Neal, John, 212, 229
Nebraska, 245
Neugebauer, Richard, 19, 21
neuroimaging techniques, 304, 335
neurointoxications, 337, 341, 344
neurological disorders. *See under* medical conditions that can cause psychiatric symptoms
neurology *versus* psychiatry, 259–269
neuropathology, 304
neuroses, 336
Nevada, 271
New Brunswick, 162–166, 189, 322, 324. *See also* public asylums (Canada)
New England Psychological Association, 270
New Hampshire, 216–217, 223, 226, 271
New Haven prevalence studies, 297, 298

New Jersey, 216, 220, 223, 245, 290
New York: asylum admissions, 319; asylum building, 204, 216, 223, 245, 248; asylum conditions, 222, 263; asylum death rates, 288, 324; asylum investigations, 262, 264–265; Blackwell Asylum/New York City Lunatic Asylum, 221–222, 225, 240, 246, 248, 257, 264; Bloomingdale Asylum, 204, 234; censuses of the insane, 204–205, 247, 248; Charles Dickens, 221; Dorothea Dix, 220–222; early provisions for the insane, 201, 204, 221; Flatbush Asylum, 222; insanity legislation, 204–205, 248, 285, 325; institutionalization of the mentally retarded, 336; Irish immigrants, 240, 241; Kings County Asylum, 222, 248; prevalence of insanity, 216, 271, 275, 288, 289; state hospitals, 279, 297; State Lunacy Commission, 268; State Medical Society, 247; Utica State Lunatic Asylum, 211, 221, 222, 248, 260, 285; Willard Asylum for the Insane, 248, 270
New York Civil Liberties Union, 307
New York Commissioners of Charity and Corrections, 265
New York Neurological Society, 261–263
Newcastle, 27
Newfoundland, 170–176, 189, 318, 319, 324. See also public asylums (Canada)
newspapers and periodicals: asylum advertisements, 210; asylum conditions, 93, 115, 166, 169, 257; asylum construction, 164, 173; asylum doctors, 256; asylum reform, 264, 266, 268; the "English malady," 46, 69–70; immigrants, 98; neurologists versus asylum superintendents, 262; rising insanity, 45, 46, 63, 75, 79, 87, 94–95, 97, 116, 165, 251, 272; violence and insanity, 75, 105, 200; wrongful confinement, 85, 86, 104
Nichols, Charles, 258
Nicholson, Margaret, 44
Nightingale, Florence, 60
Nolan, M. J., 138
Norfolk Asylum, 47

North Carolina, 210, 223, 226, 298
North Dakota, 271, 274
Northamptonshire: asylum, 65; county, 17, 121
Nottinghamshire Asylum, 47, 69
Nova Scotia, 164, 176–187, 190, 318, 322, 323, 324. See also public asylums (Canada)
nutrition, poor. See medical conditions that can cause psychiatric symptoms

Ober, William, 119
Oberhelman, David, 63, 64, 82–85
O'Brien, Patricia, 174
O'Casey, Sean, 156–157
O'Connell, Daniel, 130
O'Connor, Jacqueline, 294
O'Donoghue, Edward, 15
Ohio, 216, 223, 227, 266
Omagh Asylum, 133, 145, 319
O'Neill, Eugene, 292–293
opera, madness in, 54
Oregon, 245
organic psychosis, 335
Overholser, Winfred, 323
Oxford, Edward, 71
Oxfordshire County: asylums, 27, 70; prevalence rates, 69, 100, 102

Packard, Elizabeth, 256–257
Packard Laws, 256
Paget, Sir James, 89
Palmerston, Lord, 77
paralytic insanity. See syphilis
paranoia/paranoid schizophrenia, 337
paresis. See syphilis
Pargeter, William, 39
parliamentary investigations, 70. See also insanity legislation; Select Committees
Parry-Jones, William, 29, 48, 114
"partial insanity," 337
Partrane Asylum, 157
Paulding, James Kirke, 213–214
pauper lunatics, 24, 28, 70, 76
Pennsylvania: asylum admissions, 205, 322–323; asylum building, 197–198,

205, 223, 245; asylum cure rates, 227; early provisions for the insane, 197–198, 201; prevalence of insanity, 216, 275; sterilization legislation, 284

Pennsylvania Hospital (Philadelphia), 28, 197–199, 202, 205–206, 210, 227, 258

Pepys, Samuel, 14

Perceval, John, 83

Percival, Spencer, 71

Percy, Lord, 14

Percy, Thomas (Bishop), 12

Perfect, William, 38

periodicals. See newspapers and periodicals

Persaud, Rajendra, 198

personality disorders, 336

Peters, George, 162–163, 164

pets,exposure to, as a risk factor for insanity, 332–333

phrenitis (high fever). See medical conditions that can cause psychiatric symptoms

Piers Plowman, 9

Pinel, Philippe, 50, 227

Plater, Felix, 343

plays/playwrights. See literature; individual playwrights

Poe, Edgar Allan, 202, 228–230, 233, 234–235

poetry. See literature

poisons. See medical conditions that can cause psychiatric symptoms: toxic disorders

polio, 332

poorhouses: conditions in, 163, 219, 220, 222, 315; for confinement of the insane, 196, 246, 247; for confinement of the violent insane, 208; for overflow from asylums, 175, 219, 246, 248; for the elderly, 325; number of insane persons in, 46, 204, 238, 247, 249

Poor's Asylum/Workhouse, Nova Scotia, 177–179

porphyria. See medical conditions that can cause psychiatric symptoms

Porter, Roy, 30, 36, 311–312, 316

postpartum psychosis, 7, 9, 40, 50, 174, 254–255

Powell, Richard, 48–49

Pratt, Foster, 272, 280

Prerogative Regis, 336

prescription drugs. See medical conditions that can cause psychiatric symptoms

Prichard, James, 62

Pridgeon, Charles, 202, 203, 204, 212, 214, 228, 233, 253

Prince, William, 257

Prince Edward Island, 167–170, 318. See also public asylums (Canada)

Prior, Lindsay, 145, 319, 329

Prison Discipline Society, 216

prison populations compared to asylum populations, 320

private asylums (England): accommodations for paupers, 70; Act for Regulating Madhouses (1774), 28–30; advertisements, 28, 70; analyses of admissions, 48–49, 70; conditions in, 70; demands for regulation, 29–30, 48; Dunnington House, 70; Eastgate House, 70; foreign observers, 48; growth, 28, 48, 70, 71; Haydock Lodge, 70; Hook Norton, 70, 111; in Essex (Matthew Allen, High Beech), 65–66; in Hoxton, 34; in Kent (William Perfect), 38; in Leicestershire (Thomas Arnold), 37; licensing and inspection, 30; Northamptonshire Lunatic Asylum, 65; patient abuse, 29–30, 48, 70, 83; at St. Albans (Nathaniel Cotton, "Collegium Insanorum"), 32; Tennyson's visits, 66; Witney, 70. See also confinement of the insane; literature; public asylums (England); York Retreat

private asylums (Ireland), 131, 156

Procter, Bryan, 64

Prohibition, 289

Protestant Ascendancy, 125, 130–131

psychiatrists: as blind to real increase in insanity, 3, 58, 78–82, 107–115, 290; as "classic capitalists," 308–309; as corrupt/ineffective, 82–85, 255–256, 312;

psychiatrists (*continued*)
as supporters of efforts to prevent insanity, 286–287; as supporters of eugenics movement, 116–117, 283–285; as supporters of real increase in insanity, 139–140; as well-meaning, 310; battle with neurologists, 259–269; effects of deinstitutionalization on, 298; English *versus* Irish psychiatrists, 140–142. *See also* literature: asylum doctors; public asylums (United States): distrust of superintendents; *specific individuals and organizations*
psychosis, definition of, 335–338
Psychosis and Civilization (Goldhamer and Marshall), 296–297, 301, 306
public asylums (Canada): analyses of admissions, 319, 322; cure rates, 323–324; death rates, 175, 187, 324. *See also individual provinces*
public asylums (England): admissions criteria, 20, 25, 112–114, 322; admissions due to syphilis, 331–332; conditions in, 94–95; cost of, 95–96; County Asylum Act (1808), 47; cure rates, 110–111, 323; death rates, 69, 70, 111–112, 114, 116, 118, 324; deaths, 69, 111, 115, 118; Dickens's visits, 63, 65; displacement of patients during war, 118, 120; funding/resistance to funding, 27, 47–48, 96, 318; growth, 27, 47–48; licensing and inspection, 61, 64, 70, 87. *See also* Bethlem Hospital ("Bedlam"); confinement of the insane; literature; private asylums (England); *individual counties and asylums*
public asylums (Ireland): admissions criteria, 145–146, 322; admissions due to syphilis, 331–332; cost of, 134, 138, 152; the criminally insane, 132; cure rates, 323; death rates, 144–145, 151, 324; deaths, 137, 151; early accommodations for the insane, 125; funding/resistance to funding, 130, 134, 138–139, 318; growth, 130, 133; low suicide rate, 140; violence in, 137.

See also confinement of the insane; literature; *individual counties and asylums*
public asylums (United States): admissions criteria, 208–209, 209, 220, 251, 322, 336; advertisements, 210; asylum building, 223; conditions in, 220–222, 225, 246, 257, 263–264, 295; cure rates, 323; death rates, 244–245, 288, 324; deaths, 222, 246, 263–264, 288; Dickens's visits, 221; distrust of superintendents, 223–224, 227, 230, 255–269; effects of Civil War, 244–245, 255; exposés of, 257, 295; funding/resistance to funding, 209, 222, 223–228, 318, 325; growth, 216, 223, 245, 274; magazine descriptions, 212; patient abuse, 263–264; Quakers as staff, 295; staff turnover, 257; transinstitutionalization, 325–326; violence in, 246, 247, 256; wrongful confinement, 256. *See also* confinement of the insane; *individual states and asylums*

Quakers/Society of Friends, 28, 131, 198–199, 202, 205, 295. *See also* Tuke, Daniel Hack; Tuke, William; York Retreat
Queens County, 133
Quen, Jacques, 306–307

rabies, 8
Rainhill Asylum, 98, 113
Rand Corporation, 296
Rank, Otto, 13
Ray, Isaac, 13, 223, 231, 232, 237, 238, 239, 241–242, 256
Reade, Charles, 85–86, 257
Redlich, Frederick C., 297
Reed, H. L., 283
Reed, Robert, 13
regency crisis, 41
Reid, Alexander, 186
Reid, John, 46
religious mania, 32, 119, 213
Renshaw, Henry, 268
Renvoize, Edward, 114

Rhode Island, 216, 223, 240, 241, 245, 290

Rice, Thomas, 129–130

Richardson, Samuel, 25, 29

Richmond Asylum ("Grangegorman"), 128–129, 132, 137, 138, 151, 157

Robertson, C. Lockhart, 78–80, 82, 110, 113

Robertson, John, 250

Rosanoff, Aaron, 283

Roscommon, 135, 148, 159

Rothman, David, 301, 305–307, 316, 317, 319

Rousseau, George S., 31

Rowley, Thomas (pseudonym), 33

Rowley, William, 38

Royal College of Physicians, 34, 48

Royal College of Psychiatrists, 78

Rush, Benjamin, 199, 201–202, 212, 214, 229

Rushton, Peter, 19, 20

Ruskin, John, 104

Russo-Finnish War, 340

Saint John (city), New Brunswick, 162–164, 165, 166, 167, 189. *See also* St. John County, New Brunswick

Saint John Island (Prince Edward Island), 167

Saint Vallier, Monseigneur de, 162

Salem witchcraft trials, 3, 194–195

Salford case register, 120–121

Salmon, Thomas, 287

Sanborn, Franklin, 278

sarcoidosis, 342, 343

Sartorius, Norman, 331

Saskatchewan, 191

Savage, George, 109

schizophrenia: admission rates, 292; among immigrants, 122; among relatives of writers, 155, 293; as a brain disease, 3, 304, 335; as nonexistent, 303, 305; as part of baseline rate of insanity, 344; as rapidly increasing in the 1800s, 313; as rare in the 1700s, 198; as a rational adjustment to insane world, 305; as social deviance, 303; case studies, 9, 17–19, 20, 38, 39–40, 198; changes in diagnostic criteria, 123; cost of, 4–5, 192; gender differences, 313; genetic predisposition, 148, 327–328; in the Bible, 7; in literature, 13, 53, 65, 229, 234, 294; paranoid schizophrenia, 337; prevalence, 113, 120–121, 122–123, 158–159, 191–192, 298, 313, 344; relationship to manic-depressive illness, 335; risk factors, 16, 122, 148, 292, 327–328, 329, 332–333; romanticization of, 305; suggested causes, 290–291, 312, 313, 329–333; symptoms of, caused by other medical conditions, 339, 343–344

Scientology, 304

Scott, Sir Walter, 53–55

Scull, Andrew, 19, 49, 57, 62, 81, 99, 112, 303, 305–313, 316–317, 319, 321

season of birth as risk factor, 122

Select Committees (Canada), 167

Select Committees (England): on abuses in private London madhouses, 29–30; increase in number of, 47; on Lunatics, 75–77, 82, 87, 93; on Madhouses, 48; on Pauper Lunatics in the County of Middlesex, 59–60; on the State of Lunatics, 46–47, 58

Select Committees (Ireland), 129, 130

senile dementia. *See* Alzheimer's disease; dementia; vascular dementia

Shaftesbury, Lord. *See* Cooper, Anthony Ashley

Shakespeare, William, 12–13

Shaw, Lemuel, 232–233

Shelley, Percy Bysshe, 55, 202

Shepherd, Michael, 18, 122

Sheridan, Frances, 30

Shimer, Michael, 51, 53

ships of fools, 19

Shorter, Edward, 309, 320

Showalter, Elaine, 312–313

Shryock, Richard, 193

Sicherman, Barbara, 284

Simms, William, 213, 214

Simon, Bennett, 7

Simond, Louis, 49

Sinclair, George, 187

Skultans, Vieda, 47
Slater, Eliot, 13
Sligo, 133, 139, 158, 318
Small, Helen, 33
Smart, Christopher, 31–32, 35, 36
Smith, Elihu Hubbard, 202
Smith, Henry Nash, 233
Smith, Leonard, 47, 319
Smollett, Tobias, 29, 30
Social Security Disability Insurance
    (SSDI), 5, 299
Somerset County, 69, 102
South Carolina, 200–201, 210–211, 217,
    224, 236, 244–245, 246, 321
South Dakota, 274
Southey, Robert, 52–53
Spitzka, Edward Charles, 261–268
Spurzheim, Johann Gaspar, 63
SSDI (Social Security Disability Insur-
    ance), 5, 299
SSI (Supplemental Security Income), 5,
    299
St. Albans, private madhouse at, 32
St. Elizabeths Hospital/Government
    Hospital for the Insane, 258, 272,
    287, 323
St. John County, New Brunswick, 163.
    See also Saint John (city), New
    Brunswick
St. John of God Hospital (Dublin), 156
St. John's, Newfoundland, 167, 171, 174,
    189–190
St. Luke's Hospital/Asylum, 27, 58, 65, 93
St. Luke's Workhouse, 97
St. Mary's priory, 10
St. Pancras Workhouse, 97
St. Patrick's Hospital, 124–125, 127
Stabb, Henry, 172–176
Staffordshire: asylum, 112; county, 69
Stansfield, T.E.K., 117
Stark, William, 45
State Care Act (New York, 1890), 325
Steele, Richard, 25
sterilization, 283–284, 285. See also
    eugenics movement
Sterne, Laurence, 30
Stevenson, Robert Louis, 105

Steward, Dugald, 68
Stockton State Hospital. See California
Stoker, Bram, 106
Strype, John, 24
Suffolk County, 48, 318
suicide/attempted suicide: as equivalent
    to insanity, 59; as symptom of insan-
    ity, 2; as the "English malady," 38; by
    asylum doctors, 256; by inpatients, 95,
    246; by writers/poets and their rela-
    tives, 32, 33, 72, 119–120, 293, 294,
    302; in literature, 10; low prevalence
    of, in Irish asylums, 140; reported in
    newspapers, 105
Sumner, Increase, 237
superintendents. See literature: asylum
    doctors; psychiatrists; public asylums
    (United States): distrust of superin-
    tendents; specific individuals and
    organizations
Supplemental Security Income (SSI), 5,
    299
Sussex: asylum, 79; county, 96, 318
Sutton, John, 320
Suzuki, Akihito, 19, 20
Swift, Jonathan, 124–127
Sydenham, Thomas, 21
Synge, John, 150–151
syphilis: as cause of asylum deaths, 111,
    144, 332; as diagnosis, 112, 270, 297;
    as disease of civilization, 332; as infec-
    tious disease model for insanity,
    331–332; as medical condition that
    can cause psychiatric symptoms, 38,
    40, 265, 268, 335, 337, 339–340, 342;
    comparative rates in England and Ire-
    land, 144–145, 332; early descriptions
    of, 21; in literature, 157; paralytic
    insanity, 265
systemic lupus erythematosus, 341
Szasz, Thomas, 4, 302–305, 307, 312, 316

temporal lobe epilepsy. See epilepsy
Tennessee, 216, 223, 224, 226, 297
Tennyson, Alfred, Lord, 66–68, 89
Thackeray, William Makepeace, 72,
    131–132

theater. *See* literature; *individual play-wrights*
Thielman, Samuel, 321
Throop, Enos, 205
thyroid malfunction. *See under* medical conditions that can cause psychiatric symptoms
Ticehurst Asylum, 114
Tipperary, 129, 147
Tomes, Nancy, 320
Toms o' Bedlam, 13, 71
Toronto Lunatic Asylum, 170
Torrey, E. Fuller, 313
toxic disorders. *See under* medical conditions that can cause psychiatric symptoms
transinstitutionalization, 325–326
Trosse, Rev. George, 20, 342
Truman, Harry S, 295
tuberculosis, 111, 324, 339
Tuke, Daniel Hack, 78, 81–82, 98, 100, 109, 111, 129, 147, 164
Tuke, Harrington, 104
Tuke, William, 28, 81, 227
Turner, Trevor, 114, 317
twin studies, 327
typhoid fever, 132, 339
typhus, 111, 132, 178, 324

Ulster, 135, 138, 152
urban risk factor, 328–333; density of population, 102; early notice of, 122, 242, 329; for schizophrenia, 16, 122; household crowding, 100; immigration risk factor, 329; in Canada, 165, 329; in developing nations, 5; in England, 100; in Ireland, 135–136, 329; in the United States, 242, 252, 275, 291–292, 329; mental retardation unaffected by, 275; overcrowding *versus* pauperism, 102; recent studies, 122; rural risk factor, 99–100, 165, 243
Urmson, G. H., 115
Uwins, David, 49, 328

Vagrancy Act (1714), 23–24
vascular dementia, 291, 325

Vermont, 216, 249, 270
Victoria, Queen, 71, 116, 166
Victorian views of insanity, 63, 74, 81, 83, 116, 119, 321
Viets, Henry, 194
violence and insanity, 4, 10, 25, 44–45, 71–72, 75, 104–105, 115, 132, 182. *See also* confinement of the insane; literature
Virginia, 199–200, 201, 245, 284, 321
vitamin deficiency, 341, 343

Waddell, John, 164
Wakefield Asylum, 69
Walker, Francis, 269, 271, 281
Walker, Nigel, 28, 44
Walsh, Dermot, 158
Walton, John, 319, 321
Ward, Jane, 295
Ward, Ned, 25
Warner, Richard, 312, 331
Washington, D.C., 258
Waterford: asylum, 130, 134, 137; county, 134–135, 152, 171
Waterston, Robert, 219
Watson, Thomas, 281
Weaver, William A., 218
Webster, John, 14
Weldon, Georgiana, 104
West Riding Asylum, 94, 104
West Virginia Hospital, 245
Westmeath, 146, 152
Wexford, 171
White, William A., 250, 285, 287, 329
Whitman, Walt, 243
Wicklow, 151
Wilkins, Robert, 111
Willan, Robert, 58
Willard, Sylvester, 247–248
Williams, Roger, 194
Williams, Tennessee, 294
Willis, Thomas, 21
Wiltshire: asylum, 75, 98; county, 69, 80, 100, 102
Windham, William Frederick, 85
Wines, Frederick, 269
Winslow, Forbes, 13, 63, 116

Winston, Ellen, 290
Wisconsin, 245, 247, 292
Witney Asylum, 70
Wollstonecraft, Mary, 29
Woodward, Samuel, 219, 223, 227, 237, 238
Woolf, Virginia, 119–120
Worcestershire County, 102
Wordsworth, William, 51–53
workhouses: as government solution to social deviance, 307–308; conditions in, 70, 130, 137–138; cost comparisons with asylums, 70, 95, 211; for confinement of the insane, 46, 62, 70–71, 95–97, 109–110, 140, 177, 195–196, 210; for overflow from asylums, 70, 96, 110, 138, 140, 175; for the elderly, 145; for the mentally retarded, 70–71, 145, 336; in Ireland, 125. *See also individual workhouses*
World Health Organization, 158, 159
World War I, 117–119, 287, 289, 315–316
World War II, 4, 118, 120, 295, 316
wrongful confinement. *See* confinement of the insane
Wynter, Andrew, 308, 316

Yeats, William Butler, 154–155
Yonge, James, 14
York Retreat, 28, 48, 114, 131, 219
Yorkshire County, 17, 27–28, 70, 71, 100, 102. *See also* West Riding Asylum; York Retreat
Young, Henry, 105
Youngquist, Paul, 53

ABOUT THE AUTHORS

E. Fuller Torrey, M.D., is a research psychiatrist specializing in schizo-phrenia and manic-depressive illness. He is the executive director of the Stanley Medical Research Institute, president of the Treatment Advocacy Center, and professor of psychiatry at the Uniformed Ser-vices University of the Health Sciences. He has authored or edited six-teen books and over two hundred papers.

Judy Miller is a senior research assistant with the Stanley Medical Research Institute and a freelance editor. She lives in Bethesda, Mary-land, with her husband and four children.